International Perspectives on Self-Regulation and Health

THE PLENUM SERIES IN BEHAVIORAL PSYCHOPHYSIOLOGY AND MEDICINE

Series Editor:
William J. Ray, *Pennsylvania State University, University Park, Pennsylvania*

BIOLOGICAL BARRIERS IN BEHAVIORAL MEDICINE
　Edited by Wolfgang Linden

HANDBOOK OF RESEARCH METHODS IN CARDIOVASCULAR BEHAVIORAL MEDICINE
　Edited by Neil Schneiderman, Stephen M. Weiss, and Peter G. Kaufmann

INTERNATIONAL PERSPECTIVES ON SELF-REGULATION AND HEALTH
　Edited by John G. Carlson and A. Ronald Seifert

PHYSIOLOGY AND BEHAVIOR THERAPY
Conceptual Guidelines for the Clinician
　James G. Hollandsworth, Jr.

THE PHYSIOLOGY OF PSYCHOLOGICAL DISORDERS
Schizophrenia, Depression, Anxiety, and Substance Abuse
　James G. Hollandsworth, Jr.

International Perspectives on Self-Regulation and Health

Sponsored by the Association for
Applied Psychophysiology and Biofeedback

Edited by

John G. Carlson
University of Hawaii at Manoa
Honolulu, Hawaii

and

A. Ronald Seifert
Behavioral Institute of Atlanta
Atlanta, Georgia

Plenum Press • New York and London

Library of Congress Cataloging-in-Publication Data

International perspectives on self-regulation and health / sponsored
  by the Association for Applied Psychophysiology and Biofeedback ;
  edited by John G. Carlson and A. Ronald Seifert.
       p. cm. -- (Plenum series in behavioral psychophysiology and
  medicine)
       "First International Conference on Biobehavioral Self-Regulation
  and Health ... held at the Hawaiian Regent Hotel in Honolulu,
  November 18-20, 1987"--Pref.
       Includes bibliographical references and index.
       ISBN 0-306-43557-8
       1. Medicine and psychology--Congresses. 2. Biofeedback training-
  -Congresses. 3. Psychoneuroimmunology--Congresses. I. Carlson,
  John G. II. Seifert, A. Ronald. III. Association for Applied
  Psychophysiology and Biofeedback. IV. International Conference on
  Biobehavioral Self-Regulation and Health (1st : 1987 : Honolulu,
  Hawaii) V. Series.
       [DNLM: 1. Behaviorl Therapy--congresses. 2. Biofeedback
  (Psychology)--congresses. WL 103 I608 1987]
  R726.5.I595   1990
  616'.001'9--dc20
  DNLM/DLC
  for Library of Congress   90-14173
                                                                   CIP

ISBN 0-306-43557-8

© 1991 Plenum Press, New York·
A Division of Plenum Publishing Corporation
233 Spring Street, New York, N.Y. 10013

All rights reserved

No part of this book may be reproduced, stored in a retrieval system, or transmitted
in any form or by any means, electronic, mechanical, photocopying, microfilming,
recording, or otherwise, without written permission from the Publisher

Printed in the United States of America

Contributors

Robert Ader, Department of Psychiatry, University of Rochester School of Medicine and Dentistry, Rochester, New York 14642, USA

Kenji Akiyama, Institute for Neurobiology, Okayama University Medical School, Okayama 700, Japan

Niels Birbaumer, Psychological Institute, University of Tübingen, D 7400 Tübingen 1, Federal Republic of Germany

James G. Broton, Cresap Neuroscience Laboratory, Northwestern University, Evanston, Illinois 60208, USA

Isolde von Bülow, Psychological Institute, University of Tübingen, D 7400 Tübingen 1, Federal Republic of Germany

Anthony Canavan, Psychological Institute, University of Tübingen, D 7400 Tübingen 1, Federal Republic of Germany

John G. Carlson, Department of Psychology, University of Hawaii at Manoa, Honolulu, Hawaii 96822, USA

Thomas Elbert, Psychological Institute, University of Tübingen, D 7400 Tübingen 1, Federal Republic of Germany

Keith Fulton, Department of Neurology and Neuroscience Program, Baylor College of Medicine, Houston, Texas 77030, USA

G. F. Gebhart, Department of Pharmacology, College of Medicine, University of Iowa, Iowa City, Iowa 52242, USA

Paul Grossman, Psychophysiology Research Group, University of Freiburg, Freiburg, Federal Republic of Germany

Nicholas R. S. Hall, Department of Psychiatry and Behavioral Medicine, University of South Florida, Tampa, Florida 33613, USA

Midori Hiramatsu, Institute for Neurobiology, Okayama University Medical School, Okayama 700, Japan

Kun Hou Huang, Chinese Academy of Traditional Chinese Medicine, 100700 Beijing, People's Republic of China

Alan J. Husband, Department of Psychology, University of Newcastle, Newcastle, NSW 2308, Australia

Hideaki Kabuto, Institute for Neurobiology, Okayama University Medical School, Okayama 700, Japan

Edward S. Katkin, Department of Psychology, State University of New York at Stony Brook, Stony Brook, New York 11794–2500, USA

Robert M. Kelsey, Department of Psychology, State University of New York at Buffalo, Buffalo, New York 14260, USA

Maurice G. King, Department of Psychology, University of Newcastle, Newcastle, NSW 2308, Australia

Robert Kvarnes, Washington School of Psychiatry, Washington, D.C., USA

Michael J. Kwon, Institute for Neurobiology, Okayama University Medical School, Okayama 700, Japan

Wolfgang Larbig, Psychological Institute, University of Tübingen, D 7400 Tübingen 1, Federal Republic of Germany

Anne Linden, Psychological Institute, University of Tübingen, D 7400 Tübingen 1, Federal Republic of Germany

Werner Lutzenberger, Psychological Institute, University of Tübingen, D 7400 Tübingen 1, Federal Republic of Germany

F. J. McGuigan, Institute for Stress Management, United States International University, San Diego, California 92131, USA

Neal Miller, Department of Psychology, Yale University, New Haven, Connecticut 06520, USA

Mirna Mitra, Department of Neurology and Neuroscience Program, Baylor College of Medicine, Houston, Texas 77030, USA

Akitane Mori, Institute for Neurobiology, Okayama University Medical School, Okayama 700, Japan

Brigitte Rockstroh, Psychological Institute, University of Tübingen, D 7400 Tübingen 1, Federal Republic of Germany

J. Peter Rosenfeld, Cresap Neuroscience Laboratory, Northwestern University, Evanston, Illinois 60208, USA

Masamichi Satoh, Department of Pharmacology, Faculty of Pharmaceutical Sciences, Kyoto University, Kyoto 606, Japan

A. Ronald Seifert, Behavioral Institute of Atlanta, Atlanta, Georgia 30342, USA

Masakatsu Shimada, Institute for Neurobiology, Okayama University Medical School, Okayama 700, Japan

James E. Skinner, Department of Neurology and Neuroscience Program, Baylor College of Medicine, Houston, Texas 77030, USA

Ronald L. Webster, Department of Psychology, Hollins College, Roanoke, Virginia 24020, USA

Lang Yan Xia, Beijing College of Traditional Chinese Medicine, 100013 Beijing, People's Republic of China

Isao Yokoi, Institute for Neurobiology, Okayama University Medical School, Okayama 700, Japan

Foreword

An attractive feature of self-regulation therapies is that, instead of doing something to the patients, they teach them to do something for themselves. Furthermore, the fact that the patient is able to do something to cope with his or her health problem can produce a significant reduction in the stress that may have contributed to that problem and in the additional stress that it produces.

While the idea that the mind can play a role in the health of the body and some therapeutic techniques based on this idea are not new, remarkable scientific advances have been made recently in the area of self-regulation and health. There has been an exciting and rapidly accelerating increase in our basic science knowledge of homeostasis, or, in other words, how the body regulates itself in order to maintain health. Technical and conceptual advances are increasing our knowledge of the details of such regulation at all levels—cells, tissues, organs, organ systems, and the body as a whole. We are learning how the competing demands of different elements at each of these levels are adjusted by the brain, which, with its neural and humoral mechanisms, is the supreme organ of integration of the body.

A simple example is when the self, centered in the brain, perceives a life-or-death emergency situation that demands extreme exertion from the skeletal muscles in acts of either fighting or fleeing. Then many complex mechanisms are brought into play, a small sample of which includes an increase in blood pressure above normally regulated levels and a shunting of blood away from the skin and the digestive system to the skeletal muscles, increasing the supply they need for maximum exertion. Some of these mechanisms are known to have injurious long-term effects, but under the primitive conditions in which people evolved, the afflictions of older age were trivial compared with whether the person was killed before having children.

This book will show how some of these physiological mechanisms for adapting to primitive conditions, and even some of the responses of the immune system, can be modified by learning which has been found to have a more profound influence on bodily processes than previously had been realized. Such learning can contribute to health by helping the person to adapt the control of primitive mechanisms in the body to the changed conditions of modern life.

A picture of the brain that emerges in this book is not of a merely passive, complex switchboard but of a system that can exert self-regulatory control over its many inputs (including pain) as well as over outputs (such as peptides and hormones) as it plays a key role in integrating the physiological functions and the behavior of the person. Exciting examples of these increases in knowledge, their therapeutic applications, and promise for future advances in knowledge and therapy are presented in various chapters of this book, which is exceptional in its scope of interdisciplinary integration. Also illustrated is how modern advances in measuring instruments can be used to help people become better aware of what is happening to certain vital functions of their bodies and hence become better able to learn to control them.

The international conference on which this book is based has helped to integrate behavioral medicine as an internationally developing area of research and therapeutic application.

NEAL MILLER

Yale University

Preface

The First International Conference on Biobehavioral Self-Regulation and Health was conceived by the editors at the annual meeting of the Association for Applied Psychophysiology and Biofeedback (AAPB, formerly the Biofeedback Society of America) in 1985, and ultimately held at the Hawaiian Regent Hotel in Honolulu, November 18–20, 1987. The advisory committee—consisting of Robert Ader (USA), Niels Birbaumer (West Germany), Jasper Brener (UK), Patrick DeLeon (USA), Bernard Engel (USA), F. J. McGuigan (USA), Neal Miller (USA), and Masamichi Satoh (Japan)—endorsed the presentation of symposia in five areas of research and application in applied psychophysiology: cardiovascular regulation, neuromuscular control, psychoneuroimmunology, pain, and the central nervous system. The committee recommended 25 eminent, multinational symposia presenters and discussants in each of these areas plus seven invited speakers, including Rene Drucker-Colin (Mexico), Edward Katkin (USA), and Steven Weiss (USA), among others from the Advisory Committee itself. Contributors to the individual symposia were also invited to submit papers for this volume and to include other collaborating researchers when appropriate. Further details of the conference and the authors and chapters of this collection are presented in the following Introduction and Overview (Chapter 1).

The planning of the First Conference was also carried out by the AAPB staff, most notably Francine Butler, executive director, and the Local Conference Coordinator at the University of Hawaii, Lori Mukaida (assisted by her staff and members of the Biofeedback and Behavioral Medicine Society of Hawaii). The great success of the conference owes largely to their contributions alongside those of the Advisory Committee, to all of whom we are eternally thankful.

Gratitude for financial and moral support of the conference is owed to the Board of Directors of AAPB and former President Mark Schwartz and to the University of Hawaii, especially former Dean D. Neubauer, College of Social Sciences.

We would also like to gratefully acknowledge Eliot Werner, senior editor at Plenum, and William Ray, editor of the Plenum Series in Behavioral Psychophysiology and Medicine, for their continuing and invaluable advice, cooperation, and support, and Andrea Martin, our conscientious and remarkably patient production editor.

Perhaps the most salient evidence of a successful meeting is to be found in continuing efforts for future meetings. Accordingly, the Second International Conference in this series is now planned for September 1991, and will be held in Munich, Germany. This conference will also serve as the basis for an edited volume of papers, the publication of which we look forward to with the same high expectations as we hold for the present one.

JOHN G. CARLSON
A. RONALD SEIFERT

Honolulu and Atlanta

Contents

Chapter 1

Introduction 1

A. Ronald Seifert and John G. Carlson

The International Conference 1
Overview: The Chapters 3

PART I. CARDIOVASCULAR AND CENTRAL DISORDERS

Chapter 2

Respiratory Mediation of Cardiac Function within a
   Psychophysiological Perspective 17

Paul Grossman

Respiratory Sinus Arrhythmia 21
Hyperventilation-Related Cardiac Alterations 32
References 37

Chapter 3

Environmental Stress and Myocardial Reactivity: Implications for
   Raynaud's Disease 41

Robert M. Kelsey and Edward S. Katkin

Pathophysiological Theories and Evidence 42
Available Facts 43

The Myocardial Performance Theory 43
Method... 47
Results 50
Discussion 59
References 61

Chapter 4

Self-Regulation of Slow Cortical Potentials and Its Role
  in Epileptogenesis 65

Thomas Elbert, Brigitte Rockstroh, Anthony Canavan, Niels Birbaumer, Werner Lutzenberger, Isolde von Bülow, and Anne Linden

Behavioral Treatment of Seizure Disorders 65
Slow Cortical Potentials Indicate Cortical Excitability 68
Self-Regulation of Slow Cortical Potentials 70
Self-Regulation of SCPs in Patients Suffering from Epilepsy 73
Biofeedback of SCPs in Patients with Epilepsy 74
Method... 75
Results 79
References 91

Chapter 5

Low-Dimensional Chaos in a Simple Biological Model
  of Neocortex: Implications for Cardiovascular and
  Cognitive Disorders 95

James E. Skinner, Mirna Mitra, and Keith Fulton

Brain Regulation of the Heart 95
Model Cortical System: Olfactory Bulb 99
Measuring the Correlation Dimension 102
Methods for Studying the Correlation Dimension in the
  Olfactory Bulb 103
New Experimental Results 105
Discussion of New Results 109
Low-Dimensional Chaotic Dynamics in Biological
  Systems: Why? 111
Summary and Conclusions 113
References 114

PART II. NEUROMUSCULAR DISORDERS

Chapter 6

Control of Normal and Pathologic Cognitive Functions through Neuromuscular Circuits: Applications of Principles of Progressive Relaxation 121

F. J. McGuigan

The Problem of "Mind" 121
How Cognitive Events Are Generated 122
The Control of Cognitive Processes 124
Learning Tension Control 125
Clinical Progressive Relaxation 126
Developing Emotional Control 128
Establishing the Meaning of Tension 129
References 131

Chapter 7

Control of Convulsions by Inhibitory and Excitatory Neurotransmitter Receptor Regulators in Epileptic El Mice and Neuromuscular Junction-Blocked Rats 133

Akitane Mori, Isao Yokoi, Hideaki Kabuto, Midori Hiramatsu, Michael J. Kwon, Masakatsu Shimada, and Kenji Akiyama

Materials and Methods 134
Results 136
Discussion 139
References 142

Chapter 8

Fluency Enhancement in Stutterers: Advances in Self-Regulation through Sensory Augmentation 145

Ronald L. Webster

Definition and Measurement of Stuttering 146
Fluency-Enhancing Conditions 148
Considerations Regarding Sensory Feedback 150
Therapies at Two Fluency-Inducing Loci 151
A Development in Vocal Enhancement for Stutterers 153

Results of Clinical Trials 155
Conclusions 156
References 157

PART III. PSYCHONEUROIMMUNOLOGY

Chapter 9

Behavior in Autoimmune Mice 163

Robert Ader

Introduction 163
Effects of Immune Status on Behavior in Lupus-Prone Mice 167
Discussion 175
References 178

Chapter 10

Behavioral Intervention and Disease: Possible Mechanisms 183

Nicholas R. S. Hall and Robert Kvarnes

Introduction 183
Emotions and Health 184
Miraculous Healing, Guided Imagery, and Health 186
Adverse Effects of Imagery 188
Physiological Processes That May Link Emotions with Health ... 190
Conclusion 193
References 193

Chapter 11

Altered Immunity through Behavioral Conditioning 197

Maurice G. King and Alan J. Husband

Effective UCSs in Immunoconditioning 198
Alternative UCSs in Immunosuppression 199
Alternative UCSs in Immunostimulation 201
Biological Mediators of Immunoconditioning 202
References 203

PART IV. PAIN

Chapter 12

Opioid Analgesia and Descending Systems of Pain Control 207

G. F. Gebhart

Introduction 207
Opioids and Analgesia 208
Stimulation-Produced Analgesia 212
Organization of Descending Systems 215
Summary 217
References 218

Chapter 13

Gate Control Theory of Pain Perception: Current Status 223

Wolfgang Larbig

Introduction 223
The Gate Control Theory of Pain 224
Spinal Pain Modulation: Further Research and Criticism 225
Descending Pain Control System 230
Clinical Implications: The Psychological Management of Pain 232
Concluding Remarks 235
References 235

Chapter 14

Behavioral–Anatomical Studies of the Central Pathways
   Subserving Orofacial Pain 239

J. Peter Rosenfeld and James G. Broton

Chapter 15

Neuropeptides and Nociception in the Spinal Cord 255

Masamichi Satoh

At the Beginning 255
Experimental Methods 256
Separate Roles of Substance P and Somatostatin 259
A Role of Calcitonin Gene-Related Peptide (CGRP) 262

At the End 264
References 266

Chapter 16

Evidence for the Role of the Cerebral Cortex in Acupuncture
  Analgesia 267

Lang Yan Xia, J. Peter Rosenfeld, and Kun Hou Huang

Introduction 267
References 278

Index 281

Chapter 1

Introduction

A. Ronald Seifert and John G. Carlson

The International Conference

All but one of the first authors of the chapters in this volume were presenters at the First International Conference on Biobehavioral Self-Regulation and Health, a 3-day meeting held in Honolulu, Hawaii, in November 1987. The stated goal of the conference was "to show the convergence and potential integration of a wide variety of related research, theory, and self-regulation techniques for disorders that respond to nontraditional medical approaches—especially from the standpoint of long-term health prevention." It was our hope to bring together outstanding researchers doing both pure and applied science in the young field of self-regulation and health to foster the dissemination of their previous research as well as new efforts through the interchange of ideas. The conference, whose participants represented 12 nations and 4 continents, both east and west, was financially cosponsored by the Association for Applied Psychophysiology and Biofeedback and the University of Hawaii at Manoa.

Many of the individual participants in the conference had not met prior to their presentations. The means for their selection was simple and very effective, as evidenced by the high quality of their contributions to this volume. Initially, an advisory committee was established for the conference that consisted of a number of the eminent individuals whose chapters are included in the several sections: Niels Birbaumer in

---

A. Ronald Seifert • Behavioral Institute of Atlanta, Atlanta, Georgia 30342, USA.   *John G. Carlson* • Department of Psychology, University of Hawaii at Manoa, Honolulu, Hawaii 96822 USA.

the area of central disorders, F. J. McGuigan in the area of neuromuscular disorders, Robert Ader in the area of psychoneuroimmunology, and J. Peter Rosenfeld and Masamichi Satoh in the area of pain. (In addition, Jasper Brener assisted with participant selection and presented a conference paper in the area of cardiovascular disorders.) In turn, these and other members of the advisory committee helped in issuing invitations to distinguished researchers in their respective fields to form symposia groups around the general topics, emphasizing specific themes that were left to the symposia presenters to determine. In addition, keynote speakers were invited, and Neal Miller, another member of the advisory committee, kindly offered to provide the foreword to this volume.

The final result of this process of delegation of selection is mirrored in the outstanding chapters presented here. In the Cardiovascular and Central Disorders section, there are 4 chapters; in the Neuromuscular Disorders section, 3 chapters; in the Psychoneuroimmunology section, 3 chapters; and in the Pain section, 5 chapters. While these 15 chapters cover only some of the issues brought out in the conference, they do represent an excellent and majority sample of the individual presentations that were given. In some cases, the authors invited colleagues to contribute to their chapters. A complete listing of the contributors appears earlier in this volume.

In addition to presentation of the chapters themselves, each presenter was invited to participate in dialogue within the symposia and in "meet the speakers" sessions at other times. This afforded each contributor the chance to share data and perspectives face-to-face with others in the field—an opportunity not often available across distant national boundaries. Also, in a session early in the conference, government and private health care officials expressed their views on the status of such issues as health care policy, funding, and governmental support of nontraditional approaches to health care. Along with poster presentations and invited individual speakers, these contributions enabled this first international conference to very successfully integrate the applied and pure research aspects of the self-regulation of health. Postconference feedback from the audience was very positive on the high quality of the presentations and the rare opportunity for spirited discussion with the internationally acclaimed presenters.

This was only the first of a series of these international meetings, already tentatively scheduled at future sites in Europe and Asia, and, we hope, the basis for future volumes of this sort. If a collection such as this one can communicate to readers, especially those unable to attend the conference, some of the accomplishments of the distinguished researchers in this field, it will serve an important and useful function. If it can inspire new research and clinical applications, it will further our greatest expectations.

Overview: The Chapters

The 37 contributors to this collection give a truly international perspective on the problems of self-regulation and health, with their multiplicity of native languages, approaches, and focus on different problems. This adds to the richness and diversity of ideas, but it does not necessarily facilitate the smooth flow of the overall content or the integration of specific ideas. While we have attempted to overcome these problems through organization, commentary, and editing, we have endeavored to preserve the exciting and informative tenor of the individual contributors as nearly as possible. In short, the balance we have sought is between leaving the contributions as much as possible in their original form, and providing enough editing, editorial summary, and integration into meaningful categories to achieve a unified collection.

The sections of this book that separate the topical areas are familiar and help to systematize the presentations. However, of course, they do little to represent the complex functions of the human organism in life and in health. Nor does this topical structure fairly present the cross-relatedness of the individual areas of presentation and discussion in the conference. It is merely our best attempt to provide structure, while it is left mainly to the reader to find points of contact and cross-fertilization for ideas across the sections and the individual chapters. As was our hope with the conference, it is our hope with this collection that astute observers will discover for themselves the interrelatedness of the bodies of knowledge presented. Such integration may provide new insights and understandings into self-regulation and health and their converse, dysregulation and disease, with the guidance of some of the leading researchers of our time.

Cardiovascular and Central Disorders

In Chapter 2, Paul Grossman provides an excellent beginning for this section in his fascinating review of phenomena relating to the complex interaction between respiratory and cardiovascular functions. Grossman points out that tasks that demand physical activity may require covariation between the lungs and heart, whereas those that do not require an increase in energy usage may involve the heart alone (and an absence of respiratory–circulatory coupling). In the healthy individual, the related mechanisms are well integrated and adaptive. However, difficulties such as illness or external signs of danger may cause a failure of normal coupling of reactions in respiration and cardiac functioning. Grossman focuses upon respiratory sinus arrhythmia (RSA) and hyperventilation as two phenomena that normally demonstrate integration of respiratory and cardiac functioning but that may also be involved in dysregulation and a failure of adaptation. In the traditional view, RSA provides an index of tonic as well as phasic cardiac control. However, Grossman believes that, under conditions of varying respiration, RSA represents only phasic control from inspiration to expiration. In one study conducted in his laboratory subjects were administered a beta-blocker (to ensure parasympathetic dominance), then were exposed to a variety of stressors in successive conditions. Resting levels of RSA were unaffected by the beta-blocker, suggesting that RSA rather purely reflects phasic vagal activity. Grossman outlines some possible mechanisms and related research to confirm this relationship. He then turns to the problem of hyperventilation in both normal and anxiety-prone individuals. Hyperventilation may reduce oxygen supply to the heart, induce ECG abnormalities, and induce a higher heart rate in order to address potential metabolic needs. In heart patients, such as those with variant angina, symptoms may become more frequent with hyperventilation. In those with coronary disease who also are prone to hyperventilation, mortality rates have been shown to be much higher. Thus, again in this area, the coupling of respiration and cardiac function may be both adaptive and dysfunctional. A clear implication is that behavioral techniques may be used to train more effective breathing, reducing hyperventilation, and arterial carbon monoxide, and related symptoms.

In Chapter 3, by Robert M. Kelsey and Edward S. Katkin, existing theories of primary Raynaud's phenomenon are each shown to be unable to explain known specific aspects of the disorder. In light of these problems, Kelsey and Katkin put forth an alternative theory, a diathesis-stress model, which states that reduced myocardial performance with low cardiac output (deficient beta-adrenergic mediation) may couple with sympathetic vasoconstriction caused by psychological or physical stress. Indirect evidence that favors this theory includes (a) the known lower blood volume, blood pressure, and various cardiodynamic indices in females than in males, paralleling relative rates of Raynaud's disease, (b) the fact that Raynaud's patients exhibit below-normal blood pressures, and (c) the observation that the incidence of Raynaud's attacks are greater in patients treated with cardioselective beta-blockers. Next the authors report a study in their laboratory in which it was predicted that myocardial reactivity to stress would be lower for Raynaud's-symptomatic subjects than for normals. They found that the preejection period for the Raynaud's subjects was longer than for the controls, showing that myocardial contractility was subnormal during stress for the former group, and that deficient beta-adrenergic activation was responsible for the performance of the Raynaud's subjects. Thus, their research supports the view that Raynaud's disease owes to a deficit in myocardial contractility during stress. This research opens the way for studies of behavioral treatment regimens, such as thermal biofeedback, to determine if myocardial reactivity is a factor.

Turning to more purely central disorders, Thomas Elbert and his coworkers in Niels Birbaumer's laboratory (Chapter 4) have attempted the conditioning of slow cortical potentials (9.5–15-Hz activity) in the treatment of epilepsy. The rationale for this technique is twofold: one, that dysregulated cortical excitability characterizes epilepsy-proneness and, two, that changes in slow cortical potentials reflect changes in cortical excitability. In a study reported in their chapter, Elbert *et al.* recruited subjects with relatively serious epileptic seizure patterns averaging nine per week. One group (feedback) was given visual feedback designed to relate to slow wave potentials, while the other group (control) was without feedback. Most of the patients in the feedback group in this study did learn to control their slow cortical potentials while the control subjects did not. More important, two-thirds of the feedback patients showed some or complete alleviation of their epilepsy in terms of seizure frequency. Among other interesting effects, it appeared that anticonvulsant medications may have impaired conditioning of slow wave potentials in some patients, and that the older the patient, the more difficult it was to develop self-regulation of slow wave potential activity. The proof of these effects, and those of other treatment strategies, including pharmacological regimens, will come in the application to a larger number of subjects and continuing attempts to show benefits at longer follow-ups. A primary advantage of the behavioral strategies, such as EEG biofeedback, is that they do not appear to have deleterious side effects. Moreover, when they are successful, the EEG tends to normalize and other positive effects are often reported.

In Chapter 5, by James E. Skinner, Mirna Mitra, and Keith Fulton, a neural model is proposed for the study of the electrochemical activities of the olfactory bulb. The olfactory bulb has the same cell types, intrinsic chemistry, and physiology as the neocortex, and its total output can be represented by noninvasive recordings from multiple surface electrodes. Each mitral cell has an open field morphology resulting in a potential at the nearby surface that is proportional to its probability of spike initiation. The composite output has been observed to change from the same stimulus events, notably psychosocial stressors, that increase the risk of heart attacks through vulnerability to arrhythmias. Output from the olfactory bulb reflects a stable "chaotic attractor," which shows reliable increases with external (meaningful) stimulation. The authors speculate that from calculations of values of the chaotic attractor, abnormal values may help in predicting cardiovascular disorders in genetically predisposed individuals as well as help to articulate the related mechanisms in the brain. In an elegant analysis of a series of studies, Skinner and his colleagues demonstrate the development of their model. One potential use may be in real-time treatment procedures for the observed complications associated with autonomic functions and specific stimulus events. The study of brain–behavior relationships is beginning to describe reliable events as well as suggest possible theory-based treatments.

Neuromuscular Disorders

In Chapter 6, F. J. McGuigan maintains that mental activity results from the interaction of processes in the central nervous system, the autonomic system, and the skeletal muscles. Cognitive activity includes speech imagery, visual imagery, and somatic cognitions owing to activity in the speech musculature, the eye muscles, and bodily reactions, respectively. McGuigan argues that cognitive activity of each variety can thus be self-regulated through tension in the related musculature. Cognitions may be initiated by speech; alternatively, cognitions may be eliminated through relaxation of the musculature. For example, in Edmund Jacobson's Progressive Relaxation procedure, tension in specific areas of the skeletal muscles is reduced, and has been shown to have a positive impact on a number of clinical disorders, including phobias and anxiety. The control of emotions in general may also be effected through neuromuscular self-regulation. Conversely, with increased muscular tension, there may be increased emotionality. McGuigan speculates that every bodily tension has both meaning and effect. For example, specific inappropriate postures or specific fears and their control come through self-regulation of the musculature in the area of "stress management." The clinical relevance of the described techniques is probably accepted by most clinicians. The relationship between thought and bodily responses proposed by McGuigan is not as widely accepted and reminds us once again of arguments regarding cause–effect sequences in behavior, cognition, and physiology. It continues to be the case that a better understanding of the related processes will enable the development of better treatments. McGuigan's model offers a basis for continuing research in this area so important to human health.

In what appears at first to be a far distance from McGuigan's proposal, Chapter 7, by Akitane Mori and his fellow researchers, presents data from studies of the effects of excitatory and inhibitory neurotransmitters upon central mechanisms of neuromuscular control. Using an animal model, specifically the "El mouse," which is genetically susceptible to seizures, these investigators show that injected antagonists of excitatory amino acids as well as an inhibitory amino acid and various other receptor antagonists inhibit the animals' convulsions. In another study, the substance baclofen given to rats was shown to suppress EEG activity, an effect that was heightened by neuromuscular junction blockers, thus showing that afferent impulses may not reach the brain in some forms of seizure disorders. Besides direct disruption of neurotransmitter systems, such as in this research, it is possible that reduction of afferent contributions of muscles may act centrally to reduce seizures. In Barry Sterman's original sensorimotor rhythm (SMR) conditioning studies, behavioral "quieting" of cats along with SMR control was reported. Thus, McGuigan's suggestions for the role of muscle regulation in various disorders may implicate neural mechanisms, such as those of Mori *et al.*

In another approach to neuromuscular disorders, Ronald L. Webster (Chapter 8) reviews a wide range of methods for the enhancement of fluency in stutterers, including delayed auditory feedback, white noise, and the use of rhythmic stimuli. These methods appear to cluster into one category focusing on auditory feedback and another category involving muscle activity in the larynx and related areas. Webster favors a servomechanistic view for the effects of dysfluent speech in stuttering that emphasizes (a) the role of sensory feedback difficulties and (b) the importance of both the auditory feedback and muscle self-regulation aspects of the various effective interventions for stuttering. A fairly high rate of success of auditory feedback treatment ("precision fluency shaping") has been obtained in Webster's laboratory. However, treatments that emphasize auditory feedback are often impractical owing to the complexities of the equipment that is required as well as annoying features of the feedback for the user. By contrast, an instrument that amplifies the "vocal buzz" in one ear (thus altering normal modes of bone-conducted auditory feedback) has been found to reduce some of these problems and to improve fluency during both reading and conversation tasks. The potential for the self-regulation of dysfluent speech is being realized in Webster's laboratory.

Psychoneuroimmunology

Robert Ader continues to make significant contributions to psychoneuroimmunology, a field that has burgeoned since his 1981 book of the same title. In Chapter 9, Ader describes some of the evidence for a reciprocal relationship between behavior and immune functions based on the existence of neural and endocrine pathways linking these adaptive systems. For example, Ader and Cohen have shown that pairing saccharine taste (the conditioned stimulus) with an immunosuppressive drug (cyclophosphamide, CY) results in the later reduction of antibody production when the saccharine is presented during immunization. Moreover, mice that develop autoimmune disease (lupus) show delay of the disease when the animals are exposed to a conditioned taste stimulus drug administrations of CY—again demonstrating conditioning of an immunosuppressive response. Ader maintains that lupus-prone mice do not develop a taste aversion to saccharine paired with CY as well as normal mice because the CY is biologically advantageous to the mice. That is, it suppresses their immune system and retards the development of the disease. On this basis, Ader hypothesizes that the degree of immune dysfunction (deviation from homeostasis) in the animals should determine the effectiveness of conditioning of the drug's reactions—as the disease progresses, it should require more conditioning to induce a taste aversion in lupus-prone animals because the drug is helping to correct a homeostatic imbalance. Ader reports the results of related studies that are consistent with this hypothesis. The studies summarized in this chapter further Ader's conviction that immunity and lowered immunity are conditionable responses. Moreover, they suggest that immune functions generate stimuli that are detectable in animals and that animals somehow act on the information in these signals. It is clear from Ader's clear and well-documented discussion that there is evidence for CNS-immune system interactions and that behavior plays some part. Ader's work is extremely significant for hypotheses concerning the possibility of human self-regulation of immunity.

Nicholas R. S. Hall and the late Robert Kvarnes (Chapter 10) take a strong stand on the role of placebo treatments in both physical and psychological disease. They maintain that interpersonal, social, and environmental variables must be taken into account in evaluating treatment outcomes, but that the current medical model emphasizes a dualistic approach to disease that is not receptive to such factors. Partly, they argue, this owes to a lack of understanding of the mechanisms that transduce an emotional state into an immunomodulatory signal in behaviorally based interventions, in placebo effects, and in other phenomena. As one demonstration, they cite a study of their own demonstrating considerable improvement on several quantifiable dimensions in one cancer patient who had learned to use imagery well. On the other side of the coin, negative effects of behavioral interventions in disease may include emotional responses such as anger, as well as ineffective imagery, and preoccupation with the disease where denial may be actually more effective. Hall and Kvarnes suggest that the transduction of emotional states into an immunomodulatory signal may occur via direct pathways, including hormones that are produced as part of the pituitary-adrenal or -gonadal axes, although there is no evidence to show a direct link between emotions and the immune system. On the other hand, *in vitro* and animal models demonstrate clear connections between the brain and the immune system, and direct anatomical or functional relations have been established between the immune system and the sympathetic nervous system and pituitary gland. The possible involvement of the central nervous system in modulating an immune response implies a feedback mechanism for monitoring of immune function by the brain. Hall and Kvarnes have identified a number of chemical signals for such a mechanism in the form of interleukin 1 and thymosin peptides. A healthy behavioral outlook actually may be part of our disease-fighting milieu, but the specifics of how the system may operate have just begun to be demonstrated. This serves both to excite and to caution careful investigators involved in the process of establishing relationships involving the brain, behavior, and health through immunity.

In their chapter dealing with altered immune reactions, Maurice G. King and Alan J. Husband (Chapter 11) explore, one, the determinants of effective unconditional stimuli in the conditioned taste aversion (CTA) procedure and, two, the components of the unconditional response that renders it more readily conditionable by either CTA or Pavlovian methods. They make the point that, with animals, some immunity-altering drugs are more effective within a CTA procedure and others within a Pavlovian conditioning model. In one line of their research, for example, the immunosuppresant antilymphocyte serum has been investigated as a relatively nontraumatic drug that nevertheless is effective within the CTA procedure. In successive studies, the drug also was shown by these researchers to produce conditioned immunosuppression that persists across some length of time. Using the immunoenhancing agent levamisole, King and Husband have also demonstrated effective conditioned aversion and an elevation of the Helper:Suppressor T cell ratio when the conditional stimulus was presented by itself. The investigators have also begun studies aimed at determining the physiological pathways that function in the CS–UCS relationship in immune conditioning procedures. Essentially, with rats it was shown that cellular proliferation and immunoglobulin synthesis could be inhibited by pretreatment of conditioned groups with dexamethazone prior to CTA training. Since the dexamethazone was administered at levels that have no immunologic effects, a mechanism implicated for its effects on Pavlovian conditioning is its tendency to inhibit ACTH and beta-endophin. Thus, a central mediation process for the conditioning of sensory CSs to immunological reactions was supported. This powerful animal model serves as an effective means to test hypotheses concerning the relationship of conditioning of the immune system with nontoxic sybstances.

Pain

Of all of the clinical entities, pain is one of the most difficult to document objectively, in part owing to our failure to establish related mechanisms. However, as discussed by G. F. Gebhart in Chapter 12, recent discoveries of opiate receptors, analgesia through stimulation, and endogenous opioids have increased our understanding of the possible mechanisms for pain. Gebhart indicates that there is considerable evidence to show that opiate receptors are unevenly distributed in the brain, the spinal cord, and certain other tissues, and are somewhat opioid-specific in action. Opioid receptors are organized according to subtypes, each of which mediates different effects. Opioids appear to act by inhibiting neuronal activity and suppressing the release of neurotransmitters. Endogenous opioid peptides have been intensively studied and it has been generally believed that the different opioid peptides selectively interact with different opioid receptors. However, Gebhart points out that correspondences have not generally been demonstrated. Rather, it appears that local processing of peptide precursors is important. Specific sites in the brain that appear to be sensitive to opioids include the periaqueductal gray matter and the rostral, ventral medulla. The former has been identified as a nodal point in descending systems of pain control across species. Electrical stimulation-produced analgesia in this area inhibits pain reception in the spinal cord, apparently through the same mechanisms that produce opioid effects. However, there are apparently other structures and systems in the brain by which opioids and stimulation-produced analgesia also may modulate pain. While the work of Gebhart and others on the elusive mechanisms of pain control is helping to further our understanding, fortunately the clinical relevance of various techniques for pain control may be somewhat easier to establish.

No single theory has so dominated thinking in recent years about pain than the gate-control theory of Melzack and Wall. In Chapter 13,

Wolfgang Larbig reviews the current status of this theory in light of recent research. The gating mechanism itself is understood to be located in the substantia gelatinosa of the spinal cord, where nonmyelinated small fibers inhibit the "T-cells" (which themselves inhibit transmission) and myelinated large fibers activate the inhibitory T-cells. The "gate-opening" (T-cell inhibition) portion of the theory has been subject to some criticism, while the "gate-closing" (T-cell activation) mechanism has generally received support through recent studies of brain-stimulation-produced analgesia and endogenous opioid peptides. Larbig concludes his chapter with a discussion of the far-reaching impact of Melzack and Wall's theory upon research dealing with pain-modulating systems in the spinal cord, descending pathways, and opioids. He also describes a variety of clinical techniques for pain control that have evolved from or provided support to gate theory, including transcutaneous electrical stimulation, electrical acupuncture (see Chapter 16), and vibration. In addition, behavioral and cognitive methods for intervention with pain—distraction, refocusing of attention, relaxation, and biofeedback—may capitalize on the central control systems that modulate the "spinal gates." The quest for the mechanisms of pain goes on.

Somatosensory information from the head, face, and oral cavity are received by ganglion neurons that synapse within the Trigemina Nuclear Complex (TN) located in the brainstem. In Chapter 14, J. Peter Rosenfeld and James G. Broton present data from their laboratory and others that are inconsistent with the traditional view—that the rear (caudal) portions of this area are the center in which pain signals from the oral area of the face are processed, whereas the forward (rostral) portions of the TN (termed the Subnucleus Caudalis) receive only nonpainful somatosensory information. In Rosenfeld and Broton's initial studies, it appeared that direct electrical stimulation of the brain in the forward portion of the TN produced apparent facial pain in rats. In subsequent studies, the effects of facial pain (through heat) were observed as a function of lesions in the TN area—lesions in the forward portion significantly reduced the researchers' index of orofacial pain—again implicating the rostral area as a pain center. These and related data (such as observations of cortical EEGs reflecting arousal following lesioning of forward TN) lead Rosenfeld and Broton to conclude that important pathways for orofacial pain stimuli include those from forward portions of the Trigeminal Nucleus through efferents leading to the thalamus. Trigeminal neuralgia most often presents clinically as excruciatingly painful. To better understand the mechanism of this phenomenon can aid in the development of more effective treatments for pain. Moreover, retaining facial sensation for nonnociceptive stimuli will be an important related goal of treatment. The work of Rosenfeld and Broton offers important clues to these and other pain phenomena.

In Chapter 15, Masamichi Satoh discusses his neuropharmacological investigations on the involvement of neuropeptides in nociceptive transmission at the spinal cord dorsal horn. In the process, he fills in detail for earlier overviews of the role of neuropeptides in pain perception by Gebhart (Chapter 12) and Larbig (Chapter 13). Satoh focuses on several neuropeptides, so-called substance P, somatostatin, and calcitonin gene-related peptide (CGRP), that are contained in small cells of the dorsal root ganglia and their axons, the small primary afferents that transmit nociceptive information. In decerebrated rabbits, amounts of substance P and somatostatin during mechanical and thermal stimulation were determined. In spinal cords from rats, substance P was assessed during applications of capsaicin. Also, responsiveness of rats was determined to thermal and mechanical stimulation of the hind paws after they were given neuropeptides. With these preparations, Satoh reports that heat appears to cause the release of somatostatin but not substance P, and that the mechanical stimulation produces opposite effects. In addition, greater analgesic effects due to paw pressure and reduced effects due to heat were related to intrathecal injections of substance P; converse effects were obtained with injections of somatostatin. These effects thus implicate substance P during mechanical noxious stimulation and somatostatin during thermal noxious stimulation. Coupled with other findings reported by Satoh, the data suggest that the afferent terminals, the small-sized cells of the dorsal horn in the spinal cord, are involved in the differential modulation of nociceptive stimulation (and probably in the perception of pain). For the spinal cord patient suffering from chronic pain, this type of research cannot be extended to human applications soon enough.

Chapter 16, by Lang Yan Xia, J. Peter Rosenfeld, and Kun Hou Huang, illustrates the best of international cooperation by researchers in the fields reviewed in this volume. These investigators review both indirect and direct evidence for the role of the cortex in "acupuncture analgesia." Indirect evidence includes pain reports in patients with unilateral cerebral lesions, identification of neurons responsive to noxious stimuli in the cortex, inhibition of responses to noxious stimuli through cortical stimulation, and effects upon analgesia due to operantly conditioned changes in somatosensory cortical evoked potentials. More direct evidence derives from a number of lines of research on the effects of electroacupuncture by Xia and his co-workers at both the animal and the human level. This evidence includes the findings with cats that electrical stimulation of specific acupoints evokes somatosensory cortical evoked potentials specific to the point, and that cortical potentials evoked from painful stimulation of teeth is inhibited by stimulation of an acupoint. In several studies with human subjects, first, distinctive differences in cerebral potentials before and after stimulation is obtained when nociceptive and nonnociceptive electrical stimulation is administered at two acupoints of a finger. Second, subjects with unilateral cerebral lesions in the somatosensory area due to surgery show diminished effects and reports of pain due to electroacupuncture at two acupoints on the lesioned side when a finger is painfully simulated. Third, pain-specific portions of evoked potentials during electrical stimulation of a finger in humans are inhibited during electroacupuncture at two acupoints. These and other results suggest that acupoints of the body may have direct connections in the central nervous system. Moreover, there may be a descending influence on brainstem structures owing to electroacupuncture that results in analgesic effects. This outstanding research is testimony to the potential gain from efforts to internationalize research and clinical endeavors.

Future attempts to bring together researchers on an international scale will continue in the quests for knowledge of the biobehavioral mechanisms of pain and disease that know no national boundaries. The application of this knowledge in efforts to provide cost-effective health care may never be fast enough to meet the demand. These are exciting times for those involved in theory development, data generation, the development of clinical applications, and the provision of self-regulatory forms of treatment. This excitement is driven and tempered by the reality of what is not yet known in the area of self-regulation and health!

Part I
Cardiovascular and Central Disorders

Research in the area of cardiovascular disorders often overlaps with that dealing with central disorders owing to common underlying mechanisms. For that reason, these two areas have been combined in the present volume. The chapters in this section include one by Paul Grossman and one by Robert M. Kelsey and Edward S. Katkin, the former on respiratory mediation of cardiac processes and the latter on the role of myocardial functions in Raynaud's disease.

Grossman's fascinating presentation in Chapter 2 sets the stage for a number of hypotheses concerning the possibilities for self-regulation of cardiac functioning in relation to the strong central control that exists over respiration. Grossman focuses upon respiratory sinus arrhythmia and hyperventilation as two phenomena that normally demonstrate integration of respiratory and cardiac functioning but that may also be involved in dysregulation and a failure of adaptation. Implications for improving cardiovascular health in these and related areas are wide open for theory and research.

Kelsey and Katkin's research, outlined in Chapter 3, supports the view that Raynaud's disease is attributable to a deficit in myocardial contractility during stress. The authors propose an intriguing model, that below-normal cardiac output in certain individuals combines with normal processes of sympathetic vasoconstriction during stress to produce the symptoms of Raynaud's disease. Their work also points the way for exciting directions of additional research that may ultimately have significant implications for mechanisms and treatment of vascular diseases.

Also in this section are two chapters dealing with central processes and related disorders, including Chapter 4 from the University of Tübingen laboratory by Thomas Elbert, Brigitte Rockstroh, Anthony Canavan, Niels Birbaumer, Werner Lutzenberger, Isolde von Bülow, and Anne Linden, who demonstrate that the conditioning of slow cortical potentials may play a significant role in the treatment of epilepsy. Their view is that epilepsy involves the dysregulation of cortical excitation and that, therefore, conditioning of self-regulation of slow wave potentials should enhance the ability of epileptics to control seizure activity. This important research shows the potential clinical application of a specific training effect of biofeedback on brain wave activity and, in that regard, provides a superb example of a blend of basic and applied research in the field of self-regulation.

In the final chapter in this section, Chapter 5, James E. Skinner, Mirna Mitra, and Keith Fulton argue that mechanisms are not available to account for the apparent role of the frontal lobe in susceptibility to hypertension and heart attacks. They suggest that the functions of the frontal system may be studied noninvasively through investigations of processes in the olfactory bulb since it contains the same cell types and biochemical functions as the neocortex. The total output of the olfactory bulb reflects changes due to psychosocial stressors and, although it is relatively unstable, Skinner and his co-workers show that it reflects a stable "chaotic attractor." This exciting research and application of recent chaos theory shows the advantages of the use of an ideal laboratory model for brain activity and has immediate important clinical implications for understanding cardiovascular disorders.

CHAPTER 2

Respiratory Mediation of Cardiac Function within a Psychophysiological Perspective

Paul Grossman

In several previously published works, my colleagues and I have emphasized the importance of understanding respiratory–cardiovascular interactions in relation to behavioral adaptation (e.g., Grossman, 1983; Grossman & Svebak, 1987; Grossman & Wientjes, 1985, 1986). The basic underpinning for such a rationale has been rather simple: Many alterations in behavior appear to require accompanying changes in physiological functioning, and one of the most evident levels of biobehavioral integration would seem to involve the mobilization, utilization, and transfer of (physical) energy taking place upon performance of a behavioral act. Such exchanges of physical energy between organism and environment, furthermore, are accomplished to a large degree by integrated respiratory and cardiovascular adjustments (e.g., Berne, & Levy, 1981). Thus, behavioral tasks requiring alterations in physical activity (e.g., isometric or dynamic exercise) and/or psychological functioning (i.e., changes in specific mental processes or emotional states) ought to induce task-dependent variations in cardiovascular and respiratory regulation, and coupling between the two physiological systems that are adaptive for meeting the specific energy requirements of the behavioral circumstances. Individual differences in such behaviorally related cardiorespiratory responses also seem important, and may reflect normal

---

Paul Grossman • Psychophysiology Research Group, University of Freiburg, Freiburg, Federal Republic of Germany.

variations in healthy physiological patterning or, alternatively, dysfunctional reactions that may, in turn, lead to breakdowns in adaptation, whether psychological, physiological, or both. Likewise, underlying causes for such individual differences may be due to psychological factors (e.g., particular coping styles), physiological characteristics (e.g., respiratory or cardiovascular hyperreactivity to certain behavioral contingencies), or both. In any case, one must consider the situational and person-dependent factors, both psychological and physiological, when interested in grasping psychophysiological mechanisms.

Within such a functional biobehavioral framework, it is quite obvious that respiratory and cardiovascular systems must often coordinate rather closely in order to achieve a balance between metabolic requirements and both physical and psychological levels of performance: The respiratory system is primarily responsible for the exchange of gases between organism and environment (i.e., the drawing into the body of oxygen necessary to meet energy demands and the expulsion of carbon dioxide, a metabolic waste product). The cardiovascular system, of course, serves a vital function in transporting and appropriately distributing blood and oxygen to the different groups of cells within the body, each of which, depending upon momentary activity levels and specific variations in cell structure, may require differential degrees of oxygenation. It is also the cardiovascular system that collects and transports carbon dioxide and other waste products to the lungs. Thus, the respiratory system, almost literally communicating with the outside world, acts as a relatively nonspecific energy pump, tanking up from the external environment as well as eliminating waste products (to a large extent CO_2). The cardiovascular system is inherently more encapsulated within the body, concerned with ensuring that all systems within the organism are adequately supplied with the combustibles of physical energy and don't get backed up with wastes.

This rather crude description of the lungs as the body's communicator of gross energy requirements with external environment, and the heart and circulation as moderators of the energy demands of different and possibly sometimes competing systems within the body, may point to some ideas for understanding behaviorally relevant interactions between these two systems. For example, when overall changes in energy utilization are required for a behavioral act (e.g., exercise), one might expect a covariation between behavioral functioning, cardiovascular activity, and respiration. However, when behavioral acts require no net increase of energy usage, but rather a redistribution of energy supply to the different organ systems throughout the body, then one might expect that behavioral adjustments would be more highly related to specific groups of cardiovascular parameters than to respiratory measures. Within this conceptual framework, therefore, a lack of covariation between cardiovascular and respiratory processes under certain conditions need not necessarily reflect a disturbance of homeostasis, but rather the varying demands upon the two systems (with, after all, two highly related, but somewhat different, functions).

There are many processes that can regulate the interaction between cardiovascular and respiratory functions (see Grossman, 1983). Three important types of mechanisms include the following: (1) Central nervous system centers collect afferent information coming into the brain from the periphery and guide coordinated respiratory and cardiovascular activity via efferent neural and humoral control; (2) alterations in cardiovascular parameters via direct mechanical and autonomic mechanisms induce adaptive and corresponding changes in respiratory parameters; (3) on the other hand, variations in respiratory variables may also alter specific cardiac or circulatory functions as a result of mechanical or autonomic neural effects.

In the healthy organism, these three mechanisms seem so well integrated that they form a complex system of feedback and feedforward loops. Under a broad range of normal circumstances, they aim at a homeostatic functioning, buffering the organism from negative consequences of extreme responses of any single or group of cardiovascular or respiratory parameters: For example, a sudden extreme elevation in blood pressure (say, caused by a behavioral alteration) may be responded to by a baroreceptor, autonomically mediated slowing of heart rate, which will, in turn, reduce the amount of blood pumped into the arteries per minute and thus lower blood pressure (also contributed to by other mechanisms; see Berne & Levy, 1981). Similar mollifying changes upon the respiratory system may also be induced by baroreceptor stimulation (e.g., Eckberg, Kifle, & Roberts, 1980).

Often, integrated physiological adjustments, like those just mentioned, are the consequence of the reactivity of a rather small set of variables to some behavioral or psychological stimulus, but they may set off a broader chain of physiological events that, in fact, constitute an *attempt* at self-regulation that sometimes may be seen as largely internal (i.e., overt behavior remains unaltered) and other times as largely transactional with the external environment (i.e., overt behavior alters with physiological adjustments). Attempts at self-regulation are, however, not always successful. For example, certain normal physiological reflexes (e.g., the baroreflex) may be absent or attenuated as a function of extreme circumstances (e.g., an emergency reaction). When such responses are short-term ones, they may be useful in helping an individual to mobilize internal resources for overt physical action. On the other hand, when they are maintained over the long term, without any concomitant occurrence of physiologically appropriate overt activity, these responses may be maladaptive physiological reactions, superceding, for longer periods, the actual ongoing or impending physical requirements of the organism. Thus, cardiorespiratory reflexes or feedback loops may be set into motion but may not achieve the reestablishment of a steady-state equilibrium. One issue that may be of significance, therefore, is what happens when specific physiological responses occur that are not adaptive or homeostatic. Such a class of events might be triggered by internal events (e.g., physical illness) or by external stimuli, whether physical or psychological (e.g., overexposure to sun, or intense fear). Cardiovascular and respiratory reactions may dissociate either from each other or from behavioral responses in an apparently dysfunctional manner, producing a breakdown in biobehavioral adaptation.

In some of our work, we have focused specifically upon the cardiovascular consequences of behaviorally induced respiratory alterations, with an interest in both homeostatic and dysregulatory cardiovascular adjustments that can be produced. Our emphasis upon the respiratory system as mediator between psychological factors and cardiovascular alterations has been based upon several points. First, available physiological literature underlines the close interplay between respiratory and cardiovascular processes, and provides a great deal of evidence that alterations in respiratory parameters can exert reflexlike changes in diverse cardiovascular variables (see Grossman, 1983). Second, it is also clear that respiratory activity and alterations are importantly under higher brain cortical control during the awake state; respiratory parameters vary greatly to a range of behavioral demands, and individual differences in psychological dispositions have also been tied to breathing styles (Bass, & Gardner, 1985; Grossman, 1983; Grossman & Wientjes, 1989). Hence, it has seemed useful to look at the indirect cardiovascular changes that might occur as a response to behaviorally induced respiratory alterations. Furthermore, because respiratory patterns can be voluntarily altered so as to duplicate the breathing seen during specific behavioral demands, we assumed it would be possible to examine whether specific cardiovascular changes as a result of behavioral manipulations were actually triggered by the respiratory response or by some mechanism working in parallel (e.g., central neural control acting upon both respiration and circulation). Finally, as a rationale for our approach, the existing research literature demonstrates that variations in particular respiratory parameters can often exert dramatic effects upon cardiac variables that could be of consequence for cardiovascular competence and dysfunction: Changes, for example, in respiration rate, tidal volume (i.e., the amount of air breathed per breath), minute ventilation volume (i.e., the quantity of air breathed per minute), and end-tidal carbon dioxide pressure (i.e., the level of CO_2 in the expired air at the end of expiration, which is closely related to arterial concentration of CO_2) can often have dramatic effects upon cardiac functioning.

In this chapter we would like to review the current knowledge concerning potential respiratory mediation of behavioral influences upon cardiovascular functioning. The major focus will be upon two phenomena, respiratory sinus arrhythmia (RSA) and hyperventilation-induced cardiac alterations. These are respiratory-mediated cardiac phenomena that demonstrate a tight coupling between the cardiovascular and respiratory systems in response to alterations in behavior. Both of these respiratory-mediated phenomena were central to specific hypotheses made in previous publications concerning the manner by which respiratory processes might moderate psychological effects upon the cardiovascular system. Our own research in the last several years, as well as that of others, has provided us with a greater data base with which to evaluate our ideas and has caused us to alter our own thinking with respect to certain previous speculations.

Respiratory Sinus Arrhythmia

RSA is defined as cyclic fluctuations in cardiac interval length (the inverse of heart rate) that correspond to phase of respiration (e.g., Clynes, 1960): Heart rate acceleration is associated with inspiration, and heart rate deceleration is associated with expiration. Thus, typically the cardiac interval length, or heart period, shortens progressively during inspiration, with the shortest cardiac interval occurring around peak inspiration; likewise the duration between heartbeats progressively increases in length during expiration and usually approaches its most extreme value toward the end of expiration. This phasic waning and waxing of heart period has gained much interest in the last decade owing to the underlying mechanisms involved, which seem to reflect almost exclusively parasympathetic, or vagal, influences upon the heart. To elucidate briefly upon the origin of RSA, it appears that respiration gates the parasympathetic traffic from the brain to the heart in such a manner that vagal efferent activity is interrupted or attenuated during inspiration (corresponding to the tachycardiac phase of RSA) and facilitated during expiration (corresponding to the bradycardia occurring during that phase; Davidson, Goldner, & McCloskey, 1976; Gilbey, Jordan,

Richter, & Spyer, 1984; Katona, Poitras, Barnett, & Terry, 1970). Various human and animal investigations have demonstrated that mechanical influences, such as alterations in intrathoracic pressure with the breathing cycle, or other autonomic mechanisms play almost no role in the occurrence of RSA, apart from indirectly affecting vagal efferent outflow to the heart by altering vagal afferents or central nervous system activity (e.g., Raczkowska, Eckberg, & Ebert, 1983).

This apparently almost purely parasympathetic origin of RSA has led several investigators to conclude that RSA magnitude represents a good index of parasympathetic control of the heart: Merely by estimating the magnitude of RSA, various researchers believe that they are provided with information concerning the quantity of vagal efferent traffic influencing the heart (e.g., Eckberg, 1983), and some even go so far as to consider RSA as accurately reflecting central levels of vagal activity (e.g., Porges, 1986), although this seems very questionable under certain circumstances (see Grossman & Wientjes, 1986). However, with respect to the former assertion, there have been several pharmacological studies with both animals and humans that tend to confirm the hypothesis that RSA is a sensitive index of cardiac parasympathetic *tone* under specific circumstances in which vagal tone varies across a wide range of levels (from very low to very high vagal tone; e.g., Akselrod, Gordon, Madwed, Snidman, Shannon, & Cohen, 1985; Fouad, Tarazi, Ferrario, Fighaly, & Alicandro, 1984; Katona & Jih, 1975; Raczkowska *et al.*, 1983). Very recent evidence also suggests that RSA may reasonably index even relatively modest variations in vagal tone, provided certain experimental restrictions concerning variations in respiratory parameters are made (Grossman, Stemmler, & Meinhardt, in press a). Furthermore, these studies support the notion that RSA also reflects *phasic* shifts in parasympathetic cardiac control from inspiration to expiration, RSA being an inherently phasic phenomenon. In our definition, *tonic* parasympathetic control of heart period indicates the quantity of vagal efferent traffic affecting the sinus node per minute, being reflected by shifts in mean heart period from one period of interest to another when other nonvagal influences remain constant; *phasic* vagal activity is defined as merely the difference in quantity of vagal efferent input to the heart during very short-term fluctuations, i.e., from inspiration to expiration in the case of RSA. This distinction between tonic and phasic levels of parasympathetic influences upon heart period becomes a crucial differentiating concept when scientists employ RSA as an index of vagal influences upon the cardiac interval, and we will discuss this point in detail a bit later.

An interesting and important feature of RSA, in terms of respiratory mediation of cardiac function, concerns the well-established fact that the magnitude of the RSA, under normal circumstances, is a direct function of changes in respiration rate and tidal volume (Angelone & Coulter, 1964; Clynes, 1960; Eckberg, 1983; Grossman, Karemaker, & Wieling, in press b; Grossman & Wientjes, 1986; Hirsch & Bishop, 1981). Thus, spontaneous or voluntary changes in the rate and depth of breathing can dramatically alter RSA amplitude: Increases in respiratory period (the inverse of respiratory rate) and/or volume produce increases in RSA magnitude, whereas decreases in respiratory period and/or volume will attenuate or, with extremely rapid and shallow breathing, all but abolish the phenomenon. Within-subject correlations between respiratory period and RSA amplitude across task periods or paced respiration conditions, for example, often are .9 or higher, and inclusion of tidal volume as an additional predictor will typically increase the correlation coefficient.

This relationship between respiration and RSA magnitude in normal adults, as well as the experimental findings that RSA amplitude seems to be tied to changes in cardiac vagal tone, led us previously to hypothesize that cardiac vagal tone might be importantly under control of variations in respiratory parameters (e.g., Grossman, 1983; Grossman & Wientjes, 1986). In other words, we believed it plausible that the large alterations in RSA magnitude that occur in response to spontaneous or voluntary changes in respiration rate and/or tidal volume could reflect important shifts in tonic parasympathetic influences upon the heart. This would, in turn, suggest that shifts in vagal tone could be mediated by psychologically induced changes in breathing pattern, well known to occur with variations in emotion and mental processes. Accordingly, this would imply a handy functional tie between respiration and cardiac activity, appearing to facilitate coordination of respiratory and cardiac function under changing behavioral conditions: When, for example, metabolic increases require large increases in respiration rate, these respiratory changes could then trigger parasympathetic withdrawal, culminating in a more rapid heart rate appropriate to the demands at hand.

We additionally suggested that, should changes in breathing induce alterations in cardiac vagal tone, voluntary manipulations of respiratory parameters might be useful to employ both for therapeutic purposes with certain cardiac risk populations (for rationale, see, e.g., Verrier & Lown, 1980) and in psychophysiological experiments in order to better understand cardiac autonomic interactions with behavioral events.

However, an alternative hypothesis that we have lately come to take very seriously concerning the relation involving RSA magnitude, cardiac parasympathetic control, and respiration is that sizable changes in respiratory parameters of rate and tidal volume do not alter cardiac vagal tone but may distort the association between RSA magnitude and cardiac vagal tone (Grossman et al., in press a). RSA, in this case, would still remain a vagal phenomenon, based upon existing evidence, but one that merely represents *phasic* shifts in vagal influences upon the heart, *but not tonic alterations,* when respiratory pattern varies substantially. Only when respiratory parameters remain fairly constant would RSA reflect *tonic* parasympathetic effects upon the cardiac interval. Deviating radically from our original orientation, this suggests that respiratory variables mediate the phasic pattern of vagal efferent traffic to the heart (i.e., the differential levels of vagal influence upon the heart during expiration vs. inspiration), but without necessarily altering the total quantity of vagal outflow to the sinus node per time unit (see Figure 1a and b). Thus, when employing RSA to index cardiac vagal tone, respiratory parameters, within this conception, would be important only as control variables so that they do not confound the relationship between vagal tone and RSA. However, when one is solely interested in short-term vagal influences upon heart period, respiratory variables could be understood as substantially influencing the pattern of those phasic effects.

In fact, we recently conducted an investigation to examine the likelihood of whether respiratory variations actually induce changes in phasic and/or tonic vagal outflow to the heart (Grossman et al., in press a). Intraindividual relationships involving RSA, parasympathetic cardiac responses, and respiratory measures were examined in this study. Subjects were initially administered a large dose of a beta-adrenoceptor-blocking drug (10 mg propranolol intravenously) and shortly thereafter exposed to a variety of experimental conditions over a 1-hour measurement period; these experimental tasks were chosen because they had previously been found to significantly influence RSA, heart period, and respiratory variables and included rest phases, paced breathing at different rates, exercise, a reaction-time task, CO_2-rebreathing (a procedure for determining central respiratory responses), and the cold pressor. Betablockade was performed so that the task-related, autonomically mediated variations in cardiac interval could be assumed to be primarily under vagal control (sympathetic responses being either eliminated or greatly attenuated owing to blockade). We reasoned that if RSA magnitude always reflected variations in vagal tone, then mean levels of beta-blocked heart period should be correlated from minute to minute, or condition to condition, with mean values of RSA, independent of whether respiratory variables covaried with RSA. On the other hand, if there was merely an association between RSA and respiratory parameters, but little or none with beta-blocked heart period, then we could be

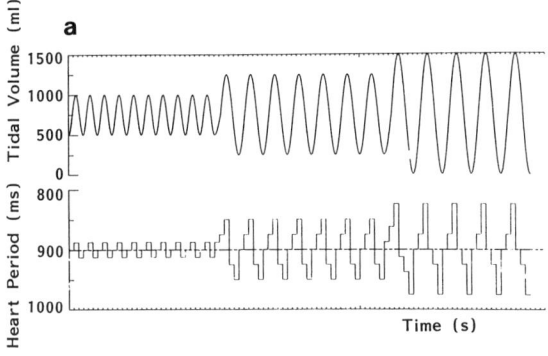

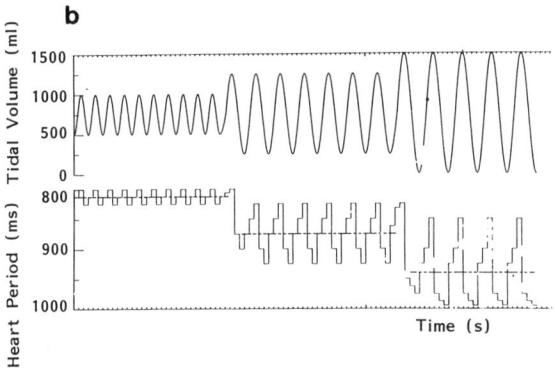

Figure 1. Contrasting hypothetical models of the relations involving respiration, RSA, and both phasic and tonic parasympathetic cardiac control. All data have been artificially generated. For the purpose of explicating the two models, in both (a) and (b) heart period data represent only vagal effects; beta-adrenergic and nonautonomic influences upon the cardiac rhythm are here considered to be theoretically eliminated. Thus, (a) provides a model in which RSA, indicative of phasic vagal effects upon the heart, covaries with respiratory parameters of cycle duration and tidal volume; but cardiac vagal tone, reflected by the mean level of heart period, depicted by the dashed line, remains unaltered and uncorrelated to the other parameters. On the other hand, model (b) suggests that respiration, RSA, phasic vagal activity, and vagal tone all covary together, since shifts in mean vagal heart period changes occur proportional to variations in RSA magnitude and respiratory variables. From Grossman et al. (in press a).

relatively certain that respiratory variables do not mediate tonic vagal responses but serve to confound any relation between RSA and cardiac vagal tone.

Results showed that although there was substantial and significant within-subject variation in mean RSA level between several conditions during betablockade, there were no corresponding alterations in mean heart period (see Figure 2a and b); thus, these findings, indeed, indicated that shifts in RSA amplitude did not track tonic vagal influences upon the cardiac interval. However, variations in RSA from condition to condition did correlate very highly with changes in respiratory cycle length and tidal volume (within-subject multiple R's across means between .87 and .97). Furthermore, in these and other analyses, mean heart period and RSA achieved a significantly positive association with

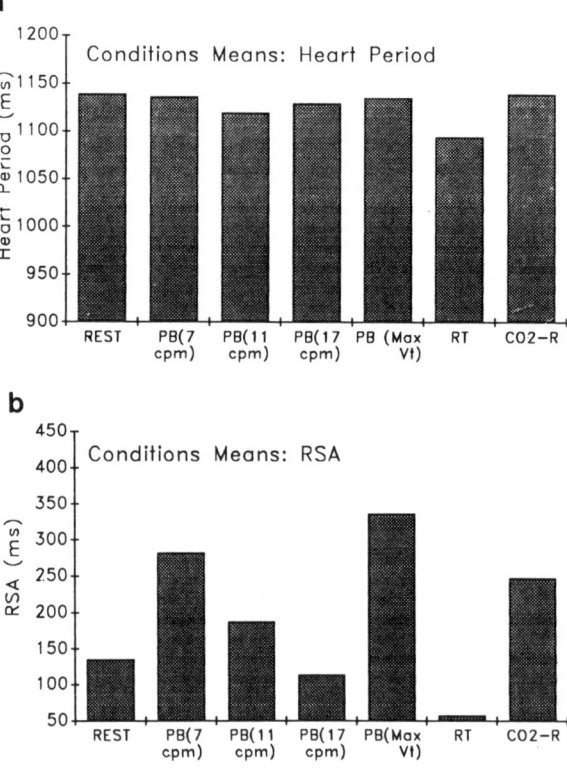

Figure 2.(a) Mean beta-blocked heart period levels across all subjects for seven experimental phases. PB = paced breathing at different rates, cycles per min (cpm); RT = reaction-time task; CO2-R = CO^2-rebreathing phase. The first three paced-breathing conditions were at a tidal volume of 1 liter; the paced breathing Max Vt, at maximal voluntary tidal volume, 7 cpm. There were no significant differences in heart period among any of the seven conditions shown here. (b) The same as (a) for respiratory sinus arrhythmia. Sixteen of the possible 21 comparisons were significantly different from each other ($p < .05$, two-tailed t tests). From Grossman *et al.* (in press a).

each other once these respiratory variables were partialed out using a multiple regression procedure, thus indicating that respiratory parameters are likely to confound the within-subject relationship between vagal tone and RSA. Nevertheless, an additional finding of this investigation, that resting levels of RSA went unaffected by beta-blockade, suggests that RSA rather purely reflects at least *phasic* vagal activity, since other research has clearly demonstrated that total parasympathetic blockade eliminates RSA (e.g., Raczkowska et al., 1983).

How can we reconcile our findings with other studies showing RSA to be a sensitive and reliable index of *tonic* parasympathetic cardiac control? First, several of the previous pharmacological validation studies used paced breathing during RSA estimation to control for respiration (e.g., Pomeranz, Macaulay, Caudill, Kutz, Adam, Gordon, Kilborn, Barger, Shannon, Cohen, & Benson, 1985; Raczkowska et al., 1983). Second, although studies that appear to have exerted no experimental control over respiratory parameters also find strong associations between cardiac vagal tone and RSA amplitude, available evidence suggests that different levels of vagal blockade do not seem to induce significant respiratory alterations (e.g., Porges, 1986). Furthermore, the fact that the range of tonic vagal activity manipulated in these experiments was very large, indeed, would imply that the effects upon RSA of any subtle shifts in respiration rate or tidal volume as a function of the drug treatments would likely to have been greatly exceeded by the dramatic variations in these experiments in cardiac vagal tone. In our study, on the other hand, the range of cardiac vagal tone could be expected to be much more modest and the range of respiratory variation was deliberately designed to be large, both levels of variation similar to what could be expected in typical psychophysiological investigations relating cardiac vagal mechanisms to alterations in behavior.

Our findings would therefore seem to indicate strongly that RSA can serve as a reliable estimate of cardiac vagal tone only when respiratory variables of rate and tidal volume are experimentally or statistically controlled, or when they do not significantly vary across experimental groups or conditions. A next logical question in this context is: why? Although we do not have sufficient information to be sure of an answer, there seem to be at least two very plausible explanations for the manner by which respiratory measures, RSA, and cardiac vagal phasic and tonic activity relate to each other. First, it is possible that the respiratory gating of vagal efferent traffic is not an all-or-nothing phenomenon, which is the basis for using RSA as an index of cardiac vagal tone. If vagal traffic occurs only during expiration, then the difference between heart period during inspiration and heart period during expiration (i.e., the magnitude of RSA) should closely correspond to the extent of vagal influence taking place during expiration. However, should it be possible that, under certain conditions, some vagal discharge also occurs during inspiration (albeit less than during expiration), then RSA would reflect a relative difference in vagal influences upon the heart from inspiration to expiration, rather than an absolute phenomenon (as suggested by Gilbey et al., 1984). Variations in respiratory rate and depth could then be hypothesized as one factor capable of inducing changes in the relation between vagal outflow during inspiration versus expiration, but not necessarily in the total quantity of vagal effects. Preliminary evidence for this notion has, indeed, been provided by Eckberg et al. (1980).

Alternatively, it would appear an even simpler and more logical explanation that respiratory cycle length would at least have to be adjusted for when using RSA as an index of cardiac vagal tone: Shorter respiratory cycles would permit fewer volleys of vagal traffic to influence cardiac interval length, even if the above-mentioned gating mechanism is an all-or-nothing event. For instance, one would expect only half the amount of vagal traffic to the heart during the expiratory period of a 3-second respiratory cycle than during the expiratory period of a 6-second respiratory cycle. Hence, the amount of expiratory cardiac slowing, represented by RSA magnitude, should also be proportionally less during the faster breathing, even though the total quantity of vagal traffic to the heart per minute would be identical.

Whatever the explanatory mechanisms involved, our findings that respiratory parameters can alter the correspondence between cardiac vagal phasic and tonic activity indicates that previous studies assuming a one-to-one correspondence between tonic and phasic vagal events were likely to be in error when they used RSA as an index of cardiac vagal tone without controlling for respiration. Therefore, the conclusions made about cardiac vagal tone in many previous publications would seem to be highly questionable when derived from RSA results in which respiratory measures have not been reported or have varied significantly (e.g., Grossman & Svebak, 1987; Pagani et al., 1986; Porges, McCabe, & Yongue, 1982). However, with regard to more positive implications of our findings, our results suggest that RSA can be applied toward understanding different facets of parasympathetic autonomic heart rate control, in interaction with respiration and other factors (e.g., sympathetic cardiac control).

In one recent study, for instance (Grossman & Svebak, 1987), we found that RSA magnitude was greatly reduced by a video-game task, particularly when the task took on a threatening element (see Figure 3). Additionally, we found that heart rate reactivity was directly associated

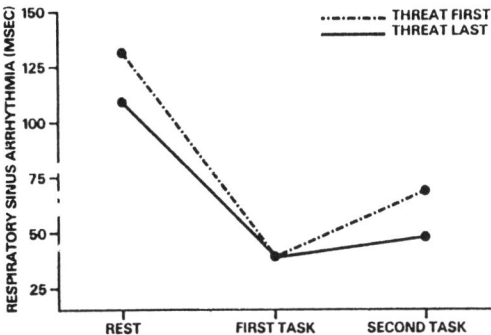

Figure 3. Mean RSA levels across experimental conditions for two groups of subjects, each performing a video-game task twice, once with and once without threat of shock (balanced order of presentation over groups). *Threat first* = the group that was presented the threat condition as first task condition; *threat last* = the group that experienced the no-threat condition first. All rest-task comparisons were significant, and a repeated-measures analysis of variance task condition X sequence of presentation interaction effect indicated that threat of shock was particularly effective at attenuating RSA when the threat was presented in the first condition. From Grossman and Svebak (1987).

with RSA responses—the greater the heart rate acceleration, the larger the diminution of RSA. At the time of publishing the paper, we, like many others, accepted the probably false notion that RSA always reflects cardiac vagal tone, and we did not provide for any control for variations across conditions in respiration. Later analysis of respiration rate and amplitude, however, revealed that RSA changes in this investigation were largely a function of these breathing parameters. This would indicate that cardiac vagal tone remained more or less constant or, alternatively, covaried with respiration rate, so that some of the changes in RSA magnitude might also have reflected alterations in cardiac vagal tone (which could be tested for only when the slope of the regression between RSA and respiratory parameters during resting paced breathing conditions would be compared with that during the task conditions, something we were unable to do). Still, the fact that RSA magnitude did vary significantly with experimental conditions clearly suggests the likelihood that phasic cardiac vagal responses to stress are mediated by respiratory changes. Just how such phasic parasympathetic effects interact with tonic ones and with sympathetic influences upon the heart remains to be studied. Nevertheless, these patterns of interaction could be of importance for issues related to biobehavioral adaptation and breakdown. It might be possible, for example, that cardiac sympathetic and both parasympathetic tonic and phasic influences covary under specific behavioral contingencies and dissociate, manifesting a variety of patterns, under others.

In another study, as yet unpublished (based on data reanalyzed from Wientjes, Grossman, & Gaillard, 1986), we, in fact, found evidence suggesting that tonic and phasic patterns of cardiac vagal activity may show diverging tendencies in response to experimental manipulations of motivational factors during performance of a task. We employed RSA as our index of phasic vagal influences upon heart period. We also used residual scores of the within-subject regression of respiration rate upon RSA to indicate tonic vagal activity; in other words, we assumed that RSA changes that were dysproportional to respiratory changes were likely to reflect alterations in vagal tone, whereas RSA changes proportional to respiratory variations might indicate just shifts in phasic patterning of vagal activity. The regressions between RSA and respiration were calculated from the means of 14 5-minute task and rest periods (4 rest and 10 task) for each of the 42 healthy young adult male subjects in the study (mean $r = .91$). All task phases utilized the same memory-search reaction-time task with a substantial monetary reward for good performance, but there were three contextual variations that were made: The task was offered (1) with feedback of performance results, (2) without such feedback, and (3) with the threat of losing all previous winnings, should performance during the last minutes not improve over that of preceding periods (here called the all-or-nothing condition). Individual performance criteria were set during a pretask training phase. RSA, respiratory, and heart period data for the different conditions are presented in Figures 4a–c. Note that RSA varied significantly from rest to task for each of the three conditions, differed among the three task conditions, and, in general, was closely inversely related to variations in respiration rate. However, statistical analyses revealed that residualized RSA differed significantly from baseline and other task levels only during the most motivating task phase, i.e., during the all-or-nothing condition; this is indicated by the dissociation of respiratory rate and RSA during the all-or-nothing task condition. This suggests that vagal tone decreased from resting values only during the most taxing behavioral condition, also the condition that showed the most pronounced decrease in heart period (Figure 4b), although conclusions must be tempered owing to possible partial covariation of respiration and vagal tone across the experimental phases. Nevertheless, comparison of the uncorrected RSA responses and the residualized responses thus indicates different patterns of reactions, each presumably reflecting specific aspects of parasympathetic cardiac control.

Future research employing RSA as an index of parasympathetic cardiac control should attend more closely to interactions among cardiac vagal tonic and phasic activity, respiratory variations, and changes in RSA. In any case, there seems to be sufficient evidence at present to indicate that respiratory parameters of rate and depth of breathing potently contribute to phasic variations in cardiac vagal activity but have little or no direct influence upon cardiac vagal tone. When respiratory

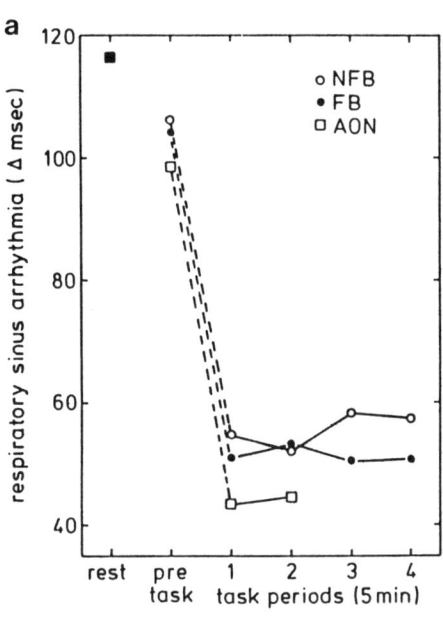

Figure 4a. Mean RSA as a function of the experimental conditions. NFB = no feedback condition; FB = feedback condition; AON = all-or-nothing condition. Rest indicates baseline level preceding task instruction, whereas pretask points represent baseline levels immediately preceding each task condition. Repeated-measures analyses of variance indicated significant rest-task effects for each task and usually differences between task conditions.

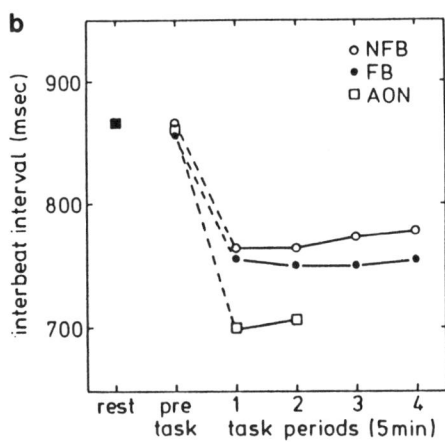

Figure 4b. Mean heart period across conditions. Heart period differences between all conditions were highly significant.

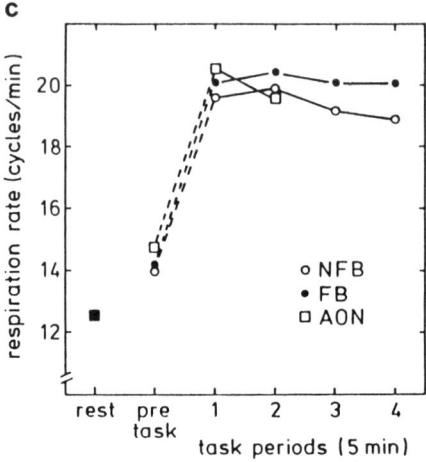

Figure 4c. Mean respiration rate across conditions. Only rest-task contrasts reached statistical significance, although several task comparisons approached significance.

parameters do covary with cardiac vagal tone, such as during exercise or hyperventilation (as we shall soon see), the responsible mechanisms for alteration of vagal tone do not appear to reside in the pattern of breathing itself. Furthermore, when employing RSA as an index of vagal tone, researchers and clinicians are advised to provide experimental control of breathing (e.g., paced respiration at a fixed rate and depth) or statistical corrections for the influence of breathing upon RSA amplitude (e.g., utilizing respiratory parameters as covariates). Using either one of these procedures appears to enable researchers to make reasonably sound conclusions concerning variations in cardiac vagal tone (Grossman et al., in press a, b).

Hyperventilation-Related Cardiac Alterations

We have also previously hypothesized that hyperventilation could play a significant role in stress-related cardiovascular disease (Grossman, 1983). In this section, we will outline the rationale for this hypothesis and attempt to examine evidence relating to it. Hyperventilation is defined as alveolar ventilation that is in excess of metabolic requirements. Thus, the amount of air breathed per minute (i.e., minute ventilation volume) is greater than that required for the concurrent metabolic state of an individual. Hyperventilation is operationalized in terms of a reduction in alveolar and arterial concentrations of carbon dioxide (CO_2). CO_2 levels may, furthermore, be measured directly and invasively from samples of arterial blood or may be accurately indexed by estimating the partial pressure of CO_2 in the expired air at the end of expiration, i.e., end-tidal CO_2.

Hyperventilation seems of importance as a potential mediator of stress-related cardiovascular function for two reasons: On the one hand, hyperventilation is known to be a relatively common respiratory response to aversive emotional stimuli, whereas, on the other hand, alterations in arterial levels of CO_2 appear to exert profound effects upon cardiac functioning. First, considering the relationship between hyperventilation and psychological factors, there are a number of investigations suggesting that emotional stress can elicit overbreathing, especially in situations that trigger fear (see Bass & Gardner, 1985; Grossman & Wientjes, 1989). One study, for example, found that 40% of aviation cadets learning to fly hyperventilated during their training flights (Balke, Ellis, & Wells, 1958), whereas several other studies show that lowering of end-tidal CO_2 is a very common reaction to the *threat* of physical pain stimuli (see Grossman, 1983). Taken as a whole, studies examining hyperventilatory responses to emotional stimuli suggest that the amount of CO_2 reduction occurring may be directly proportional to the perceived threat of the stressor. Additional evidence also indicates that there are large individual differences in the propensity to hyperventilate in specific situations, often related to psychological characteristics (Grossman & Wientjes, 1989). In particular, anxious, neurotic, and depressive individuals, as well as panic disorder patients, seem to have a tendency to lowered arterial CO_2 levels.

Turning to the cardiovascular consequences of hyperventilation, reductions in arterial carbon dioxide levels are known to produce various and often profound alterations in cardiac activity among both healthy individuals and patients with cardiac disorders (Grossman, 1983; Grossman & Wientjes, 1985, 1989). In our own research, we have examined the effects upon voluntary hyperventilation among a group of 69 25-year-old men (Grossman & Wientjes, 1985). Subjects were requested to breathe rapidly and deeply in order to induce substantial hyperventilation. The average heart rate increase from resting baseline induced by hyperventilation was on the order of 100% (range, 38–190%).

More recently, in the beta-adrenergic blockade study already briefly described, we also examined heart rate responses to hyperventilation before and after betablockade in order to approach an understanding of the autonomic effects (Grossman, Karemaker, & Wieling, unpublished results). We found no significant blockade effect upon cardiac interval shortening from resting baseline, heart period shortening 220 ms preblockade and 250 ms postblockade. Given that the level of betablockade was very large (10 mg intravenous), beta-adrenergic influences to the heart could be assumed to be absent or at least greatly attenuated. These findings suggest therefore that, since heart rate is almost solely under autonomic control, heart period responses to hyperventilation may be largely under vagal control; thus, hyperventilation appears to elicit rather profound reductions in cardiac vagal tone.

Still other research indicates that hyperventilation or increases in minute ventilation volume produce elevations of cardiac output, i.e., the amount of blood pumped from the heart per minute; Cummin, Iyawe, Mehata, and Saunders (1986), for example, found a 20% rise in cardiac output to increased ventilation that was both rapid and sustained. An interesting feature of this study is that increases in cardiac output were produced by voluntary increases in respiration rate and tidal volume, with or without changes in end-tidal CO_2, indicating that depth and frequency of breathing can exert cardiac effects independent of carbon dioxide.

Furthermore, a number of other investigations indicate that hyperventilation can alter the oxygen supply to the heart itself (via myocardial vasoconstriction and impaired oxygen availability), induce ECG abnormalities, and elicit chest pain (see Grossman & Wientjes, 1985), the last two symptoms apparently consequences of the first. These responses also are not modest: Rowe, Castillo, & Crumpton (1962) demonstrated the effects of a 15-minute period of hyperventilation upon coronary blood flow and oxygenation among six healthy subjects. The extent of hyperventilation, it should be added, was generally of the same magnitude as typical levels during naturally occurring psychological stress. Drops in coronary blood flow during the hyperventilation phase ranged from 30 to 52% in all but one subject, and a mean reduction in arteriovenous oxygen difference of 23% were indicative of a very substantial diminution of oxygen supply to the heart itself.

The current evidence concerning the cardiac effects of hyperventilation thus seems to suggest a state of cardiovascular disequilibrium: The heart is beating more rapidly and pumping more blood than is necessary to meet general metabolic requirements, yet the blood supply to and oxygenation of the heart muscle itself is, on the other hand, insufficient for specific cardiac metabolic needs. Perhaps, as has often been suggested, such a physiological pattern aims transiently to prepare the individual for physical action, the commencement of actual physical activity serving to restore balance between physiological function and metabolic requirements. However, sustained hyperventilation, with no prospect of appropriate physical action in sight, may compromise cardiovascular functioning.

Although cardiovascularly healthy young persons appear to be at no cardiac risk during hyperventilation (there are only vague suggestions in the literature that hyperventilation may in rare instances play a role in sudden cardiac death among such individuals), potential dangers of hyperventilation for certain coronary patients appear to be quite real. In one study, we examined cardiac effects of hyperventilation among different groups of patients with heart disorders, among patients with other noncardiac disorders causing chest pain (gastrointestinal and skeletal muscle disturbances), and among healthy controls (Mortensen, Nielsen, & Grossman, 1986). The major target group were patients with Prinzmetal's variant angina, a disorder characterized by anginal attacks during resting states that apparently are set off by coronary arterial spasms, dramatically reducing blood supply to the myocardium. However, patients with coronary artery disease, cardiomyopathy, and other heart disease were also studied. All subjects performed voluntary hyperventilation for a 6-minute period, during which large drops of arterial CO_2 occurred, and the ECG was continuously monitored. Results indicated that six of the seven variant angina patients responded to the hyperventilation with chest pain and ECG changes indicative of insufficient myocardial oxygen supply. Two other patients with presenting complaints of frequently occurring chest pain, but no apparent heart disease and normal coronary arteries, also responded similarly. However, all other subjects in the investigation showed no abnormal responses to the hyperventilation.

These results support the findings of previous studies suggesting hyperventilation to be a trigger of coronary arterial spasm among variant angina patients and thus suggest that a specific group of heart patients may be so hyperreactive to hyperventilation that episodes of overbreathing could place them at increased cardiovascular risk of insult or death. Furthermore, the fact that two seemingly healthy patients also manifested extreme cardiac responses to the hyperventilation suggests that certain normal individuals may also be dangerously susceptible to the coronary effects of hyperventilation.

An even more recent investigation by Rasmussen, Jull, Bagger, and Henningsen (1987) further dramatizes the potential risks of hyperventilation and provides evidence that a broader range of heart patients than previously thought may be vulnerable to the effects of hyperventilation. In this study, 190 patients with actual documented coronary disease also performed voluntary hyperventilation using a protocol similar to that described above. Patients were classified upon their ECG ST-segment response to the respiratory challenge (using criteria similar to our own). On this basis, 25% of the patients were identified as positive responders (i.e., demonstrating abnormal ECG reactions), and 75% were identified as negative responses (i.e., normal reactions). Furthermore, invasive arteriographic measurement of coronary arterial constriction during hyperventilation were taken among subsets of both groups in order to validate the classification criteria. Indeed, the positive responders demonstrated an average reduction of coronary arterial diameter during the challenge of 54%, compared with 7% among the negative responders. Thus, a large group of coronary artery patients show marked and life-threatening coronary arterial constrictive responses to hyperventilation (some up to 100% constriction), and these patients were much more susceptible to the consequences of hyperventilation than others. Of equal significance, the investigators followed all patients for a 4-year period after the initial classification and found that the positive responders to hyperventilation had a significantly higher mortality rate over the years than the negative responders. For example, at 2 years after classification, 32% of the positive responders had died versus 12% of the nonresponsive group, and this was independent of all other risk factors studied.

These findings therefore clearly indicate that factors associated with exaggerated coronary responses to hyperventilation may contribute to mortality among a rather large proportion of coronary artery patients. Just what direct role hyperventilation itself may play in relation to the increased risk of these individuals is clearly still a matter of speculation. However, the extreme consequences of hyperventilation upon coronary blood flow definitely point to potentially progressive, deleterious, and permanently damaging effects upon the cardiac muscle that can be produced by a physiological change known to commonly occur to emotional stressors. It would thus not appear too farfetched to hypothesize that emotional upset for certain cardiac patients may place them at great danger owing to the mechanism just described. Particularly vulnerable would appear to be those coronary artery patients who also concurrently suffer from anxiety disorders known to increase the likelihood of hyperventilation attacks (see Grossman & Wientjes, 1989), since it is clear that such disorders may often coexist with organic heart disease (e.g., Bass, Wade, & Gardner, 1983). So far, however, there has been little sound psychophysiological research into this matter, and obviously much more work still needs to be done to test the importance of this idea.

In any case, our original hypothesis concerning hyperventilation as a possible mediator between psychological factors and cardiovascular dysfunction and disease seems to be still viable. Hyperventilation induces profound and potentially compromising cardiovascular changes, apparently placing cardiac patients at increased risk. Unfortunately, little is yet known about the psychophysiology of hyperventilation, since the kind of intensely aversive emotional stimuli apparently triggering dramatic reductions in arterial CO_2 levels often cannot be ethically simulated in the laboratory, and since ambulatory monitoring of ventilation and carbon dioxide in more natural settings presents severe technical difficulties. Nevertheless, the challenge of studying hyperventilation in relation to psychological factors is gradually being met by the employment of innovative experimental paradigms—e.g., hypnotic suggestion of previous negative emotional experiences during physiological monitoring (Freeman, Conway, & Nixon, 1986), as well as prolonged measurement of end-tidal CO_2 in the laboratory among groups of individuals selected for their likelihood to hyperventilate (Gardner, Meah, & Bass, 1986). Future research should be extended to include important cardiovascular concomitants of emotionally induced hyperventilation among normals and cardiac patients, both with and without predispositions to hyperventilate.

References

Akselrod, S., Gordon, D., Madwed, J. B., Snidman, N. C., Shannon, D. C., & Cohen, R. J. (1985). Hemodynamic regulation: Investigation by spectral analysis. *American Journal of Physiology, 249,* H867–H875.

Angelone, A., & Coulter, N. A. (1964). Respiratory sinus arrhythmia: A respiration frequency dependent phenomenon. *Journal of Applied Physiology, 19,* 479–482.

Balke, B., Ellis, J. P., & Wells, J. G. (1958). Adaptive responses to hyperventilation. *Journal of Applied Physiology, 12,* 269–277.

Bass, C., & Gardner, W. (1985). Emotional influences upon breathing and breathlessness. *Journal of Psychosomatic Research, 29,* 592–609.

Bass, C., Wade, C., & Gardner, W. (1983). Unexplained breathlessness and psychiatric morbidity in patients with normal and abnormal coronary arteries. *Lancet, 1,* 605–609.

Berne, R. M., & Levy, M. N. (1981). *Cardiovascular physiology* (4th ed.). London: C. V. Mosby.

Clynes, M. (1960). Respiratory sinus arrhythmia: Laws derived from computer simulation. *Journal of Applied Physiology, 15,* 863–874.

Cummin, A. R., Iyawe, V. I., Mehata, N., & Saunders, K. B. (1986). Ventilation and cardiac output during the onset of exercise, and during voluntary hyperventilation, in humans. *Journal of Physiology, 370,* 567–583.

Davidson, N. S., Goldner, S., & McCloskey, D. I. (1976). Respiratory modulation of baroreceptor and chemoreceptor reflexes affecting heart-rate and cardiac vagal efferent nerve activity. *Journal of Physiology, 259,* 523–530.

Eckberg, D. L. (1983). Human sinus arrhythmia as an index of vagal cardiac outflow. *Journal of Applied Physiology, 54,* 961–966.

Eckberg, D. L., Kifle, Y. T., & Roberts, V. L. (1980). Phase relationships between human respiration and baroreflex responsiveness. *Journal of Physiology, 304,* 489–502.

Fouad, F. M., Tarazi, R. C., Ferrario, C. M., Fighaly, S., & Alicandro, C. (1984). Assessment

of parasympathetic control of heart rate by a noninvasive method. *American Journal of Physiology, 246,* H838–H842.
Freeman, L., Conway, A., & Nixon, P. (1986). Physiological responses to psychological challenge under hypnosis in patients considered to have the hyperventilation syndrome. *Journal of the Royal Society of Medicine, 79,* 76–83.
Gardner, W., Meah, M. S., & Bass, C. (1986). Controlled study of respiratory responses during prolonged measurements in patients with chronic hyperventilation. *Lancet, 1,* 826–830.
Gilbey, M. P., Jordan, D., Richter, D. W., & Spyer, K. M. (1984). Synaptic mechanisms involved in the inspiratory modulation of vagal cardio-inhibitory neurones in the cat. *Journal of Physiology, 356,* 65–78.
Grossman, P. (1983). Respiration, stress and cardiovascular function. *Psychophysiology, 20,* 284–300.
Grossman, P., & Svebak, S. (1987). Respiratory sinus arrhythmia as an index of parasympathetic control during active coping. *Psychophysiology, 24,* 228–235.
Grossman, P., & Wientjes, C. (1985). Respiratory-cardiac coordination as an index of cardiac functioning. In J. Orlebeke, G. Mulder, & L. van Doornen (Eds.), *Psychophysiology of cardiovascular control* (pp. 451–464). New York: Plenum.
Grossman, P., & Wientjes, C. (1986). Respiratory sinus arrhythmia and parasympathetic cardiac control: Some basic issues concerning quantification, application and implications. In P. Grossman, K. H. Janssen, & D. Vaitl (Eds.), *Cardiorespiratory and cardiosomatic psychophysiology* (pp. 117–138). New York: Plenum.
Grossman, P., & Wientjes, C. (1989). Respiratory disorders: Asthma and hyperventilation syndrome. In G. Turpin (Ed.), *Handbook of clinical psychophysiology* (pp. 521–556). New York: Wiley.
Grossman, P., Karemaker, J., & Wieling, W. (in press a). Prediction of tonic parasympathetic cardiac control using respiratory sinus arrhythmia: The need for respiratory control. *Psychophysiology.*
Grossman, P., Stemmler, G., & Meinhardt, E. (in press b). Paced respiratory sinus arrhythmia as index of cardiac parasympathetic tone during varying behavioral tasks. *Psychophysiology.*
Hirsch, J., & Bishop, B. (1981). Respiratory sinus arrhythmia in humans: How breathing modulates heart rate. *American Journal of Physiology, 241,* H620–H629.
Katona, P. G., & Jih, R. (1975). Respiratory sinus arrhythmia: A noninvasive measure of parasympathetic cardiac control. *Journal of Applied Physiology, 39,* 801–805.
Katona, G., Poitras, J., Barnett, O., & Terry, B. (1970). Cardiac vagal efferent activity and heart period in the carotid sinus reflex. *American Journal of Physiology, 218,* 1030–1037.
Mortensen, S., Nielsen, H., & Grossman, P. (1986). Hyperventilation as diagnostic stress test for variant angina and cardiomyopathy: Cardiovascular responses, likely triggering mechanisms and psychophysiological implications. In P. Grossman, K. H. Janssen, & D. Vaitl (Eds.), *Cardiorespiratory and cardiosomatic psychophysiology* (pp. 303–318). New York: Plenum.
Pagani, M., Lombardi, F., Guzzetti, S., Rimoldi, O., Furlan, R., Pizzinelli, P., Sandrone, G., Malfatto, G., Dell'Orto, S., Piccaluga, E., Turiel, M., Baselli, G., Cerutti, S., & Malliani, A. (1986). Power spectral analysis of heart rate and arterial pressure variabilities as a marker of sympatho-vagal interaction in man and conscious dog. *Circulation Research, 59,* 178–193.
Pomeranz, B., Macaulay, R. J., Caudill, M. A., Kutz, I., Adam, D., Gordon, D., Kilborn, K. M., Barger, A. C., Shannon, D. C., Cohen, R. J., & Benson, H. (1985). Assessment of autonomic function in humans by heart rate spectral analysis. *American Journal of Physiology, 17,* H151–H153.

Porges, S. W. (1986). Respiratory sinus arrhythmia: Physiological basis, quantitative methods and clinical implications. In P. Grossman, K. H. Janssen, & D. Vaitl (Eds.), *Cardiorespiratory and cardiosomatic psychophysiology* (pp. 101–116). New York: Plenum.

Porges, S. W., McCabe, M., & Yongue, B. G. (1982). Respiratory-heart rate interactions: Psychophysiological implications for pathophysiology and behavior. In J. T. Cacioppo & R. E. Petty (Eds.), *Perspectives in cardiovascular psychophysiology* (pp. 223–264). New York: Guilford.

Raczkowska, M., Eckberg, D. L., & Ebert, T. J. (1983). Muscarinic cholinergic receptors modulate vagal cardiac response in man. *Journal of the Autonomic Nervous System, 7,* 271–278.

Rasmussen, K., Jull, S., Bagger, J. P., & Henningsen, P. (1987). Usefulness of ST deviation induced by hyperventilation as a predictor of cardiac death in angina pectoris. *American Journal of Cardiology, 59,* 763–768.

Rowe, C. G., Castillo, C. A., & Crumpton, C. W. (1962). Effects of hyperventilation on systemic and coronary hemodynamics. *American Heart Journal, 63,* 67–77.

Wientjes, C. J. E., Grossman, P., & Gaillard, A. W. K. (1986). *Breathing and stress.* (Technical report IZF c-10). Soesterberg, The Netherlands: TNO Institute for Perception.

Verrier, R. L., & Lown, B. (1980). Vagal tone and ventricular vulnerability during psychological stress. *Circulation, 62*(Suppl. 3), 176.

CHAPTER 3

Environmental Stress and Myocardial Reactivity
Implications for Raynaud's Disease

Robert M. Kelsey and Edward S. Katkin

This study tested aspects of a new theory (Kelsey, 1986) of the etiology and pathophysiology of *primary Raynaud's phenomenon*. Raynaud's phenomenon is defined as an episode of vasoconstriction, or vasospasm, of the small cutaneous arteries and arterioles in the extremities that causes a severe reduction in blood flow and a corresponding decrease in temperature in the skin of affected areas (Coffman & Davies, 1975; Gifford & Hines, 1957). These vasospastic episodes usually affect the fingers, causing them to turn cold, numb, and white; thus, Raynaud's phenomenon is characterized as "episodic vasospastic ischemia of the digits" (Halperin & Coffman, 1979, p. 89). The phenomenon is further classified into *primary* and *secondary* forms. Primary Raynaud's phenomenon, also known as *Raynaud's disease,* refers to idiopathic manifestations of the disorder, whereas secondary Raynaud's phenomenon refers to manifestations of the disorder that are symptomatic of an underlying primary disease, such as scleroderma.

Robert M. Kelsey • Department of Psychology, State University of New York at Buffalo, Buffalo, New York 14260, USA.   *Edward S. Katkin* • Department of Psychology, State University of New York at Stony Book, Stony Brook, New York 11794–2500, USA.

Pathophysiological Theories and Evidence

There are three major classes of theory about the etiology and pathophysiology of primary Raynaud's phenomenon: (a) systemic theories, (b) local theories, and (c) rheological theories.

Systemic theories postulate that the vasospastic episodes of Raynaud's disease are attributable to sympathetic nervous system overactivation that produces enhanced vasoconstriction in response to stimuli. The available evidence concerning sympathetic overactivation as the pathophysiological mechanism of Raynaud's disease is contradictory (Blunt & Porter, 1981; Coffman & Davies, 1975; Mendlowitz & Naftchi, 1959). While Peacock (1957, 1959a,b), Jamieson, Ludbrook, and Wilson (1971), and McGrath, Peek, and Penny (1978) have found evidence of excessive sympathetic vasoconstrictive activity in Raynaud's disease patients, other researchers (Downey & Frewin, 1973; Kontos & Wasserman, 1969) have failed to identify significant evidence of sympathetic overarousal in Raynaud's patients as compared with normals. Consequently, *systemic theories of Raynaud's disease based upon sympathetic overactivation are open to question.*

Local theories postulate that the vasospastic episodes of primary Raynaud's phenomenon are due to local vascular abnormalities that cause the vessels to become hypersensitive to cold. The evidence in support of local vascular abnormality as a factor in Raynaud's disease (Burch, Harb, & Sun, 1979; Mendlowitz & Naftchi, 1959) has been criticized on the grounds that it has been gathered from observations of patients with either extremely severe, advanced Raynaud's disease or secondary Raynaud's phenomenon associated with an underlying disorder (Coffman & Davies, 1975). In addition, a number of studies have failed to find any evidence to support the local vascular hypothesis (Jamieson *et al.*, 1971; Kimby, Fargrell, Bjorkholm, Holm, Mellstedt, & Norberg, 1984; McGrath *et al.*, 1978; Porter, Snider, Bardana, Rosch, & Eidemiller, 1975). Furthermore, theories of local cold hypersensitivity may be criticized for failing to account for the role of emotional stimuli in eliciting vasospastic episodes in Raynaud's disease (Coffman & Davies, 1975).

Rheological theories postulate that the vasospastic episodes of primary Raynaud's phenomenon are due to abnormalities in blood rheology that result in increased blood viscosity. The evidence for the role of blood viscosity in the pathophysiology of Raynaud's disease is equivocal at best (Ayres, Jarrett, & Browse, 1981; Goyle & Dormandy, 1976; Jahnsen, Nielsen, & Skovborg, 1977; Jamieson *et al.*, 1971; McGrath *et al.*, 1978; Pola, Savi, Dal Lago, Flore, & Shami, 1980; Pringle, Walder, &

Weaver, 1965). As with abnormalities in vascular structure, abnormalities in blood viscosity may be significant in severe cases of Raynaud's disease and in secondary Raynaud's phenomenon, but they do not appear to be significant factors in mild and moderate cases of primary Raynaud's phenomenon. Moreover, as in the case of local theories, rheological theories fail to explain the mechanism by which emotional stimuli elicit vasospastic episodes in Raynaud's disease.

Available Facts

A number of conclusions about Raynaud's disease may be drawn from available evidence (Kelsey, 1986):

1. Episodes of primary Raynaud's phenomenon may be elicited by cold and/or psychological factors, such as mental or emotional stress.

2. Raynaud's disease patients tend to have lower resting levels of hand and finger blood flow and lower finger temperatures than do normal subjects, although levels fall within the lower normal range in some cases.

3. Patients with Raynaud's disease tend to have levels of mean arterial blood pressure, systolic blood pressure, and transmural pressure that either are lower than normal or fall toward the lower end of the normal range.

4. Patients with Raynaud's disease do not necessarily exhibit a greater than normal vasoconstrictive response to cold or stress, nor do they necessarily have greater levels of sympathetic nervous system activation and sympathetic vasomotor tone than do normal subjects.

5. Except in severe or advanced cases, Raynaud's disease patients do not necessarily exhibit local vascular abnormalities or rheological abnormalities.

The Myocardial Performance Theory

Several researchers (Coffman & Davies, 1975; Downey & Frewin, 1973; Halperin & Coffman, 1979) have hypothesized that primary Raynaud's phenomenon may result from a normal degree of sympathetic vasoconstriction "superimposed on an already low blood flow and pressure in the digits" (Coffman & Davies, 1975, p. 137). Despite the fact that researchers have not established a satisfactory explanation for the "already low blood flow and pressure" found in the fingers of Raynaud's patients (Cohen & Coffman, 1982; Downey & Frewin, 1973;

Nielsen, 1978), research efforts have continued to focus primarily upon *peripheral* sympathetic responses to environmental or psychological stress.

The present study tested an alternative theoretical perspective (Kelsey, 1986) that focuses on *cardiodynamic* factors in Raynaud's disease, specifically on the role of myocardial performance in the etiology and pathophysiology of the disorder. This theory suggests that the reduced digital blood flow and pressure associated with Raynaud's disease may result from *reduced myocardial performance*—that is, cardiac output that is below normal or at the low end of the normal range. Moreover, it suggests a diathesis-stress model of Raynaud's disease, in which the diathesis is diminished myocardial performance and the stress may be either physical (e.g., cold temperature, dampness, weather change) or psychological (e.g., cognitive, mental, emotional).

Cardiac output is, of course, a major determinant of blood flow and blood pressure; therefore, the reduced digital blood flow and pressure associated with Raynaud's disease could result from reduced cardiac output. The effects of low cardiac output would be particularly evident in the small arteries and arterioles in the skin of the extremities. Thus, the effects of diminished myocardial performance would increase the probability that sympathetic vasoconstriction in response to cold or psychological stress would precipitate an attack of vasospastic ischemia.

Indirect evidence can be summoned to support this theory of Raynaud's disease. First, there are consistent sex differences that are supportive. The incidence of Raynaud's disease is much greater in females than in males, with reported estimates of female to male incidence ranging from ratios of 2 to 1 (Agrifoglio & Agus, 1976; Heslop, Coggon, & Acheson, 1983) to 8 to 1 (Velayos, Robinson, Porciuncula, & Masi, 1971). There also are gender differences in cardiac function that are consistent with the myocardial performance hypothesis: (a) Both heart size and central blood volume are smaller in women than in men (Frey, Doerr, & Miles, 1982); (b) under conditions of rest and various levels of exercise, women exhibit significantly lower oxygen consumption, cardiac output index, and stroke volume index as compared with men (Hossack & Bruce, 1982); (c) peripheral vascular resistance is greater in women than in men (Hossack & Bruce, 1982); (d) systolic and diastolic blood pressures are lower in women than in men during the second through fifth decades of life (Rose, 1980); (e) hand and digital blood flows are significantly lower in young women than in young men (Bollinger & Schlumpf, 1976; Wouda, 1977). These normal differences in cardiovascular functioning between females and males are consistent with the high incidence of Raynaud's disease in young women, with the cardiovascular data reported for Raynaud's disease patients, and with our myocardial performance theory.

Second, it is usually assumed that peripheral vascular resistance is elevated in Raynaud's disease patients owing to excessive alpha-adrenergic vasoconstrictive activity. Elevated vascular resistance in the presence of normal cardiac output should result in elevated blood pressure; yet the incidence of hypertension in female patients with Raynaud's disease (Gifford & Hines, 1957) is less than half of that in the general population of age-matched females (Rose, 1980). In fact, Raynaud's disease patients tend to have *below* normal blood pressure (Cohen & Coffman, 1982; Thulesius, 1976), especially with respect to systolic pressure. Since myocardial performance exerts a greater effect on systolic pressure than on diastolic pressure, this evidence suggests that diminished myocardial performance may be a factor in Raynaud's disease.

Third, Raynaud's phenomenon is a frequent side effect of *beta-adrenergic blockade* in the treatment of hypertension (Eliasson, Danielson, Hylander, & Lindblad, 1984; Marshall, 1980; Marshall, Roberts, & Barritt, 1976; Poulter & Gabriel, 1979). Approximately a third of hypertensive patients treated with atenolol, a *cardioselective* beta-blocker, develop vasospastic symptoms, indicating that a decrease in beta-adrenergic activation of the heart may be sufficient to induce Raynaud's phenomenon. Finally, the reported effectiveness of terbutaline, a beta-adrenergic agonist that increases cardiac output, in the treatment of patients with primary Raynaud's phenomenon (Thune & Fyrand, 1976) suggests that reduced cardiac output might be a significant pathogenic factor in Raynaud's disease.

The myocardial performance theory provides a parsimonious explanation for the low hand and digital blood flow, low systolic blood pressure, low intravascular pressure, low transmural pressure, and enhanced vasoconstriction characteristic of Raynaud's disease. The principal parameters of myocardial performance are rate, force, and volume; therefore, a reduction in either heart rate, myocardial contractile force, or stroke volume may result in a reduction in cardiac output. Moreover, the hypothesized deficiency in myocardial performance may be evident at rest or in response to cold or psychological stress.

The available data indicate that there are no significant differences in heart rate between Raynaud's disease patients and normal controls (Freedman & Ianni, 1983). There are apparently no studies that have compared stroke volume, cardiac output, or measures of myocardial contractility in Raynaud's disease patients and normal controls.

The present experiment was designed to test primarily the *reactivity* aspects of our theory of Raynaud's disease. The cardiodynamic and peripheral vascular responses of young female subjects who reported symptoms of Raynaud's disease and young female asymptomatic control subjects were evaluated during resting conditions and during psychological stress in a normal thermal environment. The study employed female subjects because of the greater incidence of Raynaud's disease in females than in males.

The psychological stressor employed in this study was a mental arithmetic task consisting of rapid serial subtractions by steps of 13. There is substantial evidence that such mental arithmetic tasks elicit both beta-adrenergic and alpha-adrenergic effects on the cardiovascular system (Brod, Fencl, Heijl, & Jirha, 1959; Krantz, Contrada, LaRiccia, Anderson, Durel, Dembroski, & Weiss, 1987; Lane, White, & Williams, 1984; Linden, McEachern, & Madaisky, 1985). The beta-adrenergic effects include increased cardiac rate, contractility, and output, as well as peripheral vasodilation, while the alpha-adrenergic effects are reflected in peripheral vasoconstriction. Similar mental arithmetic tasks have been employed as stressors in other psychophysiological investigations of Raynaud's disease (Halperin, Cohen, & Coffman, 1983; Hugdahl, Fagerstrom, & Broback, 1984). Halperin et al. (1983) evaluated Raynaud's disease patients in warm environments versus control subjects in warm and cool environments during resting conditions and during mental arithmetic stress. They found that all subjects exhibited significant increases in heart rate and mean blood pressure in response to stress. Peripheral vascular responses to stress differentiated the patient and control groups, however, with control subjects exhibiting the expected digital vasoconstrictive response to stress, while Raynaud's patients exhibited an unexpected digital vasodilatory response to stress. Hugdahl et al. (1984) studied Raynaud's disease patients and controls under conditions of freezing cold and freezing cold plus mental arithmetic stress. They found that only the control group exhibited increased pulse rate and vasoconstriction in response to mental arithmetic stress.

The indexes of cardiovascular activity that were employed in the Halperin et al. and Hugdahl et al. studies do not provide sufficient information for an evaluation of the myocardial performance theory. Both studies relied primarily upon peripheral vascular measures, which do not provide adequate information about myocardial activity. The measures related to cardiac function that were reported (e.g., heart rate, pulse rate, and mean blood pressure) do not provide clear information about the relative sympathetic and parasympathetic influences on the myocardium, nor do they provide sufficient information about inotropic aspects of myocardial performance. The present study employed impedance cardiographic techniques in order to obtain this information.

Impedance cardiography provides a reliable, noninvasive method for assessing changes in stroke volume, cardiac output, systolic time intervals, and indexes of myocardial contractility (Miller & Horvath, 1978). It is a particularly useful method for measuring preejection period (PEP), a sensitive index of myocardial contractility and beta-adrenergic effects on the heart (Newlin & Levenson, 1979; Obrist, Light, James, & Strogatz, 1987). Thus, impedance cardiography is capable of providing clear and specific information about inotropic aspects of myocardial performance and sympathetic nervous system influences on the heart.

It was expected that all subjects would exhibit increased myocardial performance during the mental arithmetic task, as indexed by increments in heart rate and cardiac output, as well as by decrements in preejection period and left ventricular ejection time. However, we predicted that myocardial reactivity to stress would be lower for subjects with Raynaud's disease as compared with asymptomatic control subjects. Specifically, it was predicted that the increments in myocardial contractility and cardiac output elicited by the stressful task would be smaller for Raynaud's subjects than for control subjects.

Two alternative predictions were entertained with regard to finger blood flow responses to stress. The Halperin et al. (1983) data suggest that mental stress in a room-temperature environment should elicit a decrease in finger blood flow in control subjects, but a paradoxical increase in finger blood flow in Raynaud's subjects. Consistent with traditional formulations, as well as with our model, it would be expected that mental stress in a room-temperature environment should elicit a decrease in finger blood flow in Raynaud's subjects, but an increase in finger blood flow in control subjects.

Method

Subjects

A 15-item health symptom questionnaire was administered to 285 women enrolled in introductory psychology courses at SUNY/Buffalo. The age range of the students was from 17 to 31, with a mean age of approximately 18.3 years. The respondents were screened on the basis of their responses to the question "How often have you experienced episodes in which any or all of your fingers become cold, numb, and white during cold weather?" Forty-one respondents (14.4%) reported that they had experienced such episodes more frequently than once a week. Thirty-five of these respondents were interviewed by telephone in order to gather additional information and to determine whether they qualified for a diagnosis of primary Raynaud's phenomenon. Nine of the interviewees who met the diagnostic criteria for Raynaud's disease (Coffman & Davies, 1975; Gifford & Hines, 1957) were recruited to serve as experimental subjects. Ten female control subjects were recruited randomly from the large pool of survey respondents who indicated that they had rarely or never experienced episodes in which their fingers became cold, numb, and white during cold weather. All subjects were offered the option of participating in the study for either $5 or one credit toward the fulfillment of a course requirement.

Physiological Recording Apparatus and Techniques

Impedance cardiographic (ZKG), electrocardiographic (EKG), finger pulse, and respiration signals were recorded continuously with a Grass model 7D polygraph. The ZKG signals included basal transthoracic impedance (Z_0, in ohms) and the first derivative of the pulsatile change in impedance (dZ/dt, in ohms per second). All physiological signals were recorded on FM tape for later analysis.

The successful application of impedance cardiography requires attention to two potential threats to its validity. First, it is important to note that impedance cardiographic measures cannot be calibrated to yield true *absolute* stroke volume levels; therefore, the utility of this index lies in its ability to assess relative change within subjects over time (Miller & Horvath, 1978).

Second, the measure may be compromised by pulsatile impedance changes induced by the respiratory cycle; consequently, reliable use of the technique is often achieved by measuring at the same point in each respiratory cycle. This approach was not feasible in the present research paradigm. An alternative approach involves computerized sampling and averaging of EKG and ZKG signals in an ensemble averaging procedure that is analogous to signal averaging procedures employed in evoked potential (EP) research.

A number of validating studies demonstrate that within the limits of proper experimental design (i.e., repeated-measure ANOVA) and mathematical analysis (i.e., ensemble averaging), impedance cardiography is an unusually sensitive and valid technique for the assessment of changes *within subjects* in stroke volume, cardiac output, myocardial contractility, and systolic time intervals (Miller, & Horvath, 1978; Muzi, Ebert, Tristani, Jeutter, Barney, & Smith, 1985; Sheps, Petrovick, Kizakevich, Wolfe, & Craige, 1982). The present study employed both a within-subjects design and an ensemble averaging technique in order to conform to these technical constraints.

Procedure

When the subjects arrived at the psychophysiology laboratory they were met by a female experimenter who informed them of the general nature of the experiment and asked them to complete a statement of informed consent. All subjects were informed that they could withdraw from the experiment at any time without penalty. The experimenter obtained the height and weight of each subject. The subject then was seated in a comfortable chair in a soundproof, temperature-controlled chamber maintained at 71° F (+/− 1° F). The chamber also contained an unobtrusive video camera and an intercom for subject communication and monitoring. The experimenter informed the subject of the nature and purpose of the equipment to be used in the experiment. She then wrapped the four mylar tape electrodes for ZKG recording around the subject's neck and torso, attached three EKG electrodes in a Lead II configuration, placed a photoplethysmograph on the subject's left index finger, and placed a respiration transducer around the subject's abdomen. The inner ZKG recording electrodes were placed at the base of the neck and at the xiphisternal junction, and the outer ZKG current electrodes were placed at least 3 cm away from the inner recording electrodes. After all of the electrodes and transducers were placed on the subject, a series of three blood pressure measurements were taken by the experimenter using the auscultatory method. Before leaving the chamber, the experimenter instructed the subject to rest, move as little as possible, and wait for further instructions.

Following the adjustment and calibration of the physiological recording devices, the subject was instructed to relax for a 5-minute baseline rest period. At the end of the rest period, the subject was given instructions for a stressful mental arithmetic task, which consisted of counting backwards aloud from a four-digit number (e.g., 1539) by steps of 13. The subject was urged to perform this serial subtraction task as quickly and as accurately as possible for a 5-minute period. A brief example of the task was given and any questions that the subject had were answered. Following the completion of the task period, the subject was instructed to relax for another 5-minute rest period. This recovery rest period was included in order to allow evaluation of possible differences in rate of recovery between experimental and control subjects. At the conclusion of the recovery period, the female experimenter reentered the chamber and obtained a second series of three blood pressure measurements. The subject then was released from the apparatus and debriefed.

Data Reduction and Dependent Measures

The following dependent measures were evaluated throughout the experiment: (a) heart rate (HR, in beats per minute), which was derived from interbeat interval (IBI, in milliseconds); (b) stroke volume (SV, in milliliters), which was based on the standard equation developed by Kubicek and colleagues (Kubicek, Witsoe, Patterson, and From, 1969); (c) cardiac output (CO, in liters per minute), defined as the product of HR times SV; (d) preejection period (PEP, in milliseconds), defined as the interval between the initiation of ventricular depolarization and the onset of left ventricular ejection; (e) left ventricular ejection time (LVET, in milliseconds), defined as the interval between the onset and the end of left ventricular ejection; (f) pulse transit time (PTT, in milliseconds), defined as the interval between the peak of the dZ/dt wave and the peak of the finger pulse wave; (g) finger pulse amplitude (FPA, in millivolts), measured from pulse rise onset to pulse peak.

Average values for each of the dependent variables were determined for each minute of each period using ensemble averaged values obtained over 60-second intervals, with the exception of IBI and HR, which were determined from the beat-by-beat averages for the same 60-second intervals. Height, weight, mean interelectrode distance (L, the average of the front and back interelectrode distance measurements), and the resting blood pressure measurements obtained before and after the experiment also were evaluated. The blood pressure measures included systolic and diastolic pressures, defined as the mean value of three readings, and pulse pressure, defined as systolic pressure minus diastolic pressure.

Results

Anthropometric and Blood Pressure Data

Table 1 presents the means and standard deviations for height, weight, mean interelectrode distance, and blood pressure data from the pre- and postexperimental measurement periods for Raynaud's and control subjects. There were no significant differences between the groups in height, weight, or mean interelectrode distance. The systolic, di-

Table 1. Means and Standard Deviations of Anthropometric and Blood Pressure Data for Both Groups during Pre- and Postexperimental Periods[a]

Measures		Raynaud's	Controls
Height	M	65.42	63.98
(in)	SD	0.53	0.71
Weight	M	132.11	134.13
(lb)	SD	15.36	9.83
Mean L	M	29.33	28.97
(cm)	SD	1.94	1.48
SBP1	M	106.76	104.51
(mmHg)	SD	12.11	13.18
DBP1	M	61.84	69.16
(mmHg)	SD	7.02	9.13
PP1	M	44.91	35.35
(mmHg)	SD	12.64	16.02
SBP2	M	106.53	104.49
(mmHg)	SD	13.64	12.32
DBP2	M	63.68	71.34
(mmHg)	SD	12.31	7.56
PP2	M	42.86	33.15
(mmHg)	SD	19.51	15.58

[a] M = mean, SD = standard deviation, mean L = average interelectrode distance, SBP1 = average preexperimental systolic blood pressure, DBP2 = average preexperimental diastolic blood pressure, PP1 = average preexperimental pulse pressure, SBP2 = average postexperimental systolic blood pressure, DBP2 = average postexperimental diastolic blood pressure, PP2 = average postexperimental pulse pressure.

astolic, and pulse pressure values obtained before and after the experimental periods were evaluated in a 2(Raynaud's vs. controls) × 2(first and second measurements) mixed-factorial ANOVA. Two control subjects were excluded from these analyses because of incomplete data. There were no significant main or interaction effects for these measures.

Cardiovascular Data

Based on *a priori* assumptions about the critical minutes for each experimental period, the data were analyzed for 3 key minutes in a 2(Raynaud's vs. control groups) × 3(minute 5 of the baseline rest period, minute 1 of the stressful task period, minute 1 of the recovery rest period) mixed factorial ANOVA, in which the first factor was between subjects and the second factor was within subjects. The last minute of the baseline rest period was selected on the assumption that it would best represent pretask baseline resting levels, the first minute of the task period was selected on the assumption that peak myocardial reactivity effects would occur early in the task (cf. Linden *et al.*, 1985), and the first minute of the recovery period was selected on the assumption that it would best reflect the rate of recovery.[1] Significant periods main effects were probed using Newman-Keuls post hoc pairwise comparisons.

Descriptive Data

Table 2 presents the means and standard deviations of all of the dependent measures for each group for the critical minutes of each period (last minute of rest, first minute of task, first minute of recovery). The trends for the means across the three periods are consistent with the expected effects of the mental arithmetic task for all of the dependent measures except stroke volume, which decreased unexpectedly. As ex-

Table 2. *Means and Standard Deviations of All Cardiovascular Measures for Both Groups for Rest Period Minute 5, Task Period Minute 1, and Recovery Period Minute 1*[a]

Measures		Raynaud's			Controls		
		Rest min 5	Task min 1	Recovery min 1	Rest min 5	Task min 1	Recovery min 1
HR	M	74.69	95.04	74.29	71.59	98.86	73.55
(bpm)	SD	9.39	13.81	9.38	7.65	19.12	9.33
SV	M	120.80	109.77	122.08	110.93	104.61	112.30
(ml)	SD	13.95	22.80	20.44	26.82	20.37	30.95
CO	M	8.97	10.53	9.01	7.64	10.24	8.01
(l/m)	SD	1.13	3.28	1.56	2.38	4.11	2.62
IBI	M	815.22	644.44	819.11	847.40	630.10	828.00
(ms)	SD	105.39	103.82	103.36	95.95	134.33	108.50
PEP	M	103.67	92.11	101.33	106.50	77.90	102.80
(ms)	SD	8.00	14.97	8.97	7.50	23.35	7.96
LVET	M	287.78	263.33	291.89	290.40	260.50	293.60
(ms)	SD	14.80	19.69	18.19	19.77	26.54	21.06
PTT	M	183.86	176.00	183.86	188.30	175.40	185.10
(ms)	SD	16.85	15.48	15.07	17.67	12.50	16.24
$\sqrt{\text{FPA}}$	M	28.75	27.71	28.08	25.32	28.38	26.25
($\sqrt{\text{vmV}}$)	SD	3.17	2.55	2.57	5.26	6.34	5.14

[a] M = mean, SD = standard deviation, HR = heart rate, SV = stroke volume, CO = cardiac output, IBI = interbeat interval, PEP = preejection period, LVET = left ventricular ejection time, PTT = pulse transit time, $\sqrt{\text{FPA}}$ = transformed finger pulse amplitude.

[1] The results obtained from analyses based on all 5 minutes of each period were essentially the same as those reported here for analyses based on the key minutes of each period.

pected, HR and CO increased in response to the task, while PEP, LVET, and PTT decreased in response to the task. The pattern for finger pulse amplitude matches traditional expectations rather than the findings of Halperin et al. (1983), since FPA *decreased in response to the task in the Raynaud's group but increased in response to the task in the control group.* With the exception of SV, the trends in the means from rest to task suggest that *reactivity to the task was lower for the Raynaud's group than for the control group.*

PEP

The ANOVA for PEP yielded a significant Groups × Periods interaction effect, $F(2, 34) = 3.937$, $p < .03$, and a significant Periods main effect, $F(2, 34) = 21.597$, $p < .001$. In the case of the Periods main effect, post hoc pairwise comparisons indicated that PEP was significantly shorter during the task than during either the rest period or the recovery period, which did not differ from each other. The Groups × Periods interaction effect for PEP, depicted in Figure 1, was probed by comparing the two groups on the *a priori* contrast of PEP during the task period

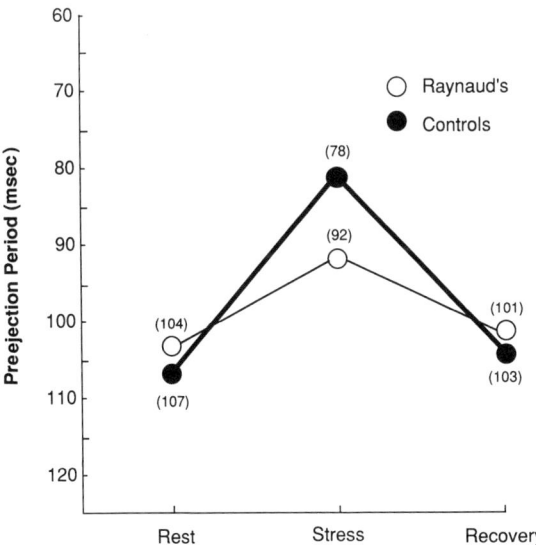

Figure 1. Mean preejection period for both the Raynaud's group and the control group during rest period minute 5 (rest), task period minute 1 (stress), and recovery period minute 1 (recovery).

versus PEP averaged over the baseline and recovery rest periods. As predicted, the difference in PEP between the task period and the mean of the two rest periods was significantly greater for the control group ($M = -26.75$, $SD = 21.11$) than for the Raynaud's group ($M = -10.39$, $SD = 11.14$), $t(14) = 2.14$, $p = .05$, two-tailed.

The results for PEP are consistent with the expected effects of the mental arithmetic task. More important, however, the Groups × Periods interaction for PEP matches predictions based on the myocardial performance theory, with Raynaud's subjects exhibiting smaller decrements in PEP during the task as compared with control subjects.

Heart Rate

The ANOVA for HR yielded a significant Periods main effect, $F(2, 34) = 55.585$, $p < .001$, attributable to significantly greater HR during the first minute of the task than during the key minutes of either rest period, which did not differ from each other. The Groups × Periods interaction was not significant.

The results indicate that HR increased during the mental arithmetic task as expected. Moreover, these results indicate that although Raynaud's subjects had slightly higher HR levels during the baseline rest period, the two groups did not differ significantly in HR increases elicited by the task.

Stroke Volume

There were no significant main or interaction effects for SV.

Cardiac Output

The ANOVA for CO yielded a significant Periods effect, $F(2, 32) = 7.725$, $p < .002$, reflecting significantly greater CO during the first minute of the task than during the key minutes of either rest period, which did not differ from each other. Thus, as expected, CO increased significantly during the mental arithmetic task. Contrary to predictions, however, the Groups × Periods interaction for CO was not significant, indicating that the two groups did not differ reliably in CO reactivity to stress.

LVET

The ANOVA for LVET yielded a significant Periods main effect, $F(2, 34) = 39.962$, $p < .001$. The Groups × Periods interaction was not significant. Post hoc testing of the Periods effect showed that LVET was significantly shorter during the first minute of the task than during the last minute of rest or the first minute of recovery, which did not differ from each other. These results are consistent with the expected effects of the mental arithmetic task.

PTT

The ANOVA for PTT revealed only a significant Periods effect, $F(2, 30) = 8.414$, $p < .001$, reflecting significantly shorter PTT during the first minute of the task than during the key minutes of the other two periods, which did not differ from each other. These results are consistent with the expected task effects.

FPA

Since the FPA signal was uncalibrated, a square root transformation was applied to the data in order to compensate for the resulting wide variability. Nevertheless, the ANOVA yielded no significant effects. Thus, the FPA results do not lend support to either of the alternative predictions described in the introduction.

Additional Post Hoc Testing of PEP Data

2 × 2 *Contingency Analyses*

These analyses examined the relationship between group membership (Raynaud's vs. control) and PEP reactivity to the task, which was defined in terms of the percent change in PEP from the rest period to the task period. Subjects were ranked on degree of PEP reactivity to the task, and the upper and lower thirds of the distribution were identified. *Five of the six most reactive subjects were in the control group, whereas five of the six least reactive subjects were in the Raynaud's group.* This distribution would not be expected by chance (Kruskal-Wallis $H = 4.89$, $p < .03$; Fisher's exact test, $p < .04$, one-tailed). These results suggest that the two groups are distinguished clearly by PEP reactivity to the task.

Preload and Afterload Effects on PEP

Changes in PEP may result from intrinsic mechanical effects, such as preload and afterload, as well as extrinsic effects, such as alterations in sympathetic nervous system influences on the myocardium (Newlin

& Levenson, 1979; Obrist et al., 1987). For example, a decrease in PEP may result from either an increase in preload, a decrease in afterload, or an increase in beta-adrenergic activation. Preload is related directly to end-diastolic ventricular pressure, which in turn is related directly to ventricular filling during diastole; increased filling causes the myocardial fibers to stretch, which reflexively enhances contractility. Thus, an *increase in ventricular filling time should lead to some increase in end-diastolic ventricular pressure and preload, which may shorten PEP*. Afterload is related directly to aortic diastolic pressure; it represents the load that must be overcome during left ventricular contraction in order to open the aortic valve to allow ejection of blood from the left ventricle into the aorta. Thus, *an increase in aortic diastolic pressure should produce an increase in afterload, which may prolong PEP*.

Although it seemed unlikely that alterations in preload and afterload could account for the decreases in PEP observed in this study, the possibility was evaluated in a 2(PEP reactors and nonreactors) × 3(rest minute 5, task minute 1, recovery minute 1) ANOVA conducted on the IBI and PTT data from the critical minutes for those subjects showing the highest and lowest degree of PEP reactivity to the task (based respectively on upper and lower thirds of the distribution for PEP reactivity to the task). IBI served as an index of preload since length of the interbeat interval should be related directly to ventricular filling time and, therefore, to end-diastolic ventricular pressure; PTT served as an index of afterload since pulse transit time should be related inversely to arterial tone and, therefore, to aortic diastolic pressure. If the differences in PEP between reactors and nonreactors were attributable to preload effects, then IBI should have been longer during the task for the reactors than for the nonreactors. If the differences in PEP between reactors and nonreactors were due to afterload effects, then PTT should have been longer (i.e., diastolic blood pressure should have been lower) during the task for the reactors than for the nonreactors. If the reactors and nonreactors did not differ in IBI or PTT, or if they differed in directions opposite to those predicted for loading effects, then it would be reasonable to conclude that the observed differences in PEP between these groups were due to greater beta-adrenergic (i.e., extrinsic neural) influences on the myocardium for reactors as compared with nonreactors.

Figure 2 presents the means of the IBI and PTT data for the two PEP reactivity groups for the three periods. The results of the ANOVA for IBI indicated that the PEP reactors were also IBI reactors, exhibiting significantly shorter, not longer, IBI in response to the task as compared with the PEP nonreactors (Reactivity Groups × Periods, $F(2, 20) = 8.696$, $p < .002$). Thus, the observed differences in PEP between the reactivity

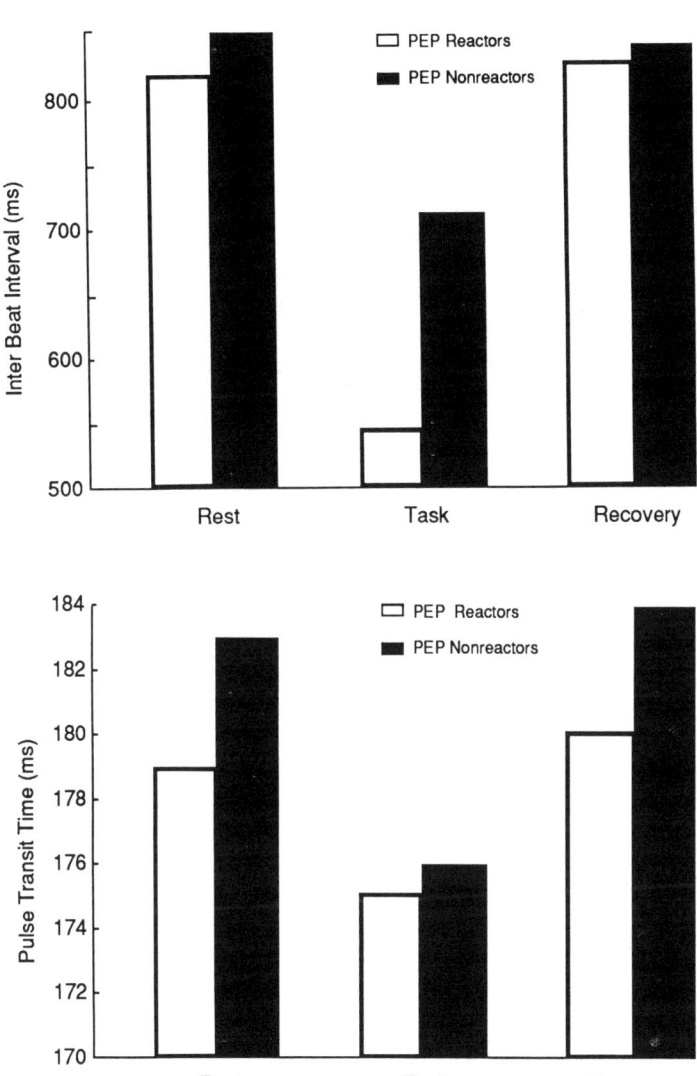

Figure 2. Mean interbeat interval and mean pulse transit time for both the preejection period (PEP) reactors and the PEP nonreactors during rest period minute 5 (rest), task period minute 1 (task), and recovery period minute 1 (recovery).

groups were apparently not due to preload effects. The results of the ANOVA for PTT indicated that the PEP reactors and nonreactors did not differ significantly in PTT across the three periods, $F(2, 16) = 0.155$). Thus, the observed differences in PEP between the two reactivity groups were apparently not attributable to afterload effects. Therefore, it may be concluded that the differences between the PEP reactors and the PEP nonreactors were not due to loading effects, but rather were due to differences between the groups in sympathetic activation during the task, with reactors exhibiting greater sympathetic reactivity than nonreactors. Moreover, since the reactive group was composed primarily of control subjects and the nonreactive group was composed primarily of Raynaud's subjects, it seems reasonable to conclude that the observed differences in PEP reactivity between the Raynaud's group and the control group were not due to loading factors, but rather were due to greater beta-adrenergic activation during the task in control subjects as compared with Raynaud's subjects.

The Relationship between PEP Reactivity and IBI Reactivity

The foregoing analyses demonstrate that the differences in PEP across periods and between groups were not due to preload or afterload effects; however, the possibility remains that the differences in PEP reactivity between the Raynaud's group and the control group may have been related to general differences in reactivity to the task, perhaps because of differences in the extent to which subjects were engaged in, or challenged by, the mental arithmetic task. That is, the Raynaud's group may have shown less PEP reactivity to the task either because of diminished reactivity associated specifically with PEP, or because of a general lack of reactivity to the task. In order to examine this possibility, analyses were conducted using IBI as a control variable to index general reactivity to the task.

A set of analyses was conducted to examine the relationship between group membership (Raynaud's vs. control) and PEP reactivity to the task independent of IBI reactivity to the task. The percent change in PEP from rest to task was divided by the percent change in IBI from rest to task to yield a ratio of PEP reactivity adjusted for IBI reactivity (PEP%/IBI%). A large value for the reactivity ratio indicates a greater change from rest to task in PEP than in IBI, whereas a small value for the ratio indicates a greater change from rest to task in IBI than in PEP. The ratios for the Raynaud's group and the control group were compared with a t test, which showed that the reactivity ratio for the Raynaud's group ($n = 9$, $M = 0.423$, $SD = 0.457$) was significantly smaller than the reactivity ratio for the control group ($n = 10$, $M = 0.929$, $SD = 0.565$), $t(17) = -2.13$, $p < .05$, two-tailed. Therefore, PEP reactivity was lower for the Raynaud's group than for the control group, even when adjusted for IBI reactivity.

Subjects were ranked on the PEP%/IBI% reactivity ratio, and the upper and lower thirds of the distribution were identified. *Five of the six most reactive subjects were in the control group, whereas five of the six least reactive subjects were in the Raynaud's group.* This distribution would not be expected by chance (Kruskal-Wallis $H = 4.89$, $p < .03$; Fisher's exact test, $p < .04$, one-tailed).

Discussion

As discussed earlier, PEP is related inversely to myocardial contractility; thus, it appears from these data that the augmentation of myocardial contractility that occurs normally in response to stress was deficient in the Raynaud's group as compared with the control group. Moreover, since the augmentation of myocardial contractility in response to stress is usually due to increased beta-adrenergic influences on the myocardium, these results suggest that beta-adrenergic reactivity to stress was lower for the Raynaud's group than for the control group. The interpretation of group differences in sympathetic activation is strengthened by the results of tests for preload and afterload effects on PEP, which demonstrated that both the task-related decreases and group differences in PEP were most likely due to neural influences rather than to loading factors.

There were no significant differences between the Raynaud's group and the control group in finger pulse amplitude reactivity to the task. Thus, the finger pulse amplitude results do not support either of the alternative predictions regarding group differences in finger blood flow, nor do they replicate the findings of Halperin *et al.* (1983). The absence of significant group differences in heart rate reactivity, however, is consistent with previous research (Freedman & Ianni, 1983) showing no significant differences in heart rate between Raynaud's disease patients and normal controls.

Although the trends in the means for cardiac output were in the predicted direction of lower reactivity to the task for the Raynaud's group as compared with the control group, the results were not significant. These negative results suggest at least two possibilities: (a) that cardiac output was not sufficiently sensitive to detect differences in myocardial performance between the groups; (b) that the differences in myocardial contractility between the groups did not extend to output, thus necessitating some revision and refinement of the myocardial performance theory. Similar comments also pertain to the results for stroke volume.

Several implications are suggested by the results of this research. First, the lower PEP reactivity to the task exhibited by the subjects who reported symptoms of Raynaud's disease as compared with the asymptomatic control subjects suggests that both myocardial contractility and beta-adrenergic activation in response to stress may be deficient in Raynaud's disease.

Second, the pattern of results is consistent with our theory of primary Raynaud's phenomenon, and suggests several refinements of the theory. The results suggest specifically that primary Raynaud's phenomenon may be characterized by a deficiency in the beta-adrenergically mediated augmentation of myocardial contractility that occurs normally in response to stress.

Third, these results suggest that it may be more appropriate to conceptualize primary Raynaud's phenomenon as a cardiovascular reactivity disorder rather than as simply a peripheral vascular disorder. Conceptualizing Raynaud's disease as a disorder involving myocardial components as well as peripheral vascular components is entirely consistent with the myocardial performance theory outlined in this chapter; conceptualizing the phenomenon as a reactivity disorder is entirely consistent with both its episodic nature and its eliciting stimuli.

Fourth, there is substantial evidence indicating that abnormally high beta-adrenergically mediated myocardial reactivity to stress may be associated with the development of essential hypertension (Obrist, 1981). The results of this study imply that abnormally low beta-adrenergically mediated myocardial reactivity to stress also may be associated with the development of cardiovascular disease. This implication and several interesting parallels between the results of this study and the results of research on myocardial reactivity and borderline hypertension (cf. Obrist, 1981) suggest the possibility that primary Raynaud's phenomenon and borderline hypertension may represent opposite extremes on a cardiovascular reactivity continuum.

The present research paradigm should be expanded in several ways: (a) It should be extended beyond warm environmental conditions to cool environmental conditions; (b) it should be replicated both with a population of medically diagnosed primary Raynaud's patients and with samples of male subjects; (c) it should be extended to evaluations of myocardial reactivity in subjects with symptoms and a family history of primary Raynaud's phenomenon as compared with subjects with symptoms and a family history of other cardiovascular disorders (e.g., essential hypertension); (d) it should be expanded to an animal model allowing direct manipulation of sympathetic nervous system activity. Finally, this investigation suggests that future research on primary Raynaud's phenomenon should incorporate measures of myocardial performance as well as measures of peripheral vascular activity, for the nature of effects observed at the myocardial level may clarify the nature of effects observed at the peripheral vascular level.

References

Agrifoglio, G., & Agus, G. B. (1976). Observations on the Raynaud's disease. *Journal of Cardiovascular Surgery, 17,* 513–518.
Ayres, M. L., Jarrett, P. E. M., & Browse, N. L. (1981). Blood viscosity, Raynaud's phenomenon and the effect of fibrinolytic enhancement. *British Journal of Surgery, 68,* 51–54.
Blunt, R. J., & Porter, J. M. (1981). Raynaud syndrome. *Seminars in Arthritis and Rheumatism, 10,* 282–308.
Bollinger, A., & Schlumpf, M. (1976). Finger blood flow in healthy subjects of different age and sex and in patients with primary Raynaud's disease. *Acta Chirurgica Scandinavica, 142* (Suppl. 465), 42–47.
Brod, J., Fencl, V. S., Heijl, Z., & Jirha, J. (1959). Circulatory changes underlying blood pressure elevation during acute emotional stress (mental arithmetic) in normotensive and hypertensive subjects. *Clinical Science, 18,* 269–279.
Burch, G. E., Harb, J. M., & Sun, C. S. (1979). Fine structure of digital vascular lesions in Raynaud's phenomenon and disease. *Angiology, 30,* 361–376.
Coffman, J. D., & Davies, W. T. (1975). Vasospastic diseases: A review. *Progress in Cardiovascular Diseases, 18,* 123–146.
Cohen, R. A., & Coffman, J. D. (1982). Reduced transmural systolic pressure promotes arterial closure in Raynaud's disease. *Clinical Research, 30,* 179a.
Downey, J. A., & Frewin, D. B. (1973). The effect of cold on blood flow in the hand of patients with Raynaud's phenomenon. *Clinical Science, 44,* 279–289.
Eliasson, K., Danielson, M., Hylander, B., & Lindblad, L. E. (1984). Raynaud's phenomenon caused by B-receptor blocking drugs. *Acta Medica Scandinavica, 215,* 333–339.
Freedman, R. R., & Ianni, P. (1983). Role of cold and emotional stress in Raynaud's disease and scleroderma. *British Medical Journal, 287,* 1499–1502.
Frey, M. A. B., Doerr, B. M., & Miles, D. S. (1982). Transthoracic impedance: Differences between men and women with implications for impedance cardiography. *Aviation, Space, and Environmental Medicine, 53,* 1190–1192.
Gifford, R. W., Jr., & Hines, E. A., Jr. (1957). Raynaud's disease among women and girls. *Circulation, 16,* 1012–1021.
Goyle, K. B., & Dormandy, J. A. (1976). Abnormal blood viscosity in Raynaud's phenomenon. *Lancet, 1,* 1317–1318.
Halperin, J. L., & Coffman, J. D. (1979). Pathophysiology of Raynaud's disease. *Archives of Internal Medicine, 139,* 89–92.
Halperin, J. L., Cohen, R. A., & Coffman, J. D. (1983). Digital vasodilation during mental stress in patients with Raynaud's disease. *Cardiovascular Research, 17,* 671–677.

Heslop, J., Coggon, D., & Acheson, E. D. (1983). The prevalence of intermittent digital ischemia (Raynaud's phenomenon) in a general practice. *Journal of the Royal College of General Practitioners, 33,* 85–89.

Hossack, K. F., & Bruce, R. A. (1982). Maximal cardiac function in sedentary normal men and women: Comparison of age-related changes. *Journal of Applied Physiology: Respiratory, Environmental, and Exercise Physiology, 53,* 799–804.

Hugdahl, K., Fagerstrom, K. O., & Broback, C. G. (1984). Effects of cold and mental stress on finger temperature in vasospastics and normal Ss. *Behaviour Research and Therapy, 22,* 471–476.

Jahnsen, T., Nielsen, S. L., & Skovborg, F. (1977). Blood viscosity and local response to cold in primary Raynaud's phenomenon. *Lancet, 2,* 1001–1002.

Jamieson, G. G., Ludbrook, J., & Wilson, A. (1971). Cold hypersensitivity in Raynaud's phenomenon. *Circulation, 44,* 254–264.

Kelsey, R. M. (1986). Raynaud's disease: A review and a proposed new psychophysiological model. In E. S. Katkin & S. B. Manuck (Eds.), *Advances in behavioral medicine* (Vol. 2). Greenwich, CT: JAI Press.

Kimby, E., Fargrell, B., Bjorkholm, M., Holm, G., Mellstedt, H., & Norberg, R. (1984). Skin capillary abnormalities in patients with Raynaud's phenomenon. *Acta Medica Scandinavica, 215,* 127–134.

Kontos, H. A., & Wasserman, A. J. (1969). Effect of reserpine in Raynaud's phenomenon. *Circulation, 39,* 259–266.

Krantz, D. S., Contrada, R. J., LaRiccia, P. J., Anderson, J. R., Durel, L. A., Dembroski, T. M., & Weiss, T. (1987). Effects of beta-adrenergic stimulation and blockade on cardiovascular reactivity, affect, and Type A behavior. *Psychosomatic Medicine, 49,* 146–158.

Kubicek, W. G., Witsoe, D. A., Patterson, R. P., & From, A. H. L. (1969). Applications of the Minnesota Impedance Cardiograph. In W. G. Kubicek, D. A. Witsoe, R. P. Patterson, & A. H. L. From (Eds.), *Development and evaluation of an impedance cardiographic system to measure cardiac output and other cardiac parameters* (NASA-CR-101965) (pp. 1–15). Houston: National Aeronautics and Space Administration.

Lane, J. D., White, A. D., & Williams, R. B., Jr. (1984). Cardiovascular effects of mental arithmetic in Type A and Type B females. *Psychophysiology, 21,* 39–46.

Linden, W., McEachern, H. M., & Madaisky, P. (1985, October). *Effect of white versus real-life noise interference during mental arithmetic on phasic cardiovascular activity.* Paper presented at the annual meeting of the Society for Psychophysiological Research, Houston, TX.

Marshall, A. J. (1980). Beta adrenoceptor blocking agents. In A. J. Marshall & D. W. Barritt (Eds.), *The hypertensive patient* (pp. 410–432). Tunbridge Wells: Pitman Medical Limited.

Marshall, A. J., Roberts, C. J. C., & Barritt, D. W. (1976). Raynaud's phenomenon as side effect of beta-blockers in hypertension. *British Medical Journal, 1,* 1498–1499.

McGrath, M. A., Peek, R., & Penny, R. (1978). Raynaud's disease: Reduced hand blood flows with normal blood viscosity. *Australian and New Zealand Journal of Medicine, 8,* 126–131.

Mendlowitz, M., & Naftchi, N. (1959). The digital circulation in Raynaud's disease. *American Journal of Cardiology, 4,* 580–584.

Miller, J. C., & Horvath, S. M. (1978). Impedance cardiography. *Psychophysiology, 51,* 80–91.

Muzi, M., Ebert, T. J., Tristani, F. E., Jeutter, D. C., Barney, J. A., & Smith, J. J. (1985). Determination of cardiac output using ensemble-averaged impedance cardiograms. *Journal of Applied Physiology, 58,* 200–205.

Newlin, D. B., & Levenson, R. W. (1979). Pre-ejection period: Measuring beta-adrenergic influences upon the heart. *Psychophysiology, 16,* 546–553.

Nielsen, S. L. (1978). Raynaud phenomena and finger systolic pressure during cooling. *Scandinavian Journal of Clinical and Laboratory Investigation, 38,* 765–770.

Obrist, P. A. (1981). *Cardiovascular psychophysiology: A perspective.* New York: Plenum.

Obrist, P. A., Light, K. C., James, S. A., & Strogatz, D. S. (1987). Cardiovascular responses to stress: I. Measures of myocardial response and relationships to high resting systolic pressure and parental hypertension. *Psychophysiology, 24,* 65–78.

Peacock, J. H. (1957). Vasodilation in the human hand. Observations on primary Raynaud's disease and acrocyanosis of the upper extremities. *Clinical Science, 17,* 575–586.

Peacock, J. H. (1959a). A comparative study of the digital cutaneous temperatures and hand blood flows in the normal hand, primary Raynaud's disease and primary acrocyanosis. *Clinical Science, 18,* 25–33.

Peacock, J. H. (1959b). Peripheral venous blood concentrations of epinephrine and norepinephrine in primary Raynaud's disease. *Circulation Research, 7,* 821–827.

Pola, P., Savi, L., Dal Lago, A., Flore, R., & Shami, J. (1980). Invariability of blood viscosity after cold testing in patients suffering from Raynaud's disease. *Journal of Cardiovascular Surgery, 21,* 211–214.

Porter, J. M., Snider, R. L., Bardana, E. J., Rosch, J., & Eidemiller, L. R. (1975). The diagnosis and treatment of Raynaud's phenomenon. *Surgery, 77,* 11–23.

Poulter, N., & Gabriel, R. (1979). Raynaud's phenomenon in hypertensive dialysis patients taking a sustained-release propranolol formulation. *Current Medical Research and Opinion, 6,* 207–208.

Pringle, R., Walder, D. N., & Weaver, J. P. A. (1965). Blood viscosity and Raynaud's disease. *Lancet, 1,* 1086–1088.

Rose, G. (1980). Epidemiology. In A. J. Marshall & D. W. Barritt (Eds.), *The hypertensive patient* (pp. 1–21). Tunbridge Wells: Pitman Medical Limited.

Sheps, D. S., Petrovick, M. L., Kizakevich, P. N., Wolfe, C., & Craige, E. (1982). Continuous noninvasive monitoring of left ventricular function during exercise by thoracic impedance cardiography-automated derivation of systolic time intervals. *American Heart Journal, 103,* 519–524.

Thulesius, O. (1976). Methods for the evaluation of peripheral vascular function in the upper extremities. *Acta Chirurgica Scandinavica, 142* (Suppl. 465), 53–54.

Thune, P., & Fyrand, O. (1976). Further observations on therapy with a beta-stimulating agent in Raynaud's phenomenon. *Acta Chirurgica Scandinavica, 142* (Suppl. 465), 84–86.

Velayos, E. E., Robinson, H., Porciuncula, F. U., & Masi, A. T. (1971). Clinical correlation analysis of 137 patients with Raynaud's phenomenon. *American Journal of the Medical Sciences, 262,* 347–356.

Wouda, A. A. (1977). Raynaud's phenomenon. *Acta Medica Scandinavica, 201,* 519–523.

CHAPTER 4

Self-Regulation of Slow Cortical Potentials and Its Role in Epileptogenesis

Thomas Elbert, Brigitte Rockstroh, Anthony Canavan, Niels Birbaumer, Werner Lutzenberger, Isolde von Bülow, and Anne Linden

Behavioral Treatment of Seizure Disorders

The prevalence of epileptic disorders is estimated to be around 1%, amounting to 1.5 million people in the United States. In at least one-third of all cases the epileptic seizures cannot be adequately controlled through antiepileptic medication. About 20% of the epileptic population is considered refractory to anticonvulsant management. And even if the seizures can be brought under control by antiepileptic medication, the side effects of the drugs put considerable strains on the patient's life (Penry & Rahel, 1986). Research has been conducted on alternative approaches relying on behavioral treatment alone or in combination with pharmacological treatment. Behavioral techniques generally have negligible side effects, which of course is highly desirable.

The following behavioral techniques have been investigated for their efficiency in controlling epileptic seizures.

Thomas Elbert, Brigitte Rockstroh, Anthony Canavan, Niels Birbaumer, Werner Lutzenberger, Isolde von Bülow, and Anne Linden • Psychological Institute, University of Tübingen, D 7400 Tübingen 1, Federal Republic of Germany.

Classical and Instrumental Conditioning of Seizure Behavior. In a widely acknowledged single case study by Efron (1957), a patient's seizures could be aborted by a strong olfactory stimulus presented during the aura (UCS). The patient was trained to connect the odor of jasmine with the sight of a bracelet (CS). This conditioning procedure allowed the patient to stop the progression of a seizure by looking at the bracelet (CR). Positive reinforcement of behavior incompatible with seizure development or immediate punishment of seizure antecedent behavior has been applied mostly in children and adolescents. A series of single case studies suggests that remarkable benefits may be achieved using classical as well as operant conditioning (e.g., Spunt, Heimann, & Rousseau, 1986); a controlled group outcome study, however, is still lacking.

Desensitization and Extinction of Reflex Epilepsy. Forster (1969, 1972, 1977) published an impressive series of studies demonstrating the usefulness of desensitization and extinction in reflex-epilepsy. Repetitive presentation of stimuli and images eliciting auras or seizures results in a considerably reduced seizure incidence.

Self-Control, Self-Perception, and Relaxation. Dahl, Melin, Brorson, and Schollin (1985) published the first well-controlled study of broad spectrum behavior therapy that was used to treat epileptic children and adolescents suffering from drug-refractory seizure disorders of varying etiology. The techniques applied were self-perception of internal and/or external cues for seizures and self-monitoring of behavior favoring seizures and relaxation as a coping response. A 1-year follow-up demonstrated a superior outcome for the experimental group compared with a matched attention placebo group and another control group receiving only pharmacological treatment.

Self-Regulation and End-Tidal Carbon Dioxide. Fried, Rubin, Carlton, and Fox (1984) published a controlled group study on the effect of biofeedback of end-tidal CO_2 on a heterogeneous group of adult epileptics. Patients in the experimental group received feedback via an infrared gas analyzer, the sensor of which was located (unobtrusively) in the right nostril. Patients were instructed to keep CO_2-level, as well as respiration frequency and depth, within optimal physiological limits using relaxation and imagery strategies. The authors report a substantial and significant improvement in seizure control in the experimental group. A validation and replication of the efficacy of this promising technique for the treatment of epileptic patients is highly desirable.

Instrumental Modification of the EEG Spectra. Instrumental conditioning of the power within distinct EEG-frequency bands has proven to be fruitful. In particular, the effects of a conditioned increase of the sensorimotor rhythm (SMR, which means frequencies in the 12- to 15-Hz band over central regions) during simultaneous suppression of activity in the low-frequency range (EEG-Theta) has been extensively investigated by Sterman and colleagues (for reviews, see Sterman, 1982, 1984, 1986) and Lubar (for reviews, see Lubar, 1982, 1984).

Sterman has developed a model that suggests considering EEG rhythmic activity a manifestation of the release of intrinsic, gated thalamocortical discharge. Rhythmic discharge is invoked when no signals are being processed. The dominant frequency generated in the thalamocortical loops depends upon cortical excitability. According to Sterman, the dominant intrinsic somatosensory frequency varies around 12 to 15 Hz and is seen most clearly during an activated but motionless state as the SMR. The SMR is associated with inhibitory processes in the sensorimotor system, having the effect of elevating seizure thresholds. This result has been obtained from studying animals challenged with convulsants. Also, the SMR probably becomes manifest in the sleep spindles appearing during non-REM sleep. Epileptic patients often exhibit EEG abnormalities that include increased power at low (3–7 Hz) and high frequencies (above 20 Hz), but a lack of waves in the range in which synchronous activity is commonly observed during the waking state (8–15 Hz). These abnormalities can be pronounced over the lateral sensorimotor cortex. Sleep EEG patterns are seriously disturbed in epileptic patients. In particular, the sleep spindles are often missing or suppressed. On these grounds, Sterman suggested that modification of such abnormalities using instrumental conditioning should yield beneficial effects on seizure frequency in otherwise poorly controlled epileptic patients. EEG feedback procedures as pioneered by Sterman and Lubar have therefore been directed at a reduction in abnormal low frequencies and a facilitation of intermediate rhythmic frequencies recorded from sensorimotor cortex.

More than a decade of elegant, well-controlled studies accomplished by these researchers has reliably documented that feedback and instrumental conditioning produces systematic changes in EEG patterns and a normalization of sleep EEG patterns, coinciding with substantial reductions in seizure frequency. Seizure frequency reduction between 35 and 50% (significant in comparison with both baseline levels and control conditions) have been achieved, this beneficial effect being maintained and even increased during follow-up periods (Sterman, Lantz,

Bruckler, & Kovalesky, 1981). In individuals with abnormal sleep EEG patterns (more than 20% paroxysmal activity during stage 2 epochs), this abnormal activity dropped below baseline levels (Lubar, 1984; Whitsett & Lubar, 1981), while patients with normal or grossly atypical spectral profiles did not show significant changes in seizure incidence following EEG control training (Sterman, 1984, 1986).

Instrumental Conditioning of Slow Cortical Potentials. As stated by Lubar, "EEG biofeedback has one very distinct advantage: the patients learn self-reliance skills. EEG biofeedback has to be practiced even when machines are not available; that is, patients should try to initiate the contingencies when they experience the beginning of a seizure" (1984, p. 125). The same holds for instrumental conditioning of other aspects of the EEG such as *slow cortical potentials* (SCP) that are considered to reflect cortical excitability (Birbaumer, Elbert, Canavan, & Rockstroh, 1990; Elbert & Rockstroh, 1987). This approach pursued by our group will be introduced in the subsequent paragraphs. However, before describing the methods and results of a program for SCP self-regulation, let us first briefly outline some core concepts.

Slow Cortical Potentials Indicate Cortical Excitability

Cortical excitability is regulated according to the constantly varying environmental and metabolic demands. If a certain piece of information or task is presented to a subject, those brain regions that are expected to become involved in the task will be preactivated by these cue stimuli. To demonstrate a phasic change in cortical excitability in the laboratory, a subject may be confronted with a tone and told that after a short interval, another acoustic stimulus is to be heard. Then a button press is required in order to avoid punishment or in order to receive positive reinforcement. One of the brain responses to this stimulus contingency, the "contingent negative variation" (CNV) represents a slow negative shift in the electrical potential. The CNV can be recorded from the scalp during the interstimulus interval, while the subject is anticipating the second event and preparing for task performance. It originates primarily in cerebral cortex, when excitatory thalamic input depolarizes the apical dendrites over extensive cortical regions (for reviews of evidence see Birbaumer, Elbert, Canavan, & Rockstroh, 1990; Rockstroh, Elbert, Birbaumer, & Lutzenberger, 1982; Rockstroh, Elbert, Canavan, Lutzenberger, & Birbaumer, 1989).

However, feedback mechanisms within the brain have to carefully control the range of this excitability: Overexcitability of cortical tissue, for instance, due to a transient failure in down-regulating mechanisms would allow an explosive chain reaction of excitation among neuronal networks. Overexcitation, meaning simultaneous firing of practically all the cell assemblies in one region, constitutes an epileptic attack (Braitenberg, 1978; Elbert & Rockstroh, 1987). If the changes in the slow cortical potential (SCP), such as the CNV, reflect changes in cortical excitability, then extreme negativities that would result from overexcitability of cortical neuronal networks should indicate a high risk for the development of seizures.

This indeed seems to be the case. As illustrated in Figure 1, seizure activity is superimposed on an extraneous slow negative potential in an unmedicated epileptic patient during hyperventilation.[1]

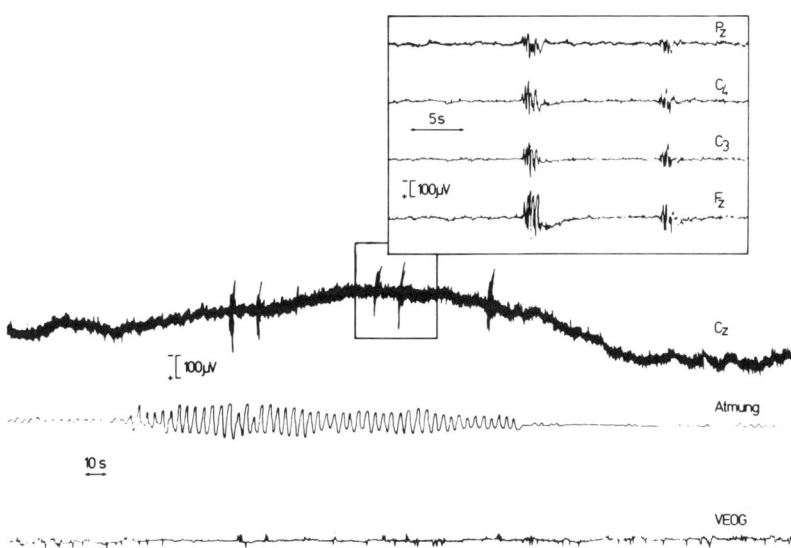

Figure 1. Vertex EEG, respiration, and vertical EOG during a 3-minute hyperventilation period obtained from a 22-year-old male epileptic patient suffering *grands maux*. Epileptiform discharges (see insert with extended time scale) are superimposed upon pronounced negative SCP shifts exceeding 100 μV.

---

[1] In clinical diagnosis, hyperventilation is used to provoke epileptiform discharges in patients presumed to suffer from epilepsy. According to Caspers and Speckmann (1974), mechanisms underlying this challenge involve changes in arterial pCO_2 and/or pH, which are able to reduce membrane stability in neuronal tissues and may thereby cause an increase in excitation.

This pattern has been repeatedly found in animals as well as in humans in the studies in which slow potentials have been recorded (Chatrian, Somasundaram, & Tassinari, 1968; von Bülow, Elbert, Rockstroh, Lutzenberger, Canavan, & Birbaumer; 1989). In the cat, the negative shift with onset of seizure activity in the EEG (induced by epileptic agents such as phenyltetrazol or penicillin) coincides with paroxysmal depolarization shifts (PDS) in cortical neurons (Caspers & Speckmann, 1969; Caspers, Speckmann, & Lehmenkuehler, 1984). In acute focal epilepsy—during the spike discharges—thousands of neurons in the focus synchronously undergo an unusually large depolarization, on which a burst of action potentials is superimposed. Widespread negativity appears during generalized tonic-clonic seizure activity followed by positive-going repolarization with termination of the seizure.

Thus, there is reason to believe that slow negative potential shifts can be considered a sign of cortical excitability, and that excitability that increases beyond control elicits an epileptic attack. The question obtrudes whether epileptic patients suffer from impaired or at least transiently failing regulation of their cortical excitability. Such a deficit should show up in an impaired capacity for self-regulation of slow cortical potentials. Hence, epileptic patients might profit from a training using feedback and instrumental conditioning, which enhances and stabilizes their ability to control SCPs. This hypothesis is currently being investigated in a large long-term project at the University of Tübingen (parts of this project are described in this chapter). A prerequisite for applying instrumental conditioning of SCPs to epileptic patients, however, is the evidence that human subjects can indeed achieve control over their SCPs.

Self-Regulation of Slow Cortical Potentials

In the paradigm that we have developed (Elbert, 1978; Elbert, Birbaumer, Lutzenberger, & Rockstroh, 1979; Elbert, Rockstroh, Lutzenberger, & Birbaumer, 1980; Roberts, Rockstroh, Lutzenberger, Elbert, & Birbaumer, 1989), subjects are reinforced for increasing or reducing their SCPs depending upon discriminative stimuli. For example, a high-pitched tone or the presentation of the letter *A* indicates that an increase in negativity as referred to pretrial baseline will be rewarded, whereas a low-pitched tone or a *B* requires negativity reduction toward or below baseline for reinforcement. Continuous visual feedback of the change in SCP is provided to the subject by means of the outline of a rocket ship appearing on a TV screen in front of the subject. The feedback interval may last for 6 s or 8 seconds (see Figure 2), with intertrial intervals varying randomly from 8 to 20 seconds. Forward movements of the rocket-ship signal the required SCP shift, while backward movements indicate inadequate performance. The visual feedback signal is a linear function of the integrated EEG referred to the mean of a 4-second prestimulus baseline interval. On-line artifact control procedures prevent movements of the signal from being affected by eye movements, muscular artifacts, or tiny electrode displacements (for details see Elbert *et al.*, 1980; Rockstroh, 1987; Rockstroh *et al.*, 1982).

Reinforcement is given by means of the feedback and monetary reward for correct SCP shifts. The effect of conditioning or "transfer of learning" is tested on transfer trials in which only the signal stimuli (e.g., A or B) are presented and no feedback is provided.

Quite a number of studies from different laboratories have demonstrated that healthy human subjects can achieve reliable control over their SCPs—i.e., significant differences between trials with required negativity and negativity suppression/positivity in this paradigm without mediation of artifactual influence from other physiological systems (Bauer & Lauber, 1979; Elbert, 1978, 1986; Elbert *et al.*, 1979; Lutzenberger, Elbert, Rockstroh, & Birbaumer, 1982; Roberts *et al.*, 1989; Rockstroh, Elbert, Birbaumer, & Lutzenberger, 1982; Trimmel, 1986; Ueda, Furumitsu, & Kakigi, 1985; Elbert, Rockstroh, Lutzenberger, & Birbaumer, 1984; Rockstroh, 1984a,b; Rockstroh *et al.*, 1989). Figure 3. illustrates the mean differentiation in SCP between trials with required negativity increase and trials with required negativity suppression achieved after two sessions of 110 trials each. This differentiation is also maintained—and even enhanced—on transfer trials without any feedback. A comparable differentiation in SCP is not exhibited by "control" subjects

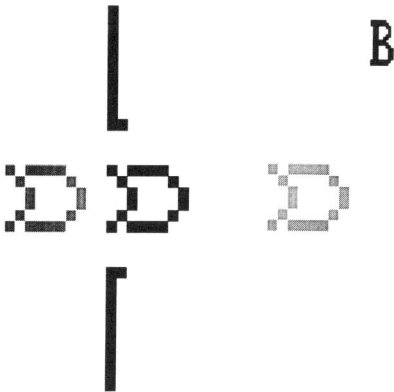

Figure 2. Graphic display of the visual feedback as it appears on the TV screen of the subject. The outline of a little rocket ship appears between the two vertical bars at the beginning of each 8-second trial. Depending on the letter presented simultaneously in the upper right corner of the TV screen, an increase in negativity above (letter *A*) or suppression below (letter *B*) pretrial baseline will move the rocket forward, traversed distance being linearly related to the achieved SCP change from baseline (gray rocket). Backward movement of the rocket signals incorrect SCP changes.

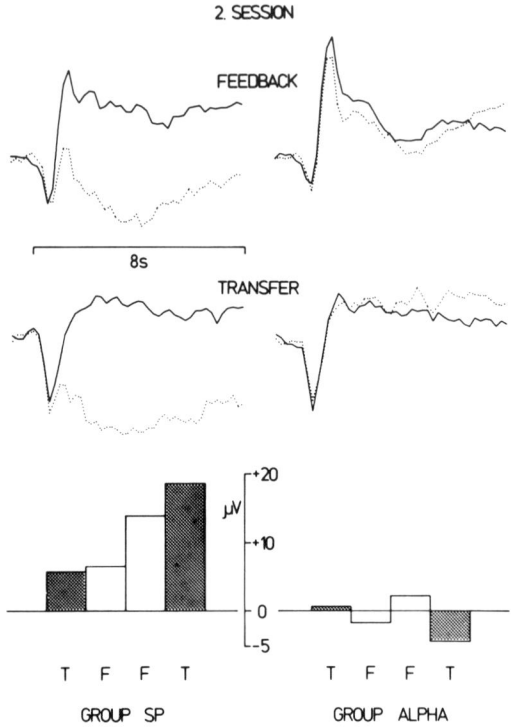

Figure 3. Grand averages for the EEG recorded from Cz in reference to linked earlobes. Negativity is up. During the second training session, trials with required negativity (solid) differ significantly from those requiring zero or positive shift (dotted) for the group receiving SCP feedback training. As illustrated in the left column, the difference achieved by this Group SP is pronounced in actual feedback (top) as well as in transfer (mid) trials. The left column indicates the SCP responses recorded from the group trained to modify EEG alpha activity (Group Alpha). Bottom graphs illustrate mean differentiation for the two groups separately for the transfer (T) and the feedback (F) trial blocks of the second session. Upright columns indicate successful control. Note that successful differentiation increases across trial blocks in Group SP, reaching its maximum during the final transfer block, while no systematic differentiation is achieved by subjects who received feedback of EEG alpha activity. (From Roberts *et al.*, 1989.)

who received feedback of their activity in the alpha frequency range (9–15 Hz) (for details see Roberts *et al.*, 1989).

SCP control can also be achieved in an area-specific manner. For example, subjects may be reinforced for producing an SCP polarity gradient between the two hemispheres—i.e., for increasing negativity in one hemisphere while simultaneously suppressing negativity in the other (Birbaumer, Lang, Cook, Elbert, Lutzenberger, & Rockstroh, 1988; Elbert, 1986; Rockstroh, 1989).

Finally, there is reliable evidence that self-induced SCP shifts affect performance on various behavioral tasks. After having achieved successful control over their SCPs, subjects respond more efficiently upon increased as compared with reduced negativity (Lutzenberger et al., 1982; Rockstroh et al., 1982), this relationship being again area-specific (Birbaumer, Rockstroh, Elbert, & Lutzenberger, 1988; Rockstroh, 1989)—i.e., performance on tasks with the left hand was more efficient following self-induced right-central negativity increase as compared with right-central negativity suppression, and vice versa.

The ability for SCP self-regulation has been confirmed (Bauer & Lauber, 1979; Bauer & Nirnberger, 1980; Trimmel, 1986; Ueda et al., 1985) and cross-validated in related paradigms (Bauer, 1984; Bauer & Nirnberger, 1981; Born, Whipple, & Stamm, 1982; Stamm, 1984; Stamm, Whipple, & Born, 1987) in a number of laboratories. Results support the relationship between area-specific SCP shifts and performance efficiency. It should be noted, however, that the relation between higher negative amplitudes and improved performance scores seems to be valid only for moderate to low SCP amplitudes. High negativities tend to increase the error rates. For instance, we observed an inverted U-shaped relationship between negativity and performance in a signal detection task (Lutzenberger, Elbert, Rockstroh, & Birbaumer, 1979), indicating that the cortical DC potential must be regulated within narrow limits ($\pm$ 2–3 μV) to achieve optimal performance.

Self-Regulation of SCPs in Patients Suffering from Epilepsy

As outlined above, epileptic patients are presumed to show impaired ability for SCP self-regulation. Therefore, they should achieve smaller or no differentiation after only one or two experimental training sessions, compared with the differentiation described above for healthy human subjects. In a first study, 11 epileptic patients were investigated in two sessions comprising 130 trials each. All of the patients responded well to pharmacological treatment, having no or only occasional seizures. The patient group did not acquire significant control over their SCPs. Only 1 of the 11 patients exhibited reliable control, and none of the patients achieved a differentiation between negativity increase and suppression comparable to that obtained for the control subjects (see Figure 4).

This result was confirmed and extended for seven drug-refractory epileptic patients. SCP differentiation after two experimental sessions (each comprising 110 trials) was compared with the differentiation ob-

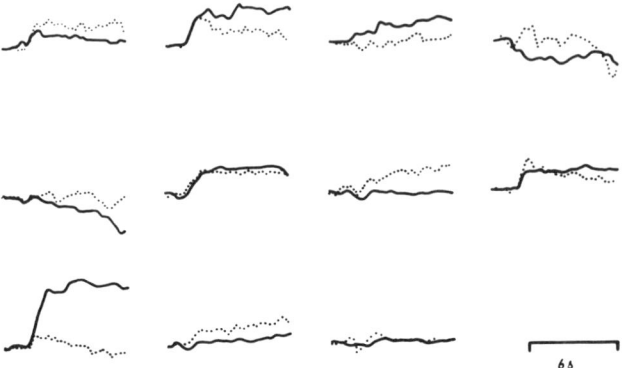

Figure 4. Single subject averages of the vertex EEG, recorded from epileptic patients during SCP feedback training. Only one of the patients achieves clear-cut control (the one in the lower left corner).

tained for healthy subjects (using the design and results illustrated in Figure 3). While healthy subjects achieved significant differentiation on feedback and transfer trials ($p < .01$), epileptic patients—no matter whether they were currently under drugs or not—failed to produce systematic SCP differentiations (the mean is actually opposite to the required difference by -5 μV but not significantly different from zero; see Figure 5). During transfer trials, in which healthy subjects usually achieve the most pronounced differentiation, the patients did not show any success. When submitted to an analysis of variance with the factors groups (patients vs. controls) and SCP differentiation, the significant two-way interaction ($p < .01$) confirms that patients do poorer than healthy subjects in regulating their SCP upon command.

Biofeedback of SCPs in Patients with Epilepsy

In light of the outlined theoretical considerations and the reported results it is currently being investigated whether or not drug-refractory patients can acquire control over their SCPs with extended periods of feedback and instrumental training and to what extent successfully acquired self-control of these brain responses might influence the patients' seizure frequency.

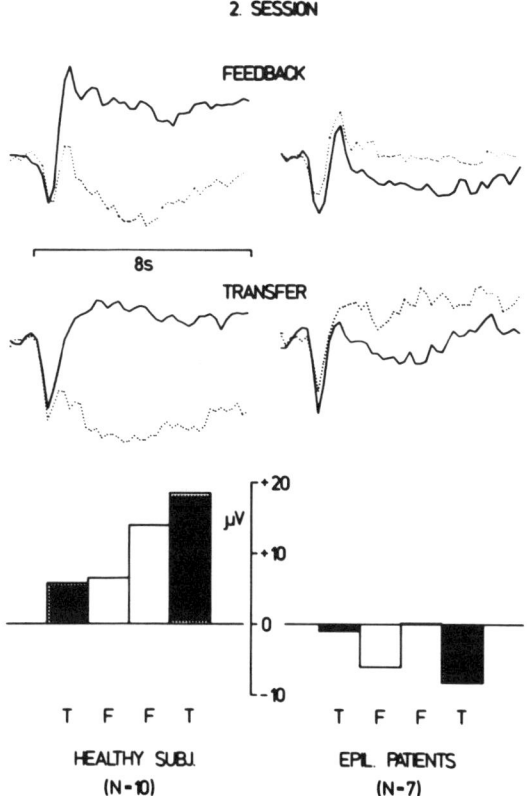

Figure 5. Identical to figure 3, the left graph shows the vertex SCP for 10 healthy subjects and its increasingly successful control in the course of a second training session (see caption of Figure 3). The right column illustrates the same response for 7 epileptic patients. Their mean differentiation is actually opposite to the type of control required.

Method

Patient Sample

So far, 14 patients (8 females, 6 males) have accomplished the standardized training program (see below). The mean age of the patients group is 26.3 years (range 15–42 years); the average duration of seizures varies between 3 and 15 years. A minimum of 1 or 2 seizures per week was required for patients to be included in the sample. The average seizure frequency varied from 1/week to more than 60/week (series of absences) around a mean of 9 (calculated from the medians during baseline). Patients mainly suffered from partial psychomotor seizures ($n = 10$), *grand mal* epilepsy ($n = 1$), and series of brief psychomotor seizures or *petit mal* seizures ($n = 3$). Individuals with progressive neurological conditions, seizures of psychological origin (psychogenic attacks), or psychiatric complications were not included in the sample, nor were patients suffering primarily from attacks during sleep.

Patients are under constant neurological supervision by the Department of Neurology, University of Tübingen. Standard EEG diagnostics are carried out prior to and following the training period. Medication regimens remain constant throughout the baseline, training, and follow-up periods, anticonvulsant blood levels being checked at regular intervals.

Design

Within a double-blind setting half of the patients are assigned to the SCP feedback group, while the others are reinforced for increasing or reducing synchronous EEG activity in the 9.5- to 15-Hz frequency range (hereafter also called Alpha). This latter group was designed as a stringent control group. Given the findings for SMR feedback (as reviewed above) we believe that patients may even profit from such a feedback.

Following the basic paradigm outlined above, continuous visual feedback is provided for intervals of 8 seconds each. For group SCP the letter *A* signals that an increase in negativity above the mean of a 4-second pretrial baseline will move the rocket ship (see Figure 2) forward, while the letter *B* asks for negativity suppression. For patients assigned to group Alpha, suppression of synchronous EEG activity is requested on *A* trials, enhancement in the 9.5- to 15-Hz band on *B* trials in order to achieve the "reinforcing" forward movement of the rocket. Each patient completes 28 sessions. Within each session blocks of 20 transfer, 60 feedback, and 30 transfer trials follow each other. Within each trial block *A* and *B* trials alternate pseudorandomly. For feedback purposes the EEG is recorded from Cz in reference to shunted earlobes, with both a time constant of 30 seconds for SCP recording and a time constant of 1 second for detection of EEG power in the extended Alpha band. Patients are told that the aim of the training is to achieve a kind of "mental gymnastic" ability, to be able to produce either response at will.

Apart from the feedback location, the EEG is also recorded from Fz, Pz, T3, and T4 during occasional sessions (2, 9, 20, 21, 28) in order to evaluate changes in scalp distribution of the generated electrical brain activity across time.

Figure 6 illustrates the design of the entire investigation. Following a baseline period of 8 weeks each patient participates in 20 training sessions of SCP/Alpha control. These training sessions are scheduled within 2 weeks (two 1-hour sessions per day with a 2-day break separating the training weeks). Following an intermission of 8 weeks, designed as a first "transfer," patients undergo another 8 sessions of training (the "booster" sessions). Sessions 10 through 28 include playing a radio program chosen by the subject in order to approach distracting conditions of real life—patients should be able not only to regulate the brain's activity when they concentrate fully on the task but also to automatize and generalize control for any time and under any circumstances. Patients are encouraged to practice the acquired SCP/Alpha control during the intermission by realizing their strategies for SCP/Alpha control on A and B trials five times per day for about 5 minutes each. During the 1-year follow-up succeeding the booster training, patients continue this home practice, which is verified by daily ratings and regular contacts with the attending staff member.

Four months after the end of the training period, generalization of SCP/Alpha control and correctness of home practice are evaluated in a session in which patients are asked to produce A and B states as they do at home, while the EEG is monitored. This testing is realized in an office in which the patient has not been before, in order to avoid possible effects of conditioning to experimental context.

Throughout the entire time period (from the beginning of baseline until the end of follow-up) patients keep diaries specifying seizure frequency, and accomplish a questionnaire on seizure characteristics, antecedents, and consequences for every attack.

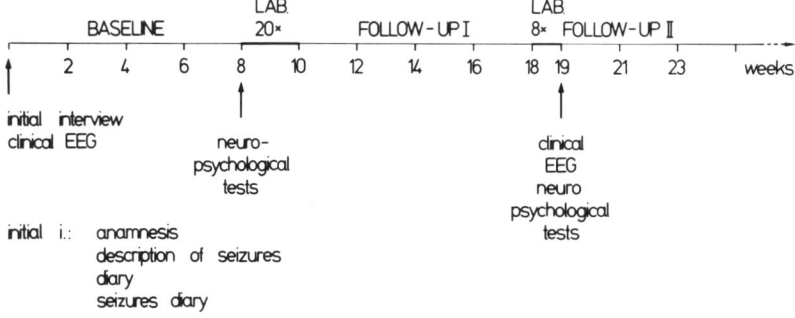

Figure 6. Sequence of training program.

Neuropsychological Tests

Each patient undergoes neuropsychological testing prior to the first and following the second training period as well as after the 12-month follow-up period. The test battery comprises tests of verbal and spatial intelligence and short- and long-term memory, a test of left-right orientation, and a test associated with frontal lobe function.

The intelligence tests were derived from the WAIS-R (Wechsler, 1981), with IQs being calculated according to Canavan, Dunn, and McMillan (1986).[2] Short-term memory for both verbal and spatial material was assessed according to standard procedures (digit span, Wechsler, 1981; block-tapping span, Milner, 1964). Immediate and delayed verbal reproduction of two stories, and verbal paired associate learning were administered in the fashion described by Powell (1979; Powell, Polkey, & McMillan, 1985) and Goldstein, Canavan, and Polkey (1988), these tests being sensitive to left temporal lobe damage. Copying and delayed reproduction of the Rey figure (Powell, 1979; Powell et al., 1985) and immediate reproduction of the Benton figures (Benton, 1985) were included as tests sensitive to apraxia (drawing components) and right temporal lobe function (memory components). Money's streetplan test of direction sense (Butters, Soeldner, & Fedio, 1972) was included as a test of left-right orientation, usually associated with parietal function. Finally, the Wisconsin card-sorting test, which proves difficult for patients with frontal lobe or neostriatal damage, was also administered (Canavan et al., 1989; Milner, 1964; Nelson, 1976).

Data Analysis

Acquisition of Control over SCP/Alpha Activity. The area below the curves for the entire 8-second interval referred to baseline was averaged for the different trial types—i.e., negativity increase and negativity suppression, or alpha suppression and alpha enhancement. For each patient the differentiation in SCP and alpha activity according to the feedback requirements was compared between the first and the second half

---

[2]These IQ scores differ from the Wechsler IQ scores in that they are based upon principal components analysis and have been found to distinguish well between patients with lesions of either the left or right temporal lobes (Powell, 1979; Powell et al., 1985), and between the various deficits in patients with frontal lobe lesions (Canavan, 1983). These IQ measures, in combination with the memory tests, applied in this study, have also recently been validated in a series of patients undergoing the sodium amytal (Wada) procedure for the lateralization of language and memory functions (Powell, Polkey, & Canavan, 1987).

of the training sessions (1–14 vs. 15–28) within an analysis of variance (ANOVA) with the factors Polarity (required negativity increase vs. suppression for group SCP, required suppression vs. enhancement for alpha activity for group Alpha), Session (averaged across 1–14 vs. 15–28), and Type of Trial (feedback vs. transfer). An additional analysis evaluated the achieved progress in differentiation of SCP/Alpha comparing the 2nd and the 28th session. The corresponding ANOVA included the factors Polarity, Session, and Type of Trial.

Seizure Frequency. For every patient the median of seizure frequency was calculated for the baseline period (8 weeks). Weekly seizure rates for the following time were then plotted in relation to, and statistically compared with, this median by sign tests.

Results

1. *Epileptic patients can learn to control their SCP by means of extended (28 sessions) feedback training.* Figure 7 illustrates the mean differentiation in SCP between trials with required enhancement of negativity and trials with required positivity.

As indicated by Figure 7 and confirmed by the corresponding two-way interaction (Polarity × Session, $p < .05$) patients achieve substantial differentiation of SCPs in the required directions by the end of the 28th session. Significant differentiation on feedback trials is already achieved in session 21, the first session following the first transfer period of 8 weeks ($t(6) = 3.2$, $p < .05$). This indicates that control can be maintained over time. Control is most pronounced during the first block of feedback trials ($t(6) = 2.5$, $p = .05$) and deteriorates toward the end of the session. This finding is supported by a closer examination of the single case data (see below) and by observations indicating that patients—as compared with healthy subjects—have more difficulties in maintaining SCP control without continuous feedback and have more difficulties in concentrating on SCP control across the session (which lasts about 45 minutes). Patients of group Alpha ($n = 7$) did not achieve significant differentiation in alpha activity, nor did they exhibit differentiation in SCP (giving rise to a significant three-way interaction, $p < .05$). In session 28, groups differ significantly on feedback trials ($t(12) = 2.4$, $p < .05$).

2. *SCP control affects seizure frequency.* Table 1 provides an overview over (a) performance on the feedback training, (b) generalization of SCP control as evaluated after 4 months, and (c) change in seizure frequency.

While only one patient of group Alpha achieved control over this

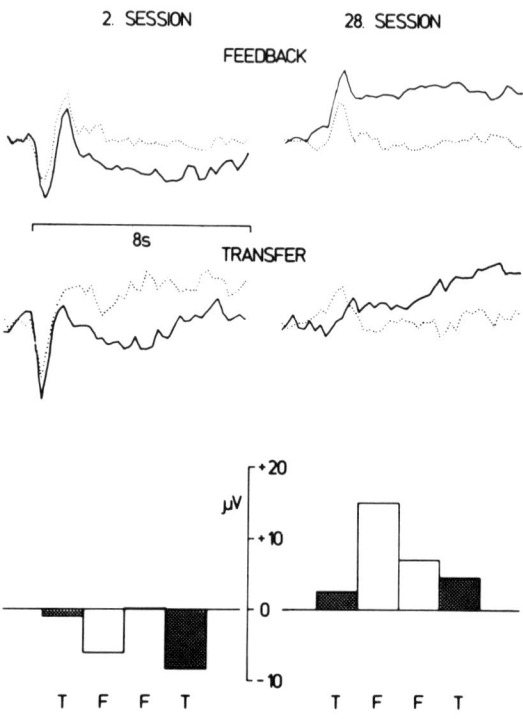

Figure 7. Learning progress in epileptic patients is illustrated comparing results from the 2nd (left) and the 28th (right) training session. As in Figures 3 and 5, the central (Cz) SCP differentiation is averaged separately for conditions. Responses were averaged separately for feedback (top) and transfer (mid) trials with required negativity (solid) and trials in which a zero or positive shift was required (dotted).

Table 1. *Ability to Achieve a Significant Differentiation in Electrical Brain Activity during the Feedback Session (Each Sign Represents One Patient)*

	Training success during feedback	
	Achieved	Not achieved
SCP feedback	✶^{a}✶^{a}✶^{a}✶^{a}✶^{a}✶^{c}✶^{b}	•
Alpha feedback	✶^{a}	••••••

$^a p < .05$.
^{b}On second training; patient first participated in Alpha training.
$^c p < .1$.

activity, six of the seven patients in group SCP achieved significant control over their electrical brain activity across the training period (with main effects of Polarity or interactions of Polarity × Session yielding $p <$ .05 in the ANOVAs comparing sessions 1–14 and 15–28). One patient of group Alpha participated in a second training after a 1-year follow-up. The second training consisted of SCP feedback. This patient learned to control the respective EEG parameter on both trainings.

It is interesting to note that all patients producing significant differentiation of SCP also showed significant differentiation in EEG synchronization; increased self-induced negativity corresponds to reduced EEG power in the 9.5- to 15-Hz band, and negativity suppression covaries with enhanced EEG synchronization. Systematic differences in SCP were observed for one patient in the Alpha group, who, however, did not exhibit systematic differentiation in EEG synchronization, but systematic differences in SCP were not observed for the patient who achieved significant control over phasic alpha activity.

Four patients of the SCP group could still produce a systematic change in their EEG potential when asked to produce the *A* or the *B* response during a test 4 months after completion of the training. As summarized in Table 2, patients of group Alpha as well as one patient of group SCP did not demonstrate such a generalized control during the testing session. The failure of subjects in the Alpha group to produce differentially the *A* and *B* responses in SCP confirms the expected specificity of SCP feedback training. The question as to whether these subjects did produce a differential pattern in EEG synchronization has not been investigated.

While only one of the patients of group Alpha has demonstrated a lasting change in seizure frequency, four patients of group SCP have become completely seizure-free. Two of them, however, became seizure-free after a change in medication regimen. Two other patients have shown reductions in seizure frequency (see Table 3). One of them, suf-

Table 2. *Generalization of SCP Control (for those Patients Tested 4 Months after Completion of Training)*

	Produce SCP upon command	
	Yes	No
SCP feedback	****	••
Alpha feedback		••••••

Table 3. Twelve-Month Follow-Up Compared with Pretraining Baseline

	Seizure incidence			
	Reduced ($p < .05$)	Unchanged	Enhanced ($p < .05$)	Dropout
SCP feedback	*[b]*[b]*[a]*[a]*[c] *[b,d]*[b,e]			•
Alpha feedback	*[b]	••••••		

[a] $p < .05$.
[b] Seizure-free for at least 6 months.
[c] On second training; patient first participated in Alpha training.
[d] In this patient the seizure frequency increased during an intense antibiotics treatment. The following treatment with anticonvulsant drugs differed considerably from the one that the patient received prior to his infection. The patient then became seizure-free.
[e] Following feedback training, seizure incidence first remained unchanged in this patient. Subsequently, the medication was changed. In the course of the year, the patient became seizure-free. It is not possible to determine whether this effect is due to pharmacological treatment alone, the feedback training, or the interaction of both, or is simply a time effect. Effects due to the first and the last possibility, however, occur with equal chance in the control group.

fering from seizures with and without loss of consciousness, reduced the incidence of the former only. No systematic change in seizure duration, intensity, or delay could be detected in any of the patients. The patient of group Alpha who experienced a decrease in seizure frequency showed systematic differentiation of SCP on the last training session. The patient who achieved control over alpha activity and —during the second training—SCP, however, showed reduction of seizure frequency below pretraining baseline only after a subsequent SCP training (case 3 below).

Single Case Reports

The results in Tables 1–3 are based on single case statistics. While the illustrated group outcome does not require sophisticated group statistics, the effects of the feedback procedures can be evaluated only by description of the single cases. The representative single case reports should serve this goal and exemplify characteristics and problems inherent in SCP/Alpha control and its effects on seizure frequency.

Case 1. Woman, age 25 years, psychomotor seizures for 5 years with a median seizure frequency of five per week. A diary, kept by the patient indicated stable seizure frequency irrespective of antiepileptic medication during the last year. The patient was free of any medication during the whole investigation. She was randomly assigned to group SCP.

Figure 8a illustrates SCP differentiation under transfer conditions for case 1 across sessions. Between-sessions comparison confirms SCP control throughout the sessions (Polarity: $F(1, 26) = 20.5$, $p < .01$). This patient already achieved reliable SCP control within the first 10 sessions, and she also maintained this control for the subsequent sessions with distracting conditions. Figure 8b illustrates the Cz versus earlobe EEG recording obtained during the generalization test, scheduled 4 months after the feedback training. As can be seen, this patient has been able to deliberately produce negative (inducing state A) and positive (inducing state B) SCP shifts demonstrating generalization of control. Figure 8c illustrates the dramatic change in seizure frequency. It dropped from a

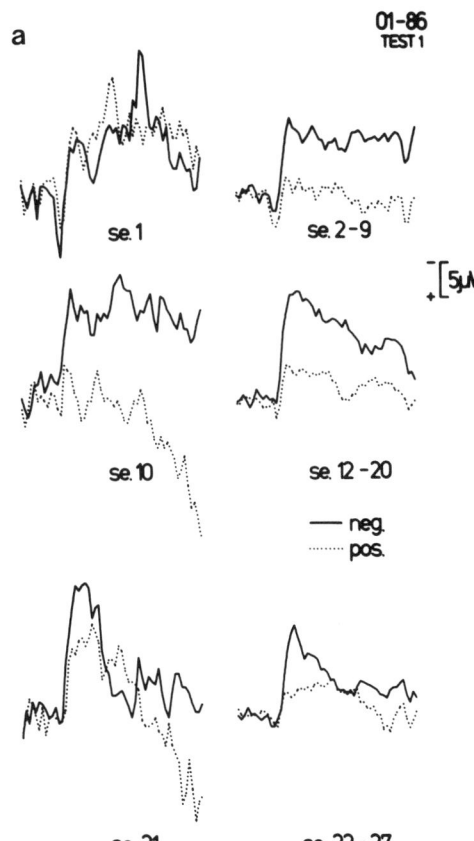

Figure 8a. SCP for case 1 for a 1-second prestimulus interval and 8-second letter presentation. The Cz-EEG traces were averaged across the first transfer trial block for session 1, mean of sessions 2–9, session 10, mean of sessions 11–20, session 21, and mean of sessions 22–27. Solid lines: trials with required negativity; dotted: trials with required negativity suppression (μV, negativity up).

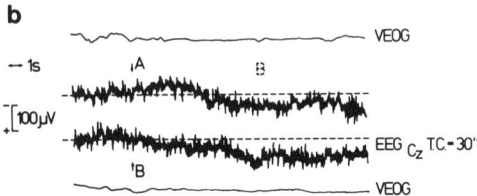

Figure 8b. Single EEG and vertical EOG traces for time segments, during which patient No. 1 deliberately induced state A (negativity increase) and then B or state B (positivity) alone. Note that deviations of the DC shift from baseline can be produced by this patient in both the negative and positive direction.

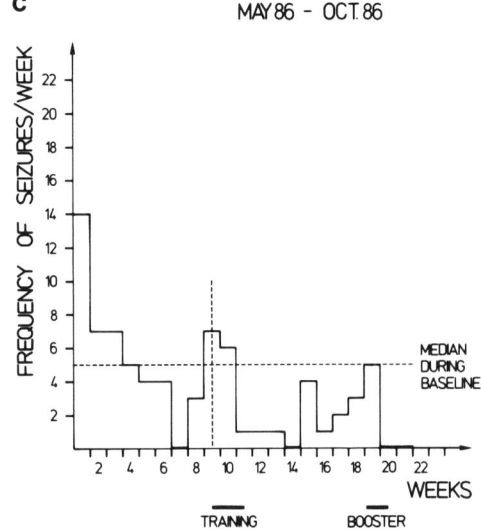

Figure 8c. Seizure frequency (ordinate) plotted across weeks (abscissa) for patient No. 1. Training periods are marked by bars below the abscissa. Dashed line: median seizure frequency for baseline (8 weeks). The patient has stayed seizure-free from week 20 on.

long-term median of five per week[3] to zero by the end of the 28th session. The patient, seizure-free ever since, keeps on practicing SCP control at regular intervals.

Posttraining neurological diagnostics confirmed a normalization of EEG patterns. Improvements on the neuropsychological test battery were found for delayed recall in both verbal and spatial memory.

This patient demonstrates that control over SCP can be successfully

---

[3]The patient kept a diary over more than half a year prior to her participation in the study. These records show that the median of weekly seizure incidence had been constantly five per week over a long time period. Seizure frequency was the same during the 8 baseline weeks illustrated in Figure 8c.

achieved within the training period, and that the ability may generalize to conditions outside the laboratory without feedback. The substantial seizure reduction appears at the time of the training procedure and hence is likely to be linked to it.

Case 2. Female, age 15 years, psychomotor seizures for 11 years, varying between two per week and three per day depending on medication regimen. Drug regimen includes carbamazepine, ethosuximide, and phenytoine. When ethosuximide was included, the weekly seizure rate dropped from 10/week to 2/week at the beginning of the baseline period. Assigned to group SCP.

Figure 9a illustrates that the patient (described herein as No. 2) quickly learned to reliably control SCPs, achieving substantial negative and positive shifts. Across training sessions, a shift toward increasing negative SCP became evident ($F(1, 26) = 19.0$, $p < .01$), but the patient maintained her ability to produce the required differentiation (accordingly, the comparison across sessions yields a significant Polarity effect, $F(1, 26) = 25.7$, $p < .01$). The patient became aware of her difficulties in producing state B (reduction of cortical negativity) especially when compared with the ease with which state A was produced, her observation being in accordance with the increasingly negative SCP levels. She reported particularly having difficulties in producing B responses prior to seizure attacks. She felt she could suppress or delay an attack several times, when she managed to create state B successfully and quickly enough during a prodromal state. On the generalization test 4 months after training, patient No. 2 quickly and reliably demonstrated negative shifts on practicing A, while it took her a couple of minutes and several attempts to achieve negativity suppression (see Fig. 9b). For 11 months following the training, there was no substantial effect on seizure frequency in this patient. During the last month of follow-up a new drug (Vigabatrin) was introduced into the medication regimen. Seizure frequency has dropped to near zero since then.

Case 2 is an example that, although control of SCPs may be successfully learned during training, effects on seizure frequency may depend especially on the ability to create positive SCPs quickly enough. (Other relations between SCP control and seizure rate will be discussed below.)

Case 3. Female, age 31 years, psychomotor seizures for 12 years, seizure frequency varying between two and six per week with occasional seizure-free weeks; medication regimen includes phenytoine and carbamazepine. Assigned to group Alpha.

Patient No. 3 did achieve control over EEG alpha activity (main

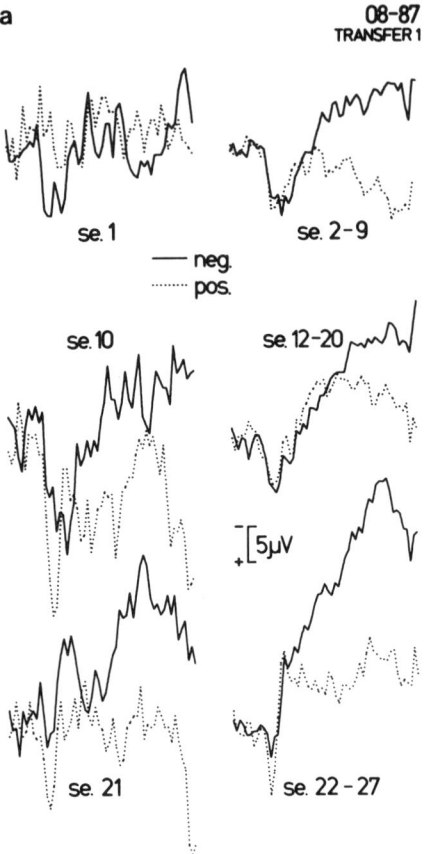

Figure 9a. Same result as in Figure 8a for Case 2.

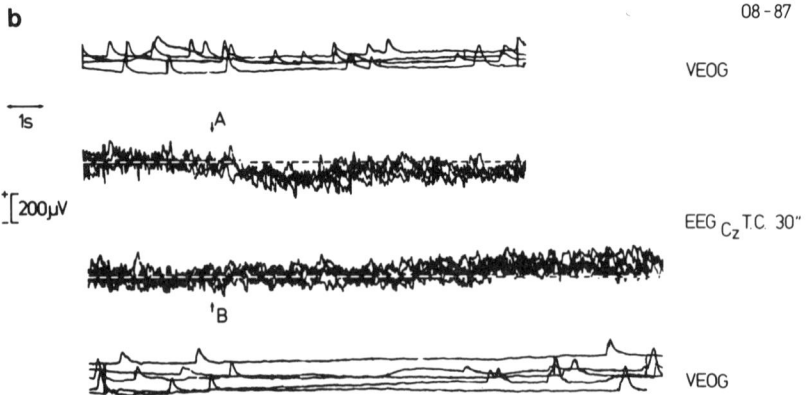

Figure 9b. Superimposed are five traces each during the generalization test. Negativity is down! Although the patient manages to produce a differential pattern for *A* and *B*, she has not learned to produce a positive shift upon command.

effect Polarity, $F(1, 26) = 11.1, p < .01$). There were no parallel systematic changes in SCPs. Correspondingly, no systematic changes in the EEG traces could be detected on the generalization test 4 months later (Figure 10a).

Following a transient reduction in seizure frequency during training periods, the patient's seizure rates increased to the baseline median again (Figure 10b). Thus, the training seemed to have no substantial effect on the seizure frequency.

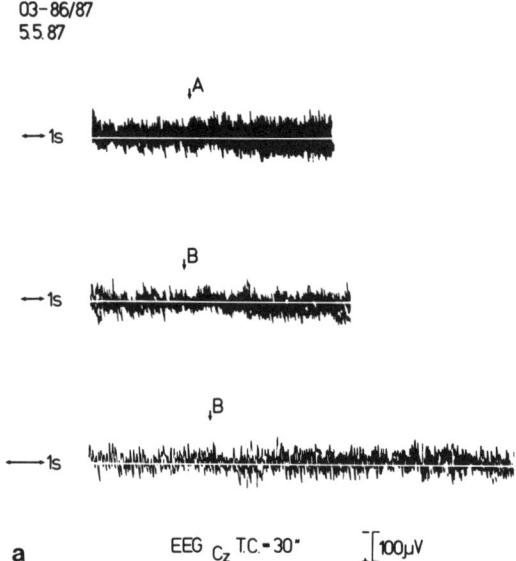

Figure 10a. The superposition of EEG traces illustrates that patient No. 3 did not produce any systematic DC changes when asked to produce response A or response B.

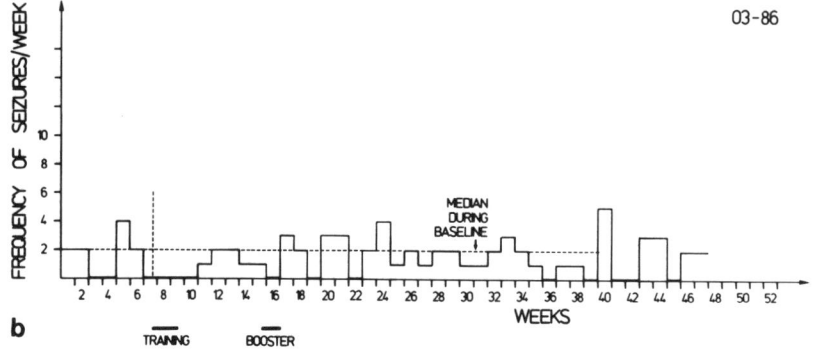

Figure 10b. Time course of the seizure incidence for case 3 indicates, if any, only a transient change. (Medication was kept constant during the period illustrated.)

Case 3 was selected as an example that training of electrical brain activity has to be specific in order to affect seizure activity. The observed transient reduction in seizure frequency may be attributed to a nonlasting placebo effect.

This patient participated in SCP training after a 1-year follow-up and acquired SCP control ($t(26) = 2.6$). Following this training, seizure frequency has remained below the median of the baseline. Conclusions should be drawn only after more data of this kind become available. Then such examples could further document the specificity of the type of electrical brain activity chosen for feedback training.

Case 4. Female, age 20 years, suffering from absences for 11 years; mean seizure frequency varying between 40 and 80 per week, increasing under stress; medication includes carbamazepine, phenobarbital, and primidone. Assigned to group SCP.

This patient gives an example that SCP control may be achieved only after extended training. Patient No. 4 produced a mean SCP differentiation of 8 μV in the direction opposite of the required differentiation during the first 10 sessions, but ended with an adequate differentiation of about 6 μV at the end of the training (Polarity × Session, $F(1, 26) = 6.2, p < .05$). During the 8 weeks of baseline the seizure incidence varied from 50 to 85 per week around a median of 64. After training, seizure incidence dropped to values as low as 10/week and has stayed below the baseline median ever since.

Variables May Influence Acquisition of SCP Control and Its Effects on Seizure Frequency.

We cannot expect that every patient will learn to reliably control his or her SCPs and that every patient achieving SCP control will benefit from this ability. But we may be able to specify and quantify determining factors. Ultimately, this task requires a very large patient sample but there are some tentative suggestions that can be derived from the present data.

Effects of Antiepileptic Medication. Two patients who became completely seizure-free following SCP training were not under current antiepileptic medication. On the other hand, those patients who did not show such substantial changes in seizure frequency were under heavy and long-term medication. It is not unlikely that anticonvulsant agents, usually central nervous depressants, might affect the brain's ability to learn and to adequately bring into action the learned regulation of SCP/cortical excitability. Apart from various impairing side effects of antiepileptic medication on learning and cognitive processing (as, for example, described by Penry & Rahel, 1986), we ourselves have demonstrated dampening effects of a commonly used anticonvulsant, carbamazepine (CBZ), and of a benzodiazepine (Clonazepam) used as an anticonvulsant, on EEG and SCP regulation in healthy human volunteers (Rockstroh et al., 1987).

A "traditional" paradigm for investigating SCP is the two-stimulus reaction time paradigm, in which a first stimulus (S1) signals a second, response-requiring stimulus (S2) to occur after a distinct time interval. In our study, the quality of the S1 (white 65-dB noise of different frequency mixture) indicated whether the S2 (a 65-dB tone to which a speeded button press was required) would follow after 2 seconds or after 6 seconds. In a double-blind setting, 20 male volunteers (mean age 24 years) received either 600 mg CBZ or the respective amount of a placebo.

While placebo subjects exhibited the negative SCP shift (CNV) typical in waveshape for a short and a longer preparatory interval (Rockstroh et al., 1982), CBZ significantly reduced anticipatory negativity (mean reduction: 7.5 μV; $t(18) = 2.3$, $p < .05$). Comparable effects were found in a more recent study (Rockstroh, Elbert, Lutzenberger, & Alteumüller, in press) for the benzodiazepine Clonazepam.

When medicated patients of the present sample were studied in the same paradigm, it turned out that the CNV was unusually small in the 2-second anticipatory interval and developed only late in the 6-second interval (see Figure 11, dashed lines).

It cannot be excluded that anticonvulsants, apart from their general dampening effects, also delay SCP development, an effect that would indicate a retarded, slowed regulation of cortical excitability. This assumption fits with the self-reports of case 2, who, in the generalization test, required several consecutive attempts and several minutes to produce a positive SCP shift—a time interval that would be too long to stop the progression of cortical overexcitation in a developing epileptic attack. It also fits with this patient's report of being unable to suppress negativity in the proximity of an attack.

Medication must be considered a serious intervening variable for SCP regulation.

Age. A detrimental effect of age on the ability to achieve self-control over brain activity has been suggested by observations of Sterman. Data from the present sample, though much smaller, confirm such an effect. The three patients exceeding 40 years in age did not acquire reliable control over their SCPs/Alpha activity (and also did not benefit from the training). The age effect may be confounded with intellectual deterioration: Sterman (personal communication, 1987) found age–IQ correlations with treatment success.

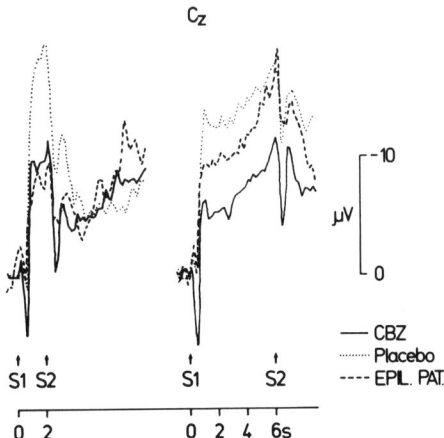

Figure 11. SCPs, recorded from the vertex, during a 2-second (left) and a 6-second (right) anticipatory (S1–S2) interval. (The SCP during the shorter ISI intervals has been also termed CNV). SCPs are averaged separately for 9 healthy subjects under carbamazepine (solid lines), 10 subject under placebo (dotted lines; data from Rockstroh *et al.*, 1987), and 8 medicated epileptic patients (dashed lines). Note that negativity in epileptic patients is reduced during the 2-second S1-interval and early in the 6-second S1 interval, while it reaches amplitudes comparable to those of placebo subjects during the last second of the 6-second interval.

Time Spent for Training/Number of Sessions. Twenty-eight training sessions within 2 months have been chosen for the Tübingen study. For successful SMR training 18 sessions (Sterman *et al.*, 1981) and training periods of 4 months (Lubar, 1984) have been reported. The time needed to learn a specific task varies a great deal from subject to subject, but unlike motor-skill learning, the simple rule "the more extensive the training, the higher the skill" seems not to apply for operant learning of EEG parameters. The present data suggest that learning occurs in steps rather than smoothly across the time. Eventually the subject seems to detect a strategy that can successfully modulate the EEG activity. And it may require time to apply this acquired tool in order to prevent epileptic fits. As reported by Sterman *et al.* (1981), benefits from SMR training increased during the period *following* treatment.

It is likely that other factors play important roles in determining the outcome of SCP feedback in epileptic patients. Of course, the specific type of the epileptic disease, the locus of an eventual focus, and other factors might be relevant. And there are a number of psychological factors, known to affect any type of learning, such as the design of the feedback or the motivation of the subject. But the present design would allow a starting point for further investigations.

In conclusion, this study indicates that epileptic patients suffer from impaired ability to regulate cortical excitability. There is, for the first time, evidence that extended training for SCP control may lead to substantial seizure reduction. The effects of SCP feedback deserve further investigation, which, for the moment, might concentrate on younger patients free of or low on medication.

References

Bauer, H. (1984). Regulation of slow brain potentials affects task performance. In T. Elbert, B. Rockstroh, W. Lutzenberger, & N. Birbaumer (Eds.), *Self-regulation of the brain and behavior* (pp. 216–226). Berlin/Heidelberg: Springer.

Bauer, H., & Lauber, W. (1979). Operant conditioning of brain steady potential shifts in man. *Biofeedback and Self-Regulation, 4,* 145–154.

Bauer, H., & Nirnberger, G. (1980). Paired associate learning with feedback of DC-potential shifts of the cerebral cortex. *Archives of Psychology, 132,* 237–238.

Bauer, H., & Nirnberger, G. (1981). Concept identification as a function of preceding negative or positive spontaneous shifts in slow brain potentials. *Psychophysiology, 18,* 466–469.

Benton, A. L. (1985). *The Revised Visual Retention Test.* New York: Psychological Corporation.

Birbaumer, N., Rockstroh, B., Elbert, T., & Lutzenberger, W. (1981). Biofeedback of slow cortical potentials. *International Journal of Psychophysiology, 16,* 389–415.

Birbaumer, N., Lang, P., Cook, E., Elbert, T., Lutzenberger, W., & Rockstroh, B. (1988). Self-regulation of slow brain potentials and imagery. *International Journal of Neuroscience, 39,* 101–116.

Birbaumer, N., Elbert, T., Canavan, A., & Rockstroh, B. (1990). Slow potentials of the cerebral cortex and behavior. *Physiological Reviews, 70*(1), 1–41.

Born, J., Whipple, S., & Stamm, J. S. (1982). Spontaneous cortical slow potential shifts and choice reaction time performance. *Electroencephalography and Clinical Neurophysiology, 54,* 668–676.

Braitenberg, V. (1978). Cell assemblies in the cerebral cortex. In R. Heim & G. Palm (Eds.), *Theoretical approach to complex systems* (pp. 171–188). Berlin/Heidelberg: Springer.

von Bülow, I., Elbert, T., Rockstroh, B., Lutzenberger, W., Canavan, A., & Birbaumer, N. (1989). Effects of hyperventilation on EEG frequency and slow cortical potentials in relation to an anticonvulsant and epilepsy. *Journal of Psychophysiology, 3,* 147–154.

Butters, N., Soeldner, C., & Fedio, P. (1972). Comparison of parietal and frontal lobe spatial deficits in man: Extrapersonal versus personal (egocentric) space. *Perceptual and Motor Skills, 34,* 27–34.

Canavan, A. G. M. (1983). Stylus maze performance in patients with frontal lobe lesions:

Effects of signal valency and relationship to verbal and spatial abilities. *Neuropsychologia, 21*, 375–382.

Canavan, A. G. M., Dunn, G., & McMillan, T. (1986). Principal components of the WAIS-R. *British Journal of Clinical Psychology, 25*, 81–85.

Canavan, A. G. M., Passingham, R. E., Marsden, C. D., Quinn, N., Wyke, M., & Polkey, C. E. (1989). The performance on learning tasks of patients in the early stages of Parkinson's disease. *Neuropsychologia, 27*, 141–156.

Caspers, H., & Speckmann, E.-J. (1969). DC-potential shifts in paroxysmal states. In H. H. Jasper, A. A. Ward, & A. Pope (Eds.), *Basic mechanisms of the epilepsies*. Boston: Little, Brown.

Caspers, H., & Speckmann, E.-J. (1974). Cortical DC-shifts associated with changes of gas tension in blood and tissue. In A. Remond (Ed.), *Handbook of electroencephalography and clinical neurophysiology* (Vol. 10, pp. 41–65). Amsterdam: Elsevier.

Caspers, H., Speckmann, E.-J., & Lehmenkuehler, A. (1984). Electrogenesis of slow potentials of the brain. In T. Elbert, B. Rockstroh, W. Lutzenberger, & N. Birbaumer (Eds.), *Self-regulation of the brain and behavior* (pp. 25–41). Berlin/Heidelberg: Springer.

Chatrian, G. E., Somasundaram, M., & Tassinari, C. A. (1968). DC-changes recorded transcranially during "typical" 3/sec spike and wave discharges in men. *Epilepsia, 9*, 185–209.

Dahl, J., Melin, L., Brorson, L.-O., & Schollin, J. (1985). Effects of a broad-spectrum behavior modification treatment program on children with refractory epileptic seizures. *Epilepsia, 26*, 303–309.

Efron, R. (1957). Conditioned inhibition of uncinate fits. *Brain, 80*, 251–260.

Elbert, T. (1978). *Biofeedback langsamer kortikaler Potentiale*. Munich: Minerva.

Elbert, T. (1986). Externally and self-induced CNV patterns of the brain hemispheres—A sign of task-specific preparation. *Human Neurobiology, 5*, 67–69.

Elbert, T., & Rockstroh, B. (1987). Threshold regulation—A key to the understanding of the combined dynamics of EEG and event-related potentials. *Journal of Psychophysiology, 1*(4), 317–333.

Elbert, T., Birbaumer, N., Lutzenberger, W., & Rockstroh, B. (1979). Biofeedback of slow cortical potentials: Self-regulation of central and autonomic patterns. In N. Birbaumer & H. D. Kimmel (Eds.), *Biofeedback and self-regulation* (pp. 321–342). Hillsdale, NJ: Erlbaum.

Elbert, T., Rockstroh, B., Lutzenberger, W., & Birbaumer, N. (1980). Biofeedback of slow cortical potentials. *Electroencephalography and Clinical Neurophysiology, 48*, 293–301.

Elbert, T., Rockstroh, B., Lutzenberger, W., & Birbaumer, N. (Eds.). (1984). *Self-regulation of the brain and behavior*. Berlin/Heidelberg: Springer.

Forster, F. M. (1969). Conditioned reflexes and sensory-evoked epilepsy: The nature of the therapeutic process. *Conditional Reflex, 4*, 103–114.

Forster, F. M. (1972). The classification and conditioning treatment of the reflex epilepsies. *International Journal of Neurology, 9*, 73–86.

Forster, F. M. (1977). *Reflex epilepsy, behavioral therapy, and conditional reflexes*. Springfield, IL: Thomas.

Fried, R., Rubin, S. R., Carlton, R. M., & Fox, M. C. (1984). Behavioral control of intractable idiopathic seizures: I. Self-regulation of end-tidal carbon dioxide. *Psychosomatic Medicine, 46*, 315–332.

Goldstein, L. H., Canavan, A. G. M., & Polkey, C. E. (1988). Verbal and abstract designs paired associate learning after unilateral temporal lobectomy. *Cortex, 24*, 41–52.

Lubar, J. (1982). EEG operant conditioning in severe epilepsy. Controlled multidimensional studies. In L. White & B. Tursky (Eds.), *Clinical biofeedback* (pp. 288–310). New York: Guilford Press.

Lubar, J. (1984). Application of operant conditioning of the EEG for the management of epileptic seizures. In T. Elbert, B. Rockstroh, W. Lutzenberger, & N. Birbaumer (Eds.), *Self-regulation of the brain and behavior* (pp. 107–125). Berlin/Heidelberg: Springer.

Lutzenberger, W., Elbert, T., Rockstroh, B., & Birbaumer, N. (1979). Effects of slow cortical potentials on performance in a signal detection task. *International Journal of Neuroscience, 9*, 175–183.

Lutzenberger, W., Elbert, T., Rockstroh, B., & Birbaumer, N. (1982). Biofeedback of slow cortical potentials and its effects on the performance in mental arithmetic tasks. *Biological Psychology, 14*, 99–111.

Milner, B. (1964). Some effects of frontal lobectomy in man. In J. M. Warren & K. Akert (Eds.), *The frontal granular cortex and behaviour* (pp. 313–334). New York: McGraw-Hill.

Nelson, H. E. (1976). A modified card sorting test sensitive to frontal lobe defects. *Cortex, 12*, 313–324.

Penry, K., & Rahel, R. E. (1986). *Epilepsy: Diagnosis, management, quality of life.* New York: Raven Press.

Powell, G. E. (1979). The relationship between intelligence and verbal and spatial memory. *Journal of Clinical Psychology, 35*, 336–340.

Powell, G. E., Polkey, C. E., & McMillan, T. (1985). The new Maudsley series of temporal lobectomy. I: Short-term cognitive effects. *British Journal of Clinical Psychology, 24*, 109–124.

Powell, G. E., Polkey, C. E., & Canavan, A. G. M. (1987). Lateralisation of memory functions in epileptic patients by use of sodium amytal (Wada) technique. *Journal of Neurology, Neurosurgery, and Psychiatry, 50*, 665–672.

Roberts, L., Rockstroh, B., Lutzenberger, W., Elbert, T., & Birbaumer, N. (1989). Self-reports during feedback regulation of slow cortical potentials. *Psychophysiology, 26*, 392–403.

Rockstroh, B. (1987). Operant control of slow brain potentials. In J. N. Hintgen, D. Hellhammer, & G. Huppmann (Eds.), *Advanced methods in psychobiology* (pp. 179–190). Toronto: Hogrefe.

Rockstroh, B. (1989). Area-specific self-regulation of slow cortical potentials. In E. Basar & T. Bullock (Ed.), *Dynamics of sensory and cognitive processing by the brain* (pp. 467–476). Berlin/Heidelberg: Springer.

Rockstroh, B., Elbert, T., Birbaumer, N., & Lutzenberger, W. (1982). *Slow brain potentials and behavior*. Baltimore: Urban & Schwarzenberg.

Rockstroh, B., Elbert, T., Lutzenberger, W., & Birbaumer, N. (1984a). Operant control of slow brain potentials: A tool in the investigation of the potential's meaning and its relation to attentive dysfunction. In T. Elbert, B. Rockstroh, W. Lutzenberger, & N. Birbaumer (Eds.), *Self-regulation of the brain and behavior* (pp. 227–239). Berlin/Heidelberg: Springer.

Rockstroh, B., Birbaumer, N., Elbert, T., & Lutzenberger, W. (1984b). Operant control of EEG, event-related and slow potentials. *Biofeedback and Self-Regulation, 9*, 139–160.

Rockstroh, B., Elbert, T., Lutzenberger, W., Altenmüller, E., Diener, H.-C., Birbaumer, N., & Dichgans, J. (1987). Effects of the anticonvulsant carbamazepine on event-related brain potentials in humans. In R. Nodar, C. Barber, & T. Blum (Eds.), *Evoked Potentials* (Vol. 3, pp. 361–369). London: Butterworths.

Rockstroh, B., Elbert, T., Canavan, A., & Lutzenberger, W. (1989). *Slow cortical potentials and behavior* (2nd ed.). Munich: Urban & Schwarzenberg.

Rockstroh, B., Elbert, T., Lutzenberger, W., & Altenmüller, E. (in press). Effects of the anticonvulsant benzodiazepine Clonazepam on event-related brain potentials in humans. *Journal of Electroencephalography and Clinical Neurophysiology*.

Spunt, A., Heimann, B. P., & Rousseau, A. M. (1986). Epilepsy. In M. Hersen (Ed.), *Pharmacological and behavioral treatment* (pp. 178–198). New York: Wiley.

Stamm, J. S. (1984). Performance enhancements with cortical negative slow potential shift in man and monkey. In T. Elbert, B. Rockstroh, W. Lutzenberger, & N. Birbaumer (Eds.), *Self-regulation of the brain and behavior* (pp. 199–215). Berlin/Heidelberg: Springer.

Stamm, J. S., Whipple, S., & Born, J. (1987). Effects of spontaneous cortical slow potentials on semantic information processing. *International Journal of Psychophysiology, 5,* 11–18.

Sterman, M. B. (1982). EEG biofeedback in the treatment of epilepsy: An overview circa 1980. In L. White & B. Tursky (Eds.), *Clinical biofeedback* (pp. 311–330). New York: Guilford Press.

Sterman, M. B. (1984). The role of sensorimotor rhythmic EEG activity in the etiology and treatment of generalized motor seizures. In T. Elbert, B. Rockstroh, W. Lutzenberger, & N. Birbaumer (Eds.), *Self-regulation of the brain and behavior* (pp. 95–106). Berlin/Heidelberg: Springer.

Sterman, M. B. (1986). Epilepsy and its treatment with EEG feedback. *Annals of the Behavioral Medicine Society, 8,* 21–25.

Sterman, M. B., Lantz, D., Bruckler, R. M., & Kovalesky, R. A. (1981). Effects of sensorimotor EEG normalization feedback training on seizure rate in poorly controlled epileptics. Proceedings of the Biofeedback Society of America, 12th Annual Meeting, Louisville.

Trimmel, M. (1986). DC potentials of the brain. In D. Papakostopoulos, S. Butler, & I. Martin (Eds.), *Clinical and experimental neuropsychology* (pp. 312–338). London: Croom Helm.

Ueda, M., Furumitsu, I., & Kakigi, S. (1985). Self-regulation of contingent negative variation (CNV) using immediate feedback. *Japanese Journal of Physiology, Psychology and Psychophysiology, 3,* 1–9.

Wechsler, D. (1981). *Wechsler Adult Intelligence Scale-Revised.* New York: Psychological Corporation.

Whitsett, S., & Lubar, J. (1981). Evidence of changes in the sleep EEG following biofeedback treatment of epilepsy. Proceedings of the Biofeedback Society of America, 12th Annual Meeting, Louisville.

CHAPTER 5

Low-Dimensional Chaos in a Simple Biological Model of Neocortex
Implications for Cardiovascular and Cognitive Disorders

James E. Skinner, Mirna Mitra, and Keith Fulton

Brain Regulation of the Heart

Our laboratory has been interested in understanding the neural mechanisms involved in information processing in neocortex, especially in those structures that regulate the sensory and cardiovascular systems. Studies in comparative physiology suggest a theoretical basis for the regulation of the cardiovascular system by the brain. Following his life's work, Cannon (1931) hypothesized the existence of a cerebral mechanism in which sensory input and autonomic output were simultaneously orchestrated; this orchestration, he suggested, became a focus for natural selection and evolved to enable the higher mammal to attend to its environment and simultaneously to prepare autonomic support in *anticipation* of the occurrence of certain survival behaviors that might be released.

Our laboratory has shown that the frontal lobes are likely to be the orchestrator hypothesized by Cannon. This bilateral structure controls

---

James E. Skinner, Mirna Mitra, and Keith Fulton • Department of Neurology and Neuroscience Program, Baylor College of Medicine, Houston, Texas 77030, USA.

sensory input by inhibiting the thalamic relay of irrelevant sensory information, and it simultaneously regulates patterns of autonomic activity during behavioral attention (Skinner, 1988; Skinner & Yingling, 1976, 1977; Yingling & Skinner, 1976, 1977). The implications of this cerebral orchestration for the cardiovascular disorders are now being widely recognized. Blockade of the descending cerebral pathway that mediates the anticipatory autonomic activities will prevent the lethal consequence of coronary artery occlusion (heart attack), even in stressed animals (Skinner & Reed, 1981). Such blockade will also normalize blood pressure elevations in several models of experimental hypertension (Szilagyi, Taylor, & Skinner, 1987).

Figure 1 shows a summary of our experiments that together indicate

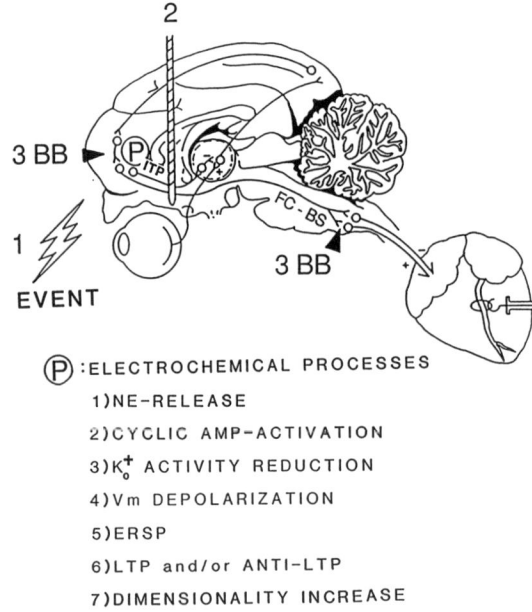

Ⓟ : ELECTROCHEMICAL PROCESSES
1) NE-RELEASE
2) CYCLIC AMP-ACTIVATION
3) K_o^+ ACTIVITY REDUCTION
4) Vm DEPOLARIZATION
5) ERSP
6) LTP and/or ANTI-LTP
7) DIMENSIONALITY INCREASE

Figure 1. Event-related cortical responses transform the information in an environmental event into a pattern of sensory gating (via the inferior thalamic peduncle, ITP), and autonomic perturbation (via the frontocortical-brainstem pathway, FC-BS). This event-related cortical process (P) selectively inhibits the thalamic relay of irrelevant sensory information and prepares the autonomic nervous system to support behavioral reactions to the remaining sensory influx. The known electrochemical correlates of process P are listed, and each is discussed in the text and illustrated in the next figure. Three independent interventions in this cerebral system are known to have salutary effect in experimental models of sudden cardiac death and hypertension: (1) learned adaptation to stressor events, (2) tractotomy in the FC-BS pathway, and (3) intracerebral beta-receptor blockade, (BB). (Adapted from Skinner, 1984).

how the frontal lobes regulate sensory input and autonomic output and, as a consequence, also control the vulnerability of the cardiovascular system to dysfunction. Each of three independent manipulations of the brain prevents the occurrence of the lethal arrhythmia (ventricular fibrillation) following acute coronary artery occlusion: (1) behavioral adaptation (i.e., learning about a novel environment), (2) neurophysiological intervention (i.e., blockade of the frontocortical-brainstem pathway), and (3) cerebral beta-receptor blockade (i.e., blockade in the brain, but not in the peripheral nervous system). The theory that links these observations stems in part from Cannon's hypotheses, but it also incorporates our own findings concerning the electrochemical transactions evoked in the frontal lobes following any type of meaningful stimulus event.

Our investigation of these electrochemical transactions began with the event-related slow potential (ERSP), an extracellularly recorded voltage evoked in the frontal lobes during all types of selective attention and autonomic regulation. This response is generated by the frontal cortex following presentation of events such as novel objects or conditioned signals (Skinner, 1971, 1984). Figure 2 summarizes the electrochemical responses associated with the occurrence of the ERSP (Skinner, 1971, 1984; Skinner & King, 1980; Skinner & Molnar, 1983; Skinner, Reed, Welch, & Nell, 1978). This accumulated evidence suggests that a meaningful stimulus event produces a sequence of actions, each of which is independently known to be causally linked to its successor: (1) First, norepinephrine is released; (2) then the beta-adrenergic receptor is stimulated (i.e., unless propranolol, its competitive inhibitor, is present); (3) adenylyl cyclase is activated (i.e., cyclic AMP accumulation is enhanced); (4) potassium-ion conductance is decreased (i.e., a calcium-dependent potassium conductance); (5) the membrane potential is depolarized (i.e., because the G_K/G_{Na} ratio that determines the potential is reduced); and finally, (6) the extracellular negative potential (the ERSP) is produced.

These linked correlates, however, do not explain how the learning-dependent noradrenergic mechanism in the frontal lobes actually processes information (process P, in Figure 1). We therefore reasoned that a simpler biological system and a more appropriate conceptual approach were needed if we were to understand the spatial and temporal dynamics of the underlying cortical network. The olfactory bulb was chosen because it has both the cell types and neurochemicals intrinsic to neocortex, but it has a much simpler and better understood neurophysiological structure (Shepherd, 1970). Furthermore, the amplitude of the field potential that occurs on the surface above each columnar unit (spaced at

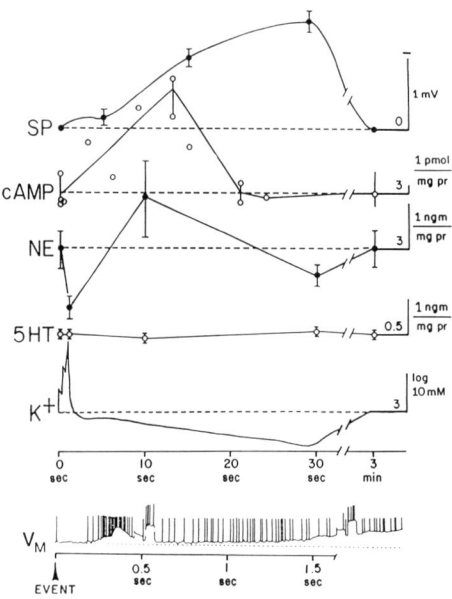

Figure 2. Some electrochemical responses in rostromedial neocortex evoked by meaningful events, such as novel or conditioned stimuli. Abbreviations: SP = extracellular event-related slow potential recorded with platinum-black electrodes from the same specific subjects (rats) in which the cAMP levels were determined (error bars indicate SD of 8 rats); cAMP = cyclic 3′,5′-adenosine monophosphate (labeled antibody assay) in rapidly frozen blocks of tissue adjacent to the platinum-black electrode (data from 14 animals are shown with each value expressed relative to the protein content); NE = norepinephrine content (high performance liquid chromatography) in tissue from another group of rats treated in an identical manner (means and standard deviations are indicated, $N = 3$ or 4 at each point); 5HT = 5-hydroxytryptamine content in same block used to determine NE (blood vessels on cortical surface were removed from each block, accounting for the relatively small mean and low variance); K± = extracellular potassium-ion activity (using 2-micron-diameter micropipettes filled with ion-selective resin, Corning); V_M = intracellular membrane potential from a frontocortical neuron in a conscious cat (input impedance = 10 megohms, using an inward, 0.5-nanoamp, 50-msec, current-pulse); outward depolarizing pulses were used to evoke hyperpolarizing afterpotentials (i.e., a calcium-dependent potassium current), which were completely blocked by 1.5 seconds after the event). Calibrations: Each baseline level and unit calibration is indicated at the right of each trace; the resting V_M was minus 55 mV. All events were novel stimuli, with the exception of V_M, which was evoked by a tone forewarning a cutaneous shock; the latter was identical to a response evoked 60 seconds earlier by a novel stimulus. (Adapted, in part, from Skinner, 1984; Skinner & King, 1980; Skinner, Reed, Welch, & Nell, 1978.)

0.5-mm intervals) is linearly related to the firing probability of the immediately underlying output neuron (mitral cell), as shown in Figure 3a and b. This tight correlation enables multiple surface electrodes to provide knowledge of the total output of the bulb without having to make massive numbers of microelectrode penetrations to reach the mitral cells (Freeman & Schneider, 1982; Gray, Freeman, & Skinner, 1984, 1986). Microelectrode recordings of the individual mitral cells illustrate that conditioned odors, but not unconditioned ones, evoke spatially dependent changes in firing probability (Wilson & Leon, 1988; Wilson, Sullivan, & Leon, 1987). Some cells fire faster following the meaningful odor, while others are inhibited, but all of this happens only in the specific parts of the bulb where the specific odor being used is known to increase metabolic activity (i.e., increase 2-deoxyglucose uptake).

Model Cortical System: Olfactory Bulb

Bulbar output, as represented by the pattern of surface activity, is illustrated in Figure 3c. The larger the dot, the larger the amplitude of the voltage recorded by that specific electrode in the 8 × 8 array. Because of the tight correlation, the larger the dot, the higher the firing probability of the underlying mitral cell. This correlation occurs because each mitral cell has an open field morphology. When the soma manifests a depolarization leading to an action potential, source current is drawn from the long apical dendrite, a low resistance process that extends toward the surface. The potential at the surface is due to this source current and is therefore indicative of the firing probability of the cell. Other cells in the bulb have radial symmetry and do not form open field dipoles. They do not contribute significantly to the surface potentials.

The spatial pattern representing bulbar output changes following the presentation of either a novel or conditioned odor. To the unaided eye this change is difficult to perceive. For example, in Figure 3c, compare Control with Novel Odor; they look nearly the same. The use of statistics, however, enables clear distinctions to be made. In Figure 3d, compare the pattern-change measure (% log Chi-square > 2.2) that follows a conditioned stimulus (i.e., CS+, under Vehicle) with that which follows an unreinforced odor (CS−, under Vehicle); the latter does not result in a statistically significant pattern change, nor does a control airodorant (A, Air). The reinforced odor (CS+), in contrast, produces a highly statistically significant pattern change ($P < .01$) (Gray et al., 1986). This same statistically significant increase in the pattern-change measure also follows a *novel* stimulus, with the amplitude being at least as large

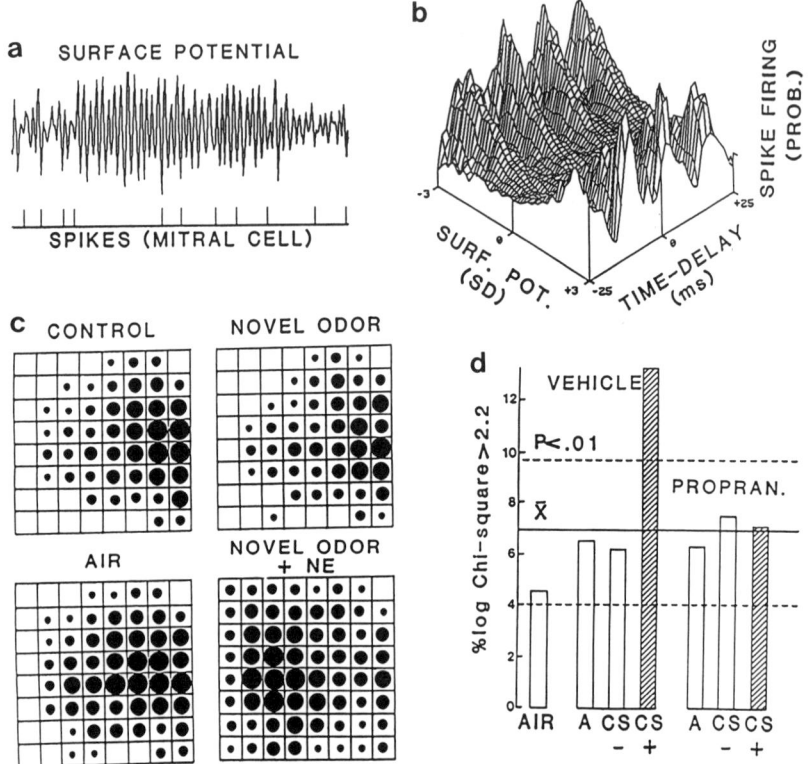

Figure 3. Composite data illustrating the patterns of electric activity recorded from the surface of the olfactory bulb of the conscious rabbit. (a) A surface potential simultaneously recorded with the extracellular spike activity of an immediately underlying mitral cell. (b) A three-dimensional plot of the probability of firing of the extracellular spike with the surface potential amplitude for all time delays just before and after each spike. (c) Activity recorded from the bulbar surface by an 8 × 8 electrode array (each surface potential is linearly related to the size of the dot within the box representing the electrode); CONTROL = nothing injected into the nose cone; AIR = air injected; NOVEL ODOR = faint odor of n-butyl alcohol injected; NOVEL ODOR + NE = n-butyl alcohol injected a week later during bulbar perfusion with norepinephrine. (d) The spatial pattern change is measured by the percentage of log Chi-square values of t tests greater than 2.2; t tests were for each electrode just before and after odor, with 10 replicated observations (i.e., 10 odor trials); 2.2 is the cutoff value for 95% of the scores during the control condition (i.e., air compared to air); this measure (% log Chi-square > 2.2) is a sensitive indication of the evoked pattern changes, such as those shown in (c); the $P < .01$ confidence interval is indicated for data collected during both vehicle and propranolol perfusions through the bulb; A = air odorant; CS− = unreinforced odor; CS+ = reinforced odor. (Also see Gray, Freeman, & Skinner, 1986.)

as that which follows a CS+. Propranolol perfused through the bulb, however, prevents this event-related pattern change (Figure 3d), and, in contrast, exogenous norepinephrine makes the change so apparent that the need for statistical analysis is not necessary (Figure 3c, Novel Odor + NE).

The stabilization of the spatial pattern brought about by propranolol may be important in explaining how centrally acting cardiac-antiarrhythmic drugs work. Long-term potentiation (LTP) is a synaptic mechanism in which high-frequency use leads to persistent enhancement of the postsynaptic potentials. LTP is a beta-receptor-mediated process (Bliss, Goddard, & Rives, 1983; Hopkins & Johnston, 1984) that is dependent upon cyclic AMP activation (Hopkins & Johnston, 1988). Ethmozine (moricizine), another antiarrhythmic drug, also blocks LTP, but it is a muscarinic agonist (Krontiris-Litowitz, Skinner, & Birnbaumer, 1985); other muscarinic agonists also block LTP (Williams & Johnston, 1988a,b). Cyclic AMP formation is inhibited by both muscarinic agonists and beta antagonists in a variety of cells containing both receptor types (Watanabe, McConnaughey, Strawbridge, Fleming, Jones, & Besch, 1978; Hildebrandt, Sekura, Codina, Iyengar, Manclark, & Birnbaumer (1983). Thus, blocking cyclic AMP accumulation in the output cells of the frontal lobes could prevent event-related LTP and thus limit activity in the frontocortical-brainstem pathway.

Both beta-antagonists (Skinner, 1988; Thompson, Newton, Pocock, Cooper, Crow, McCallum, and Papakostopoulos, 1978) and Ethmozine (Skinner & Pratt, 1982) block or reduce the amplitude of the ERSP in humans. These findings suggest that indeed both types of cardiovascular drugs have a common site of central action and that this site is the frontal lobes, the generator of the potential. For one of these drugs, propranolol, it is its central action, and not its peripheral cardiovascular influence, that mediates the antimortality (Skinner, 1984, 1988) and antihypertensive (Reid, Lewis, Myers, & Dollery, 1974; Tackett, Webb, & Privitera, 1985) effects.

The clinical action of the centrally acting cardiovascular drugs may be to counter a genetically based, overreactive, noradrenergic mechanism in frontal lobe. A nonlethal single-gene mutation has been shown in mice to lead to hypertrophy of the cerebral noradrenergic system (Levitt & Noebels, 1981). Neurotech Laboratories, Inc. (1988) has recently reported preliminary results showing that the ERSP is enhanced in preclinical subjects with family history of cardiovascular disease compared with individuals without such a genetic background. There is no longer any question that genetics play an important role in hypertension and sudden cardiac death; even the traditional cardiovascular physiologists have come to this conclusion independently of the neuroscientists (Folkow, 1982). The question remains, however: What is the neural mechanism? We expect that the study of the spatial patterns on the bulbar surface (the output) during controlled stimulus events (the input) will lead to an understanding of how information is acquired and stored in a cortical system. A problem, however, still exists in the conceptual approach. Although statistically significantly different during the pre- and postodor intervals, the spatial patterns on the bulbar surface are quite noisy and require statistical analysis, over trials, to observe the change. Such noise, operationally defined as signal, suggests that a low-dimensional *chaotic* process may be generating the observed dynamical patterns (Farmer, 1982). If this is the case, then a *breakthrough* could be at hand in our ability to construct a theoretical model of a biological system composed of numerous, highly interconnected, neural elements. That is, we could know the *dimension* of a mathematical function whose time-series behavior is the same as that of the generator of the surface potentials; that is, we could know the value of n in the n-dimensional function that is a mathematical model of the biological system. Knowing this dimension, we would then know the number of independent variables involved in the dynamical process in the tissue (i.e., the variables involved in process P, in Figure 1). The purpose of the present study is to determine the dimensions of the field potentials on the bulbar surface that collectively represent its pattern of output.

Measuring the Correlation Dimension

The trick that enables the estimate of the dimension of a generator from a sample of its time series, such as a sample of a surface potential, is that the phase space of any function can be constructed in *two* ways: (1) from the orthogonal derivatives, if the function is known (e.g., by plotting dx/dt vs. d^2x/dt^2, etc.) or (2) from orthogonal time-delay axes constructed from the time series, if the function is unknown. Takens (1981) has shown that the dimensions of these two phase portraits (i.e., their correlation dimensions, D_2) are the *same in the limit*—that is, as the number of sample points in the time series becomes sufficiently large. In the case of the unknown function, D_2 is estimated by Nu (V) in the expression, $C(r,N) = r^V$, where n is the cumulative number of r values and r is the range of vector *differences* in a multidimensional phase portrait (m) of the time series being analyzed; N is the number of sample points observed in the epoch. Saturation (convergence) of Nu must occur at higher values of m (e.g., $m > 2D_2 + 1$) if the time series is to be successfully represented by a low-dimensional chaotic attractor. The criteria for determining convergence for finite data from a biological system have not yet been clearly established.

For example, some investigators have reported low-dimensional chaotic processes in scalp-recorded EEG potentials from neocortex (Babloyantz & Destexhe, 1986, 1987; Graf & Elbert, 1988; Roschke & Basar, 1988). These studies, however, have not considered (1) the effects of signal *filtering* on the calculation of the D_2 estimate, (2) alterations in the *shape* of the correlation integral due to finite data samples, and (3) the problem of *stationarity* of the dynamical process during the data sampling. Highly filtered white noise, as we will show, can appear to be convergent. Although the effects of N and Tau (the time delay for constructing the axes) have been examined empirically, the issue regarding the distribution of the sample points over the presumed attractor have not yet been investigated. And finally, the problem of stationarity of the generator process has been recognized as the central problem in the application of nonlinear dynamics to neurobiology (Mayer-Kress, 1986), but this issue has not yet been studied systematically. Addressing some of these issues in our model cortical system is another aim of the present investigation.

Methods for Studying the Correlation Dimension in the Olfactory Bulb

Dimensional Analysis

The algorithms of Grassberger and Procaccia (1983), Packard, Crutchfield, Farmer, and Shaw (1980), Takens (1981), and Theiler (1988) were used to analyze the data. Adjustments to correct the autocorrelation effect (i.e., to discount the spatial near-neighbors resulting from a temporal correlation) were made, in some cases, according to the algorithm of Theiler (1986). The estimate of the saturated correlation dimension (D_2) was calculated by a Masscomp computer (WS-500) for each of the chosen data epochs. In most cases, 1 to 15 embedding dimensions were used to visualize the convergence; in some cases 1 to 30 embedding dimensions were employed to verify the D_2 saturation. Epochs of 500 msec to 6 sec were recorded from the bulb and each consisted of 320 to 10,000 digitized voltages produced by a Masscomp AD12FA converter capable of running at 500k Hz. As stationarity must be presumed, 500-msec epochs were used initially, to increase the likelihood that stationarity would be maintained during data acquisition.

To calculate the D_2 estimate we first established a time delay, Tau. The initial Tau interval chosen was the first zero crossing of the autocorrelation function of the surface potential for each specific epoch analyzed. Other Tau intervals were investigated, such as the interval of the digitizing rate and ¼ cycle of the predominant frequency. According to the prescription of Packard et al. (1980), vector differences were determined from serial digitized voltages located at integer-multiples of Tau, in which case the integer specifies the embedding dimension (m). Each voltage vector was subtracted from the value of all the rest to provide a set of absolute differences for D_2 dimensional analysis at each specific embedding dimension (Grassberger & Procaccia, 1983). Recall that the number of absolute vector differences, n, accumulated within a range, r, of a given embedding dimension, m, is related to the estimate of the correlation dimension, Nu (V), by the expression, $n = r^V$. If a linear relationship is detected in a plot of log(n) versus log(r), then V is quantifiable, since it is the slope. Nonlinearities due to near-neighbor effects were eliminated in some cases by the Theiler (1988) algorithm, C(r,N,W), where W was usually the number of data points within 1 Tau unit. When the embedding dimension was increased, the slope representing V will eventually saturate; that is, it will converge if a low-dimensional attractor exists. This *saturated value* of V is the *estimate* of D_2 (the correlation dimension), of the generator of the data set.

Approximately N^2 vector differences are required for each embedding dimension. It would take a fast computer months to calculate D_2 estimates for large numbers of embedding dimensions for long epochs of data. For large N calculations, we used the box-assisted algorithm developed by Theiler (1988); this algorithm calculates D_2 over specified ranges of r (i.e., r_o), a procedure that eliminates the necessity for calculating the correlation integral over *all* values of r and thus speeds up the estimate. The Theiler algorithm, however, only operates at the moment with Tau = 1 (i.e., the digitizing rate), so N must be large.

Besides estimating D_2 for the biological data, we also used narrow-band filters (Krohn-Hite) applied to Gaussian noise to create control data with the same spectral band as our biological data. The objective here was to distinguish clearly the biological D_2 estimate from that of noise filtered at the same spectral bandpass. The null hypothesis tested was that the sampled data was filtered noise.

Behavioral Paradigm

Behavior state was changed by presenting a rabbit with a faint novel odor delivered through a nose cone. All subjects were *highly adapted* to the experimental apparatus before any data were collected. This included adaptation to having novel odors presented in the recording chamber. The respiratory behavior of the rabbit was monitored with a thoracic bellows and strain gauge to determine accurately the first inspiration during which odor detection occurred. This inspiration invariably has a briefer cycle than those during the preceding interval ($P < .01$, Gray et al., 1986). This same paradigm has been used by us in other publications (Gray et al., 1986; Gray and Skinner, 1988).

Data Acquisition

Olfactory bulb surface potentials were recorded by an 8 × 8 array of stainless steel electrodes (0.23 mm dia.), each of which was separated from the others by the observed spatial frequency of the bulb (0.5 mm). The array was first constructed and then implanted under sterile surgical conditions, as described previously (Gray et al., 1986; Gray & Skinner, 1988). Each surface potential was amplified by a high-gain preamplifier with variable bandpasses (2-microvolt noise level at a bandpass of 20 to 200 Hz, 3-dB roll-off). The multiple amplified signals were digitized by a 500k Hz A/D burst (12 bit) at the selected sampling rate (i.e., 640 to 10k Hz), streamed to a 2-megabyte RAM, offloaded to a 70-megabyte hard disk and saved on digital tape.

New Experimental Results

Figure 4 shows several observations of new and unpublished data from the olfactory bulb. First, the occurrence of the ERSP on the surface of the bulb is demonstrated in Figure 4a. Note that this large-amplitude slow wave has been filtered out in all other data acquisitions. The spatial uniformity of the D_2 estimates and their event-related changes are exhibited in Figure 4b. An attractor of approximately 5.02 dimensions generates activity during the control condition (pre-novel odor); this attractor then shifts to 1 of approximately 6.02 dimensions following the presentation of a novel odor. The scale of values between 5.0 and 6.1 are shown beneath the diagrams and indicate calculated values from 32 simultaneously recorded electrodes. The deviant values at the upper left borders were recorded from electrodes observed at postmortem not to be in close contact with the bulbar surface because of its curvature. The epoch length was 500 msec ($N = 320$, $m = 15$), and the calculated slopes of $\log(n)$ versus $\log(r)$ for embedding dimensions 1 through 15 are shown in Figure 4c. The slope was determined for the visually selected linear portion of each curve, which had a least-squares linear regression of at

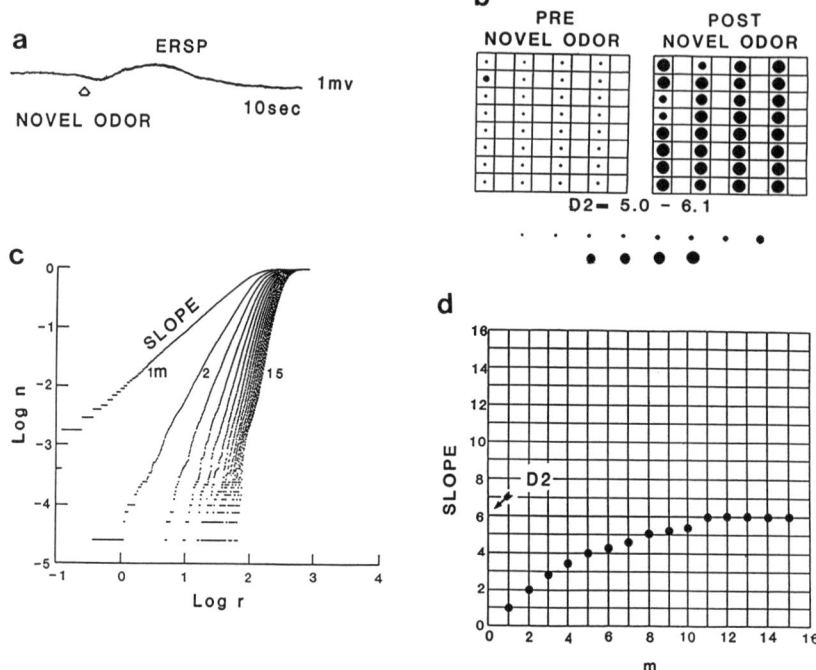

Figure 4. Event-related changes in the correlation dimension (D_2) of the surface patterns of activity recorded from the olfactory bulb of the conscious rabbit. (a) Event-related slow potential recorded from a bulbar surface-electrode using a DC amplifier. (b) Surface pattern of D_2 values for 500-msec epochs of digitized data recorded by each electrode in an 8 × 8 array; the scale for the D_2 values between 5.0 and 6.1 is indicated beneath the two array patterns; note the spatial uniformity of D_2 just before and after the presentation of the novel odor (n-butyl alcohol). (c) An example of log(n) versus log(r) plots for each of 15 embedding dimensions (m); the data were recorded from one of the electrodes illustrated in (b) during Novel Odor; the slope (SLOPE) is measured for each m, by least-squares linear regression, in the part of the curve where $R > 0.991$. (d) The plot of SLOPE versus m for the data shown in c; note that at the 11th embedding dimension the slope has converged and no longer increases and is therefore an estimate of D_2. (Also see Skinner et al., 1988.)

least $R > .991$ (SLOPE). Convergence was detected as the asymptotic value of the plot of SLOPE versus m, as shown in Figure 4d. Note that the event-related change in the spatial pattern of activity shown in Figure 4b, which is based on *single-trial* D_2 values at each electrode, is a much clearer change than that of the spatial amplitude changes, detected over 10 trials, shown in Figure 3c.

We compared rabbit bulbar data with those from the low-dimensional Lorenz attractor ($D_2 = 2.05$ in the limit), as shown in Table 1. For

Table 1. Comparison of the D_2 Estimates for the Lorenz Attractor (Continuous Set) and the Olfactory Bulb: Investigation of Effects on Accuracy of the Order of the Number of Data Points (N), Number of Cycles of the Predominant Frequency of the Attractor (C), and the Tau Interval[a]

C predominant-frequency cycles	N data points	Lorenz attractor Tau = 1 D_2 estimate[b]	Olfactory bulb Tau = 1 D_2 estimate[b]	Olfactory bulb Tau = 74 D_2 estimate[c]
30	320	3.54	5.97	5.17 ± .18
30	5,000	1.96	2.34	
30	10,000	1.89	2.10	
120	320	2.54	7.75	7.10
120	5,000	2.16	6.90	4.54[d]
120	10,000	2.03	4.52[d]	
Inf.	Inf.	2.05 ± .01		

[a] Tau = 1 indicates an interval of 0.05 msec, which is the A/D rate (i.e., 20k Hz); Tau = 74 indicates 3.7 msec, the approximate interval of the first zero crossing of the autocorrelation function or 1/4 cycle of the predominant frequency.
[b] The D_2 estimations were made using the Theiler (1988), box-assisted, algorithm, where r_0 = approximately 30% of the small-r vector differences, w was set at 74 points (i.e., to minimize the near-neighbor autocorrelations, see Theiler [1988]; p. 211.), and m = 20. This very fast algorithm currently works only for a Tau = 1.
[c] The D_2 estimations were made using the Grassberger and Procaccia (1983) algorithm, where m = 1 through 15.
[d] Best estimates of the D_2 of the olfactory bulb.

the Lorenz attractor, the D_2 estimate is seen to be a function of both the number of data points (N) and the number of cycles of the predominant frequency of the attractor (C). The question then arises, is the D_2 estimate for the brief (and presumed stationary) epochs illustrated in Figure 4 very *accurate*? The mean D_2 from three rabbits with five estimates each is D_2 = 5.17 ± 0.18 SD (epoch length = 500 msec, N = 320 data points, C = 30). This stable result suggests the existence of a reliable between-subject biological process, but it does not attest to the *accuracy* of the D_2 estimate itself.

Analysis of the Lorenz attractor, using comparable cycles of the predominant frequency (Table 1), suggests that the bulbar D_2 estimate described in Figure 4 is probably too *large*, because the sample size (N = 320) is too small. Using 10,000 data points in the same 500-msec epoch, however, the bulbar data were found to have D_2 = 2.10, again with good convergence, as shown in Figure 5. This latter estimate was made using

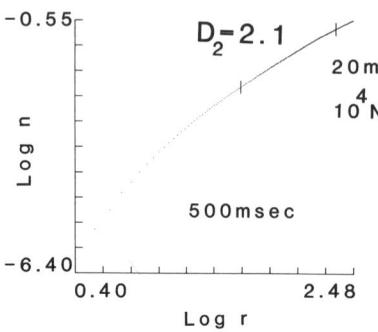

Figure 5. Effects on D_2 of oversampling. Example of the $\log(n)$ versus $\log(r)$ plot (correlation integral), for biological data recorded from the surface of the olfactory bulb of a conscious rabbit in which $C = 30$ and $N = 10^4$. Epoch length was 500 msec. The animal was highly adapted to the recording environment. The box-assisted algorithm of Theiler (1988) was used for all calculations ($m = 20$, Tau = 1 and $W = 74$).

the Theiler (1988, p. 211) algorithm, where $m = 20$ and $w = 74$, Tau = 1, and $\log(r_o) = 2.5$. This estimate, however, may be erroneous because, in comparison with the Lorenz attractor, the sample size relative to the predominant frequency cycles is too large. Our best estimate, based on comparison with the Lorenz attractor, would require 100 cycles and 10,000 data points; this dictates an epoch length of approximately 1.5 seconds. Using these algorithm values we found $D_2 = 4.52$ when Tau was selected to be 1, as shown in Figure 6. When Tau was selected to be ¼ cycle of the mean predominant frequency, a one order smaller N was required to approach the same value, as shown in Table 1.

The majority of epochs longer than 2 seconds generally did not manifest linear slopes and did not converge within 15 embedding dimensions. This seemed to be the case, even in the highly adapted rabbits. Even with no overt behavioral reactions, the olfactory processes appeared nonstationary over epochs more than a few seconds long.

Table 2 shows that filtering Gaussian noise brings its D_2 value down from infinity to a lower value. Filtering white noise to the same spectral range as the rabbit surface potentials (i.e., 50 to 200 Hz) gives a noise estimate of $D_2 > 9.0$ (no saturation observed at 15 embedding dimen-

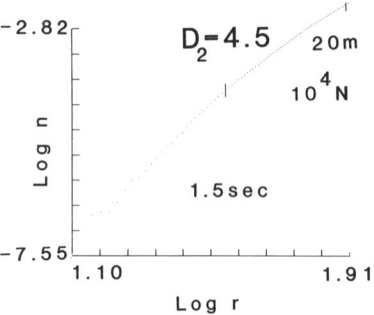

Figure 6. Best estimate of D_2. Example of the correlation integral for biological data recorded from the surface of the olfactory bulb of a conscious rabbit in which $C = 100$ and $N = 10^4$. The same animal as in the previous figure was used, but with the epoch length extended to 1.5 seconds to accumulate more cycles of the attractor. The box-assisted algorithm of Theiler (1988) was used for all calculation ($m = 20$, Tau = 1 and $W = 74$).

Table 2. Separation of D_2 Values for White Noise and Olfactory Bulb Surface Potentials at Various Signal Bandpasses (Bandpass)[a]

	Bandpass		
	50–2000 Hz	20–200 Hz	50–80 Hz
D_2 of white noise	>>10.0[b]	>>9.0[b]	6.5
D_2 of rabbit bulb	5.6	5.6	4.6

[a] D_2 was calculated (Grassberger & Procaccia, 1983) for epoch lengths of 500 msec. Signals were amplified to 1 volt RMS and passed through a Krohn-Hite filter. Each result was determined two times, using separate epochs, and found to be identical within 2-digit precision. Embedding dimensions of m = 1 to 15 were used in all cases to assure convergence.
[b] >>, No saturation occurred in the plot of slope versus m; the value indicated was at 15 embedding dimensions.

sions). This value is noticeably greater than that observed for the same bandpass of the bulbar data. Further filtering of the noise (50 to 80 Hz) brings D_2 down to the level of the rabbit data. In this case the convergence is quite satisfactory. Such narrow-band filtering of the rabbit data, however, also brings its D_2 down. That is, the filtered noise and the bulbar data are distinguishable even though their spectra are similar.

Discussion of New Results

Our main findings are that (1) D_2 estimates of the bulbar surface potentials indicate a low-dimensional chaotic attractor with long linear ranges in the log(n) versus log(r) plots and good convergence of their slopes versus the embedding dimensions; (2) D_2 is sensitive to a change in the state of the system (i.e., D_2 is event-related); stationarity is achievable for brief epochs ranging from 0.5 to 1.5 seconds only if sufficient behavioral control is applied; (3) D_2 is spatially uniform within the tissue, with all surface electrodes showing essentially the same values at all times; (4) D_2 is not yet known to be accurately estimated, because the choices of N, Tau, m, attractor cycles, and epoch length have not yet been clearly established for finite data sets of bulbar signals; in analogy with the Lorenz attractor, the dimension of which is known, our best estimate for the bulbar data, using 100 cycles of the predominant frequency of the attractor (approximately 1.5-second epochs) and 10,000 sample points, is $D_2 = 4.5$; and (5) the bulbar surface potential cannot be regarded as highly filtered noise to explain its low dimension.

The problems of stationarity and accuracy have been recognized as the central issues in the application of nonlinear dynamics to neurobiology (Mayer-Kress, 1986). Our current data from a model cortical system suggests that if the epoch lengths are brief, but enable the occurrence of at least 100 cycles of the predominant frequency, and if behavior is carefully controlled, then accuracy and stationarity may be reasonably presumed and D_2 estimates declared valid. If behavior is not highly controlled, then the presumption of stationarity is not reasonable. Our data show that the presentation of a faint novel odor to an animal highly adapted to such presentations will interrupt a stationary process and within 500 msec evoke an increase in the D_2 estimate of the new process.

Small N is dictated when recording from many electrodes for many seconds; that is, the capacity of the data acquisition system is limited. As indicated in Table 1, such undersampling leads to an overestimate of D_2, at least for the Lorenz attractor. On the other hand, oversampling (i.e., too large an N for the number of cycles of the predominant frequency) leads to an underestimate. We do not know why the underestimate occurs, but we speculate that it may be associated with too much emphasis by the algorithm related to the "fine grain" relative to the "long period" of the attractor. For the Lorenz attractor, the algorithm values leading to the best estimate of D_2 (i.e., the value closest to its known dimension) was 10,000 data points with 100 cycles. This suggests that 1.5-second epochs at 7000-Hz A/D would be the optimum for the bulbar data. Therefore, our best estimate for the bulbar data, using these values and a Tau = 1, was D_2 = 4.52. If Tau = 74 was used (i.e., the first zero crossing of the autocorrelation function), then the same D_2 value occurred with N being 1/10th the size.

Theiler (1988) has suggested an estimate for the sample size, $N - N_o e^{k(V+4)}$, where k is $-1/4 \log$ (error/V). For the estimated D_2 = 5.0, the estimate of N is approximately 10^4, which is what we used for our best estimate. For D_2 = 2.0, this value for N is perhaps several orders of magnitude too large, given the small number of predominant cycles of the attractor. Our present analyses of the Lorenz attractor indicate that N alone is not sufficient to determine accuracy. The number of cycles of the long period of the attractor must also be considered.

It would be very unlikely that 32 simultaneously recorded electrodes on the bulbar surface would manifest the same D_2 values unless they were connected to the *same* system. Bullock and Basar (1988), in a comparative study in invertebrates through mammals, suggested that during evolution the field potentials in a neuropile become spatially more coherent. Our finding in the bulb, representing a mammalian cortical system, supports this view. If the system were not coherent, then it would not manifest the same D_2 at virtually all locations. The opposite, however, is not the case; high coherence (i.e., linear predictability of activity between 2 electrodes, for all time delays) does not dictate that the D_2 estimates at each location will be the same. For example, if the underlying neural generators are loosely coupled, then they will have high coherence, but if they subserve different information processes, then they are not likely to have similar D_2s. The nonlinear deterministic D_2 estimate enables a different type of neuroanatomical "mapping" than does the linear stochastic coherence measure.

The single-trial variance of D_2 is small, even though its estimate many be inaccurate owing to over- or undersampling (Table 1). This *sensitivity* of the measure, however, suggests several important uses. For example, it could be used to determine the boundaries between different information processors within apparently homogeneous neuroanatomical tissues, such as those that exist within the visual cortices. Furthermore, D_2 seems to be so sensitive that it easily reflects event-related changes in neural processing within a *single* trial.

Low-Dimensional Chaotic Dynamics in Biological Systems: Why?

It is generally the event-related increase or decrease of D_2 that seems to be the focus for current neurobiological applications. The fact that the D_2s generally appear to be *fractions* may also be of importance. "Fractional dimension" has recently become associated with "fractal dynamics" as the characteristic descriptor of the system. Fractal dynamics often, but *not always,* is associated with fractional D_2s (Mandelbrot, 1983).

Self-similarity of phase-plane trajectories independent of scale is the hallmark of a truly fractal system (Mandelbrot, 1983). Empirical findings show that phyisicochemical reactions (Bak, 1985, 1986), enzymatic processes (Hess & Markus, 1987; Markus, Kuschmitz, & Hess), membrane potentials (Chay & Rinzel, 1985), and single ion-channel kinetics (Liebovitch, Fischbarg, Koniarek, Todorova, & Wang, 1987; Liebovitch & Sullivan, 1987) all manifest behaviors characteristic of low-dimensional chaotic attractors. If these molecular processes all have the same D_2 as the bulbar output, then they are likely to be part of the process. Thus, a "mapping" along a continuum of increasingly larger scales may enable the anatomical identification of the so-called nuts and bolts a single specific process. Is this perhaps why reductionism works?

The "nuts and bolts" explanations do not tell us *why* the "fractal" processes, as opposed to *n*th-order integer processes, occur in cognitive mechanisms—was this selection by nature merely adventitious or was there a strategy involved? For example, only two coordinates placed in a fractal function (e.g., the one generating the Mandelbrot set) can be transformed deterministically into 10 megabytes of exact pixel information. The biological problem, however, is the *inverse*—that is, how to compress the enormous amount of pixel information back into the two coordinates before either transmission or storage of the information. We propose that the existence of fractal processes in cognitive systems might occur because only this type of dynamics enables such *data compression*.

In support of our proposition, Barnsley, Massopust, Strickland, and Sloan (1987) have shown that *geometric affine-mapping* applied to graphics data depicting "natural" objects (e.g., fern leaves, steam clouds, tree branches) leads to the construction of different attractors for the data set depending upon where one starts. These abstracted attractors of the inherently fractal data can then be stored or transmitted at reduced bit rates and then later used to reconstitute, deterministically, the original data set. The data-compression ratio can be as high as 10^6 to 1. We propose that this property (i.e., the "inverse" process) may explain why nature selected fractal dynamical systems in biological tissues to process cognitive information. A lot of information transfer and storage is involved, which can be handled efficiently only if compressed.

A stimulus (e.g., an odorant) has fixed physical attributes, but its accompanying context (e.g., the trial number) is variable each time the stimulus is presented to the subject. When the stimulus-plus-context is novel, more information must be stored than when the stimulus exists within a familiar context. This is because the thalamic gating mechanism *lets more information through* to the cortex when the stimulus is novel than when it is familiar (Skinner & Yingling, 1977). Once the stimulus is either completely conditioned or habituated, evidence shows, inhibitory thalamic gating suppresses the ascent of irrelevant sensory information (Skinner & Yingling, 1977). We propose that when the stimulus is novel, a higher dimensional chaotic attractor is required to store the greater amount of information. This untested hypothesis is based on our present biological observations in which a novel stimulus is associated with a higher D_2 estimate for the bulbar activity.

The affine-mapping and attractor-reconstitution mechanics described and demonstrated by Barnsley and Sloan (1988) require a relatively massive parallel processor to handle the fractal data. Cortical tissues, including the olfactory bulb, are well-known parallel processors (Shepherd, 1970). Parallel processing could be a mechanistic feature, and not present in cortex merely for "backup" in case some circuits are damaged. Massive parallel processing by highly interconnected elements (i.e., "connectionist models") are claimed to have emergent properties that resemble real behavioral learning (Hopfield & Tank, 1986; Sejnowski & Rosenberg, 1987). Skarda and Freeman (1987) suggested (and perhaps we have shown) that fractal dynamics occur in the olfactory bulb that cannot be attributed to strictly connectionist models. They propose that making linear connectionist models operate as nonlinear dynamical systems may yield even more realistic emergent properties. When neuroscientists gain a clearer understanding of the biological significance of fractal processes comparable to that of some physical systems (Gleick, 1987), then we may come to a completely different (perhaps even revolutionary) view of what the basic cognitive process is.

Summary and Conclusions

In summary, we conclude that several potential applications exist for the clinical and nonclinical uses of D_2 estimates—that is, if the time-series data can be recorded in such a manner that the presumption of stationarity is valid. (1) It may be that both control and event-related values, accurately calculated, will deviate from a norm, and thus predict pathology. This is analogous to the finding that the ERSP is enlarged in preclinical subjects who have a genetic background of cardiovascular disorder (Neurotech, 1988). (2) Studies directed at defining what a D_2 variable is may lead to discovery in a previously unapproachable mechanism. For example, it seems from Figure 4b that one variable is added during an event-related slow potential (i.e., D_2 shifts from 5.02 to 6.02, exactly one variable appears to be added to the total). In Figure 3d, it would appear that this one added variable may involve beta-receptor stimulation. Since propranolol infusion seems to prevent both the spatial pattern change and the ERSP, both of which are correlates of the event-related D_2 alteration. (3) The sensitivity of the D_2 measure, both between and within subjects, may enable "mapping" studies to define the location of the anatomical boundaries of a single process. The "mapping" applied to the single process, at different scales of resolution, may lead to discovery of intermediate (reductionistic) processes with the same D_2. (4) If rapid computer algorithms or devices can be developed, then perhaps on-line "biofeedback" of D_2 could result in a significant therapy, as has been found for some physiological measures related to cardiovascular dysfunction (see Steptoe, 1988). (5) D_2 estimation may be the only valid observation in "fractal" information-processing systems that deal with compressed data.

References

Babloyantz, A., & Destexhe, A. (1986). Low-dimensional chaos in an instance of epilepsy. *Proceedings of the National Academy of Sciences of the USA, 83,* 3513-3517.
Babloyantz, A., & Destexhe, A. (1987). Strange attractors in the human cortex. In L. Rensing, U. an der Heiden, & M. C. Mackey (Eds.), *Temporal disorder in human oscillatory systems.* Springer Series in Synergetics (Vol. 36, pp. 488-456). Berlin: Springer-Verlag.
Bak, P. (1985). Mode-locking and the transition to chaos in dissipative systems. *Physica Scripta, T9,* 50-58.
Bak, P. (1986). The devil's staircase. *Physics Today, 86,* 38-45.
Barnsley, M. F., & Sloan, A. D. (1988). A better way to compress images. *Byte, 1,* 215-223.
Barnsley, M. F., Massopust, P., Strickland, H., & Sloan, A. D. (1987). Fractal modeling of biological structures. *Annals of New York Academy of Sciences, 504,* 179-194.
Bliss, T. V. P., Goddard, G. V., & Rives, M. (1983). Reduction of long-term potentiation in the dentate gyrus of the rat following selective depletion of monoamines. *Journal of Physiology (London), 334,* 475-491.
Bullock, T. H., & Basar, E. (1988). Comparison of ongoing compound field potentials in the brains of invertebrates and vertebrates. *Brain Research, 472,* 57-75.
Cannon, W. B. (1931). Again the James-Lange and the thalamic theories of emotion. *Psychological Review, 38,* 281-295.
Chay, T. R., & Rinzel, J. (1985). Bursting, beating, and chaos in an excitable membrane model. *Biophysical Journal, 47,* 357-366.
Farmer, J. D. (1982). Dimension, fractal, measures, and chaotic dynamics. In H. Haken (Ed.), *Evolution of order and chaos.* Heidelberg: Springer-Verlag.
Folkow, B. (1982). Physiological aspects of primary hypertension. *Physiological Reviews, 62,* 347-504.
Freeman, W. J., & Schneider, W. S. (1982). Changes in spatial patterns of rabbit olfactory EEG with conditioning to odors. *Psychophysiology, 19,* 44-56.
Gleick, J. (1987). *Chaos: Making a new science.* New York: Viking Penguin.
Graf, K. E., & Elbert, T. (1989). Dimensional analysis of the waking EEG. In E. Basar & T. H. Bullock (Ed.), *Brain Dynamics Progress and Perspectives* (pp. 174-191). Berlin: Springer-Verlag.
Grassberger, P., & Procaccia, I. (1983). Measuring the strangeness of strange attractors. *Physica 9D,* 183-208.
Gray, C. M., & Skinner, J. E. (1988). Centrifugal regulation of neuronal activity in the olfactory bulb of the waking rabbit as revealed by reversible cryogenic blockade. *Experimental Brain Research, 69,* 378-386.
Gray, C. M., Freeman, W. J., & Skinner, J. E. (1984). Associative changes in the spatial amplitude patterns of rabbit olfactory EEG are norepinephrine-dependent. *Society for Neuroscience Abstracts, 10,* 121.
Gray, C. M., Freeman, W. J., & Skinner, J. E. (1986). Chemical dependencies of learning in the rabbit olfactory bulb: Acquisition of the transient spatial pattern change depends on norepinephrine. *Behavioral Neuroscience, 100,* 585-596.
Hess, B., & Markus, M. (1987). Order and chaos in biochemistry. *Trends in Biochemical Science, 12,* 45-48.
Hildebrandt, J. D., Sekura, R. D., Codina, J., Iyengar, R., Manclark, C. R., & Birnbaumer, L. (1983). Stimulation and inhibition of adenylyl cyclases is mediated by distinct proteins. *Nature, 302,* 706-709.
Hopfield, J. J., & Tank, D. W. (1986). Computing with neural circuits: A model. *Science, 233,* 626-633.

Hopkins, W. F., & Johnston, D. (1984). Frequency-dependent noradrenergic modulation of long-term potentiation in the hippocampus. *Science, 226,* 350–352.
Hopkins, W. F., & Johnston, D. (1988). Noradrenergic enhancement of long-term potentiation at mossy fiber synapses in the hippocampus. *Journal of Neurophysiology, 59,* 667–687.
Krontiris-Litowitz, J., Skinner, J. E., & Birnbaumer, L. (1985). A muscarinic agonist (Ethmozine) prevents long-term potentiation in the hippocampal slice. *Society for Neuroscience Abstracts, 11,* 781.
Levitt, P., & Noebels, J. L. (1981). Mutant mouse tottering: Selective increase of locus ceruleus axons in a defined single-locus mutation. *Proceedings of the National Academy of Sciences of the USA, 78,* 4630–4634.
Liebovitch, L. S., & Sullivan, M. J. (1987). Fractal analysis of a voltage-dependent potassium channel from cultured mouse hippocampal neurons. *Biophysical Journal, 52,* 979–988.
Liebovitch, L. S., Fischbarg, J., Koniarek, J. P., Todorova, I., & Wang, M. (1987). Fractal model of ion-channel kinetics. *Biochimica et Biophysica Acta, 896,* 173–180.
Mandelbrot, B. B. (1983). *The fractal geometry of nature.* New York: W. H. Freeman.
Markus, M., Kuschmitz, E., & Hess, B. (1985). Properties of strange attractors in yeast glycolysis. *Biophysical Chemistry, 22,* 95–105.
Mayer-Kress, G. (1986). Introductory remarks. In G. Mayer-Kress (Ed.), *Dimensions and entropies in chaotic systems* (pp. 2–5). New York: Springer-Verlag.
Neurotech. (1988). Supporting data for the "Stress Analyzer." Neurotech Laboratories, Inc., Suite 340, 1120 Medical Plaza, The Woodlands, Texas 77380.
Packard, N. H., Crutchfield, J. P., Farmer, J. D., & Shaw, R. S. (1980). Geometry from a time-series. *Physical Review Letters, 45,* 712.
Reid, J. L., Lewis, P. J., Myers, M. G., & Dollery, C. T. (1974). Cardiovascular effects of intracerebroventricular d-, l-, and dl-propranolol in the conscious rabbit. *Journal of Pharmacology and Experimental Therapeutics, 188,* 391–399.
Roschke, J., & Basar, E. (1989). Correlation dimensions in various parts of cat and human brain in different states. In E. Basar & T. H. Bullock (Eds.), *Brain dynamics progress and perspectives* (pp. 131–148). Berlin: Springer-Verlag.
Sejnowski, T. J., & Rosenberg, C. R. (1987). Parallel networks that learn to pronounce English text. *Complex Systems 1,* 145–168.
Shepherd, G. M. (1970). The olfactory bulb as a simple cortical system: Experimental analysis and functional implications. In F. O. Schmitt (Ed.), *The neurosciences: Second study program* (pp. 539–552). New York: Rockefeller University Press.
Skarda, C. A., & Freeman, W. J. (1987). How brains make chaos in order to make sense of the world. *Behavioral and Brain Sciences, 10,* 161–173.
Skinner, J. E. (1971). Abolition of a conditioned, surface-negative, cortical potential during cryogenic blockade of the nonspecific thalamo-cortical system. *Electroencephalography and Clinical Neurophysiology, 31,* 197–209.
Skinner, J. E. (1984). Central gating mechanisms that regulate event-related potentials and behavior. In T. Elbert, B. Rockstroh, W. Lutzenberger, & N. Birbaumer (Eds.), *Self-regulation of the brain and behavior* (pp. 42–58). New York: Springer-Verlag.
Skinner, J. E. (1988). Brain involvement in cardiovascular disorders. In T. Elbert, W. Langosch, A. Steptoe, & D. Vaitl (Eds.), *Behavioural medicine in cardiovascular disorders* (pp. 229–253). London: Wiley.
Skinner, J. E., & King. G. L. (1980). Contribution of neuron dendrites to extracellular sustained potential shifts. In H. H. Kornhuber & L. Deecke (Eds.), *Motivation motor and sensory processes of the brain. Progress in brain research* (Vol. 54, pp. 89–102. Amsterdam: Elsevier/North-Holland Biomedical Press.

Skinner, J. E., & Molnar, M. (1983). Event-related extracellular potassium-ion activity changes in the frontal cortex of the conscious cat. *Journal of Neurophysiology, 49*, 204–215.
Skinner, J. E., & Pratt, C. M. (1982). Ethmozin reduces the amplitude of the cerebral event-related slow potential in patients with ischemic heart disease. *Abstracts of the American Heart Association*.
Skinner, J. E., & Reed, J. C. (1981). Blockade of a frontocortical-brainstem pathway prevents ventricular fibrillation of the ischemic heart in pigs. *American Journal of Physiology, 240*, H1156–H1163.
Skinner, J. E., & Yingling, C. D. (1976). Regulation of slow potential shifts in nucleus reticularis thalami by the mesencephalic reticular formation and the frontal cortex. *Electroencephalography and Clinical Neurophysiology, 40*, 288–296.
Skinner, J. E., & Yingling, C. D. (1977). Central gating mechanisms that regulate event-related potentials and behavior: A neural model for attention. In J. E. Desmedt (Ed.), *Progress in clinical neurophysiology* (Vol. 1, pp. 30–69). Brussels: Karger-Basel.
Skinner, J. E., Reed, J. C., Welch, K. M. A., & Nell, J. H. (1978). Cutaneous shock produces correlated shifts in slow potential amplitude and cyclic 3', 5'-adenosine monophosphate level in the parietal cortex of the conscious rat. *Journal of Neurochemistry, 30*, 699–704.
Skinner, J. E., Martin, J. L., Landisman, C. E., Mommer, M. M., Fulton, K., Mitra, M., Burton, W. D., & Saltzberg, B. (1988). Chaotic attractors in a model of neocortex: Dimensionalities of olfactory bulb surface potentials are spatially uniform and event-related. In E. Basar & T. H. Bullock (Eds.), *Brain dynamics progress and perspectives* (pp. 168–173). *Dynamics of sensory and cognitive processing by the brain*. Berlin: Springer-Verlag.
Steptoe, A. (1988). The processes underlying long-term blood pressure reductions in essential hypertensives following behavioural therapy. In T. Elbert, W. Langosch, A. Steptoe, & D. Vaitl (Eds.), *Behavioural medicine in cardiovascular disorders* (pp. 139–148). London: Wiley.
Szilagyi, J. E., Taylor, A. A., & Skinner, J. E. (1987). Cryoblockade of the ventromedial frontal cortex reverses hypertension in the rat. *Hypertension, 9*, 576–581.
Tackett, R. L., Webb, J. G., & Privitera, P. J. (1985). Site and mechanism of the centrally mediated hypotensive action of propranolol. *Journal of Pharmacology and Experimental Therapeutics, 235*, 66–70.
Takens, F. (1981). Detecting strange attractors in turbulence. In Warwick (Ed.), *Dynamical systems and Turbulence, 1980, Vol. 898 of Lecture Notes in Mathematics*. Berlin: Springer-Verlag.
Theiler, J. (1986). Spurious dimension from correlation algorithms applied to limited time-series data. *Physical Review A, 34*, 2427–2432.
Theiler, J. (1988). *Quantifying chaos: Practical estimation of the correlation dimension*. Doctoral dissertation, California Institute of Technology, Pasadena.
Thompson, J. W., Newton, P., Pocock, P. V., Cooper, R., Crow, H., McCallum, W. C., & Papakostopoulos, D. (1978). Preliminary study of pharmacology of contingent negative variation in man. In D. A. Otto (Ed.), *Multidisciplinary perspectives in event-related brain potential research* (pp. 25–55). Washington, DC: U.S. Environmental Protection Agency.
Watanabe, A. M., McConnaughey, M. M., Strawbridge, R. A., Fleming, J. W., Jones, L. R., & Besch, H. R., Jr. (1978). Muscarinic cholinergic receptor modulation of B-adrenergic receptor affinity for catecholamines. *Journal of Biological Chemistry, 253*, 4833–4836.
Williams, S. H., & Johnston, D. (1988a). Muscarin depresses an APV-sensitive form of LTP in CA3 hippocampal neurons. *Abstracts Society for Neuroscience, 14*, p. 564.

Williams, S. H., & Johnston, D. (1988b). Muscarinic depression of long-term potentiation in CA3 hippocampal neurons. *Science, 242,* 84–87.
Wilson, D. A., & Leon, M. (1988). Spatial patterns of olfactory bulb single-unit responses to learned olfactory cues in young rats. *Journal of Neurophysiology, 59,* 1770–1782.
Wilson, D. A., Sullivan, R. M., & Leon, M. (1987). Single-unit analysis of postnatal olfactory learning: Modified olfactory bulb output response patterns to learned attractive odors. *Journal of Neuroscience, 7,* 3154–3162.
Yingling, C. D., & Skinner, J. E. (1976). Selective regulation of thalamic sensory relay nuclei by nucleus reticularis thalami. *Electroencephalography and Clinical Neurophysiology, 41,* 476–482.
Yingling, C. D., & Skinner, J. E. (1977). Gating of thalamic input to cerebral cortex by nucleus reticularis thalami. In J. E. Desmedt (Ed.), *Progress in clinical neurophysiology* (Vol. 1, pp. 70–96). Brussels: Karger-Basel.

PART II

Neuromuscular Disorders

This section, on the self-regulation of neuromuscular functions, includes a general paper by F. J. McGuigan on the role of the musculature in cognitive functions, an experimental report by Akitane Mori and his colleagues at the Okayama University Medical School—Isao Yokoi, Hideaki Kabuto, Midori Hiramatsu, Michael J. Kwon, Masakatsu Shimada, and Kenji Akiyama—on neurotransmitter regulation of convulsions in epileptic mice, and a chapter by Ronald L. Webster on the use of a new "sensory augmentation" method for work with stutterers.

Across his career, McGuigan has consistently argued for and demonstrated the close relationship between muscle tension and experiential states, as he does in Chapter 6. McGuigan maintains that cognitive and emotional activity can be self-regulated through tension in the related musculature. Owing to the considerable central control we normally exercise over our musculature, this aspect of self-regulation has perhaps the strongest clinical utility for alleviating a wide variety of stress-related disorders and achieving health.

In Chapter 7, Mori *et al.* show with an animal model that injections of various receptor antagonists inhibit convulsions and, with another procedure, that afferent impulses may not reach the brain in some forms of seizure disorders. Although the research of Mori and his colleagues does not directly demonstrate a method of self-regulation for seizure control, their identification of two forms of control through neurotransmitters—control of excitatory receptors and enhancement of inhibitory receptors—suggests mechanisms for seizure control that perhaps could be influenced through as yet unspecified behavioral interventions.

By contrast, Webster's Chapter 8 reviews a variety of known behavioral methods for the measurement and definition of another neuromuscular disorder, stuttering. On the treatment side, Webster reviews a wide range of methods for the enhancement of fluency and points out that treatments that emphasize auditory feedback are often impractical.

However, an instrument that amplifies the "vocal buzz" in one ear has been found to overcome some of these problems. Webster's ongoing attempts to make use of a wide variety of behavioral methods in the treatment of stuttering is a model for the applications of self-regulation techniques in the improvement of health.

CHAPTER 6

Control of Normal and Pathologic Cognitive Functions through Neuromuscular Circuits
Applications of Principles of Progressive Relaxation

F. J. McGuigan

The Problem of "Mind"

Everyday language is replete with a variety of mentalistic terms, such as *dreams, hallucinations, ideas, images, thoughts, fears, anxieties, depressions,* and *emotions,* that refer to functions of the "mind." While these mentalistic (cognitive) terms vary, the subjective experiences to which they refer are all quite similar. The different terms merely indicate similar experiences that occur under various environmental and organismic conditions. For instance, night dreams, daydreams, and rational thought all differ, in part, because of the degree to which they are influenced by environmental input. During sleep, the images of our night dreams are chaotic since they are not directed by external reality. In contrast, problem-solving processes are more systematic and are directed to a greater extent by reference to cues in the external environment, such as in notes and calculations. While hallucinations are (mistakenly) ascribed to external factors, they are controlled by internal stimuli such as those generated

---

F. J. McGuigan • Institute for Stress Management, United States International University, San Diego, California 92131, USA.

by covert speech (McGuigan, 1966). Perceptual processes probably represent the extreme of cognitive events that are directly controlled by external stimuli. Even so, our awarenesses of what is happening in our immediate world constitute subjective experiences that themselves do not seem to differ from those of night dreams or hallucinations. They merely occur under different circumstances. It is not unusual, in fact, for us to confuse the content of night dreams with actual perceptions, not being sure whether something happened in our dreams or in our waking life.

Organismic variables constitute another kind of factor that influences our mental activity. An example is a brain lesion which causes hallucinations that, again, themselves do not differ in nature from true perceptions.

These and other mentalistic terms refer to experiences that have generated our classical problem of the nature of the mind.

How Cognitive Events Are Generated

In addressing the problem of the mind, our primary thesis has been that mental processes occur when bodily systems selectively interact (e.g., McGuigan, 1978, 1981, 1984, 1989). Those systems include the receptor organs (e.g., eyes, ears), the central nervous system, striated musculature, the autonomic system (e.g., the gastrointestinal tract, the cardiovascular system), and their neural interconnections. Considering the tremendous complexity of the human body and of these individual systems, the interactions among them must be extremely complex, exceeding those of all of the computers in the world if they were connected in a network.

The initial processing of information during cognitive activities occurs within neuromuscular circuits principally involving the brain and the striated musculature (Figure 1). Given the fact that there are some 10 billion neurons in the brain and that, by weight, almost half the body is striated muscle, there must be thousands of neuromuscular circuits functioning in parallel channels to process information during any cognitive activity. Because they are slower, the autonomic activities of the body come into play in interactions somewhat later.

Extensive research using psychophysiological methods has established that a variety of events occur in different systems throughout the body during any cognitive activity. Principally, these include brain events measured through electroencephalography, striated muscle events measured through electromyography, and eye responses mea-

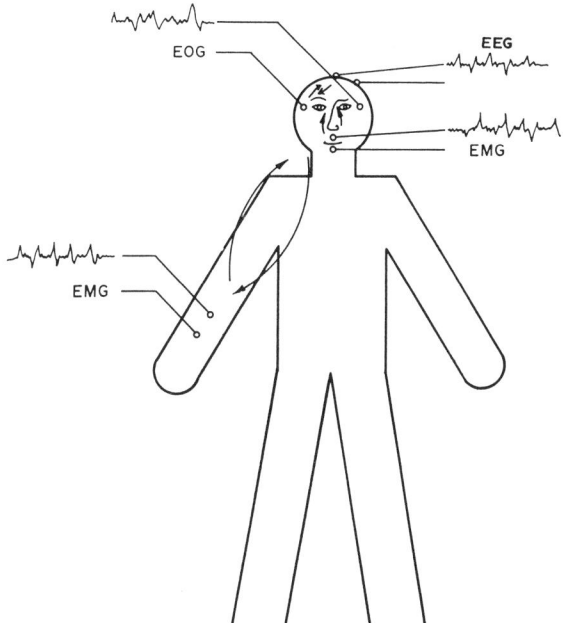

Figure 1. A representation of three classes of neuromuscular circuits by which we control ourselves. Subclasses of cognitive phenomena include speech imagery generated by speech–brain circuits, visual imagery generated by eye–brain circuits, and somatic imagery generated by interactions between various bodily regions such as the arm and the brain. Components of the circuits may be recorded through electrical methods indicated, i.e., EOG, EMG, and EEG.

sured through electrooculography. Of the several hundred studies summarized by McGuigan (1978), some of the more important works have been as follows. Excellent accounts of brain functioning during thought may be found in Delafresnaye (1954), Eccles (1966), and Young (1970). The eye has been of unique importance as, for instance, Hebb (1968), in analyzing perception and imagery, held that peripheral activity, especially eye movement, is essential during the formation of images. A general treatment of visual system functioning during cognition may be found in Chase (1973). Visceral activity has been empirically and theoretically implicated in cognitive processes in a variety of ways; we should especially mention work on the esophagus (e.g., Jacobson, 1925), on electrodermal activity (e.g., Grings, 1973), and on the autonomic system in general (e.g., Lacey & Lacey, 1974). Indeed, the entire body is active during any kind of cognitive process. The extensive list of these psychophysiological events that occur in close temporal proximity during cognition leads to the inference that they are interrelated. The ways in which they interact, by our model, is by means of neuromuscular circuits that have cybernetic characteristics.

Two general strategies document this conclusion. The first is a positive one, as discussed above—i.e., the general finding that a variety of muscular, eye, brain, etc., events have been recorded when any of a wide variety of cognitive activities do occur. The reverse, negative strategy yields the fact that when the striated muscles are well relaxed, cognitive events disappear (Jacobson, 1929/1938). Thus, normal individuals who have been taught to relax well universally report that they have no mental processes when they reach a sufficiently low degree of relaxation. The same phenomenon occurs with patients who have psychiatric difficulties. When any component of the neuromuscular circuits ceases to function, the circuits stop reverberating, whereupon mental processes also terminate. Thus, any interruption of the neuromuscular circuits will eliminate thoughts and prevent them from appearing. The first strategy is principally a scientific one, while the second is principally a clinical one, the data for each stretching over many decades.

In an approximate sense, most cognitive processes have three components: speech imagery, which is generated by contraction of the speech musculature in conjunction with processes in the linguistic regions of the brain; visual imagery, which is generated by the eyes and eye musculature in conjunction with events in the visual regions of the brain; and somatic cognitions involving selected differential reactions throughout the body, depending upon the nature of the somatic imagery, in conjunction with events in somasthetic regions of the brain.

The Control of Cognitive Processes

The neuromuscular model is quite explicit as to how we can control our cognitive processes. When the body volitionally runs itself, the striated musculature is the component of interacting neuromuscular circuits over which we have direct control. Whatever act you wish to perform is carried out by that system in coordination with neural systems. Whether you get up to walk out the door or elevate your pulse rate with exercise, the direct controlling system is the striated musculature. Conversely, one can quiet the body, including producing a lower pulse rate, by reversing the process and relaxing the striated muscles. The overt and covert functions of the body can all be controlled through striated muscle tensions whether they be large or minuscule. Early scientists recognized this principle of self-control when they used the synonymous term *voluntary muscles* to refer to the striated muscles. The voluntary muscles were quite correctly regarded as "the instrument of the will."

In controlling cognitive activity, then, we can instruct ourselves to engage in whatever kind of cognition we wish. As we shall shortly develop, this is accomplished principally by *covert* speech behavior (McGuigan, 1981). If we wish to be more emphatic, we can instruct ourselves by means of *overt* speech. Most of our problems in control of cognitive activity, however, come when we have unwanted thoughts, such as when we worry or experience phobias. Our general principle is that to eliminate undesired thoughts, we merely relax our muscles. More specifically, by relaxing the speech muscles, the speech imagery components of thoughts can be eliminated. By relaxing the complex set of muscles around the eyes, the visual imagery involved in thoughts can be relaxed away. Somatic imagery can be eliminated by relaxing the remainder of the muscles of the body. In short, by relaxing all of the muscles of the body, all mental processes can be brought to zero.

It is not unusual for students in the early stages of learning progressive relaxation to observe that when they do relax, they become unaware of an arm's existence. A medical student once made this report after class, whereupon I asked him why that should be. After a little reflection he correctly answered that relaxed muscles do not generate tension (control) signals so that, with no neural impulses being transmitted from the arm to the brain, he did not receive information as to the location of his arm in space, or even that he had an arm. The next question I asked him was: What would happen if *all* of the muscles of the body relaxed? A little further thought led him to the obvious conclusion that a totally relaxed person would be unaware of any aspect of the body and thus unaware of anything. This reasoning has been repeatedly confirmed by reports of totally relaxed individuals who state that they had been completely unconscious—no thoughts at all. In short, we can use the striated muscles to control activities of the body, and that includes mental processing. By learning to systematically control our striated muscles, we can efficiently guide our thoughts, and as we shall shortly develop, our emotions too.

Learning Tension Control

In clinical work, as with "normal" individuals, patients first develop a highly cultivated ability to observe their internal sensory muscle signals (the classical muscle sense of Bell). By studying all of the muscle groups specified in the program (see McGuigan, 1981) these become *control* signals. The method of progressive relaxation starts by learning to control the tensions in the arm. First, one learns to identify a localized tension and then one relaxes it away. By systematically repeating the process of identifying a localized tension and repeatedly relaxing it away, one comes to effectively control tension in that region. The learner repeatedly contrasts the previous state of tension and the ensuing state of relaxation.

There are six different control signals in each arm that are studied. After sufficient practice with them, the muscles in the arms can come under excellent control. At that point the learner moves on to control the tension throughout the legs, then the trunk, progressing on through the neck muscles to the eyes, and finally to the speech muscles. At this point the learner has gained control over all of the major muscles of the body. However, the procedure has been practiced lying down in a quite room and our goal is to learn to relax in the hustle of everyday life. Consequently, more advanced lessons are taken in which the learner practices tension control in the same order but while sitting up. Eventually, the method carries the learner to automatically relax during various activities in everyday life, such as reading, writing, and even sleeping.

Clinical Progressive Relaxation

Those individuals who have complaints of a mental nature go through the stages of practicing, as discussed above. They are given specialized training in observing the small muscle tensions present when they experience their particular complaints. Those muscle tensions are the ones that control the neuromuscular circuits that are activated when their disturbing or unwanted mental acts are generated. By consistently relaxing covert striated muscle components, the resultant tranquillity of the neuromuscular circuits eliminates the worry, phobia, or depression.

To illustrate these procedures for a typical case of depression, note that progressive relaxation is specific for this disorder. After the body is thoroughly trained, the clinician usually focuses attention on the eyes to control visual imagery. The depression often can be triggered by the visualization process or by some bodily substitute for visualization. The clinician sleuths carefully through the patient's extremely detailed introspective reports for the imagery associated with the depression, for the patient seldom, if ever, is aware of those images prior to extensive training. These visual images are often extremely fleeting, having a duration of perhaps only one- or two-100ths of a second. Eventually, by first reporting in detail on the tensions throughout the body and then on the resulting visualizations or their bodily substitutes, the clinician can gain insight into the problem. The therapist can then reinstate the visualizations that help trigger depression for the patient by instructions to imagine the depressing scene uncovered through introspection. Thereupon, the patient studies the control signals throughout the eye musculature and elsewhere. By systematically relaxing the muscular control signals, the patient can diminish and eventually eliminate the visualizations that trigger depression. This same general process is applicable to the other psychiatric disorders, such as phobias.

The procedure developed by Wolpe (1975), known as systematic desensitization, resembles in many respects the clinical application of progressive relaxation for phobias. For instance, one classic case reported by Jacobson (1934) was of a man who feared heights. He was first taught the elements of progressive relaxation so that he acquired good control over his bodily tensions. Then he was instructed to imagine minimal height-related activities, such as a feather floating to the table. During the imagination act the patient described the location of the control signals and then the imagery of the imagination act in great detail. Such detail includes even items like what color imagined objects are, their size, and their location. Then, following the general principles, the control signals were relaxed away, at which time the mental processes also ceased. Gradually, the phobic intensity of the imagination act was systematically increased, each time the controlling tensions being located and relaxed away. Finally, the instruction was given to imagine hanging out of a window of a tall building. Control signals in this activity could be expected to be not only in the eyes for visualizing the experience, but elsewhere too, such as in the arms, for the purpose of imagining holding onto the windowsill. To abbreviate the case history, the man eventually rented an office in a tall building where he could overlook Chicago in a relaxed manner with no fears at all.

Individuals who are excessively anxious, often continuously rehearse their griefs, their worries, their difficulties with life. If they can acquire control of the striated muscle tensions that key such internal speech, they can consequently control these negative mental processes along with accompanying unwanted emotions. These controls occur principally in their speech muscles for verbalizing their problems, as well as in the eyes for visualizing their difficulties, though the remaining mass of skeletal musculature also contributes to such mental processes. By thorough training in progressive relaxation it is possible to gradually change from a habit of continuously attending to difficulties, and to habitually turn attention away from those issues. One thus becomes better able to verbalize relevant contingencies and to react more rationally to problems. Thus, instead of reacting reflexively to a difficulty, one can stop, reason about the problem, and pursue a wise course of action.

Developing Emotional Control

As one's learning to relax progresses, emotional control increases. As the body becomes relaxed, the patient attends less frequently to troubling issues, becoming less emotionally disturbed about problems. One time a lady asked what she should do about her husband, who had a habit of verbally berating her immediately when he stepped in the door at night. I suggested that she should stop, relax, and assess the situation, verbalizing to herself that "this man seems to be yelling and screaming at me, and it is to his advantage as well as to mine if I do not yell and scream back at him." Of course, merely answering her question did not provide her with the ability to engage in such reasonable emotional behavior. Perhaps she had learned what she *should* do, but she still could not be expected to know *how* to do it.

How *does* one develop control over one's emotions? Again, the paradigm for controlling one's bodily processes, including emotions of fears, joys, and worries, relies on the model that they are generated when neuromuscular circuits are selectively activated. Research has established that cerebral events are involved in emotions, principally hypothalamic and cortical. We also know that striated muscle events are rampant and that there is a variety of autonomic events, including changes in the smooth muscle in the viscera, throughout the cardiovascular system, as in changes of the pulse and blood pressure, respiratory changes, glandular changes, such as in the sweat glands, and throughout the endocrine system. Cerebral and striated muscle events are extremely rapid, occurring within milliseconds of a stressful event, while the autonomic system is much slower to react. Changes throughout the viscera occur in a matter of seconds following semantic processing of a stressful situation. But the point is that the cerebral and autonomic events are *directly controlled* by changes in the striated musculature.

Patients and experimental subjects also find it impossible to be emotional, as they do in other mental processes, while relaxing (Jacobson, 1938). For instance, it is impossible to engage in visual imagery while simultaneously relaxing the eye muscles. Similarly, patients and experimental subjects alike report a lack of emotionality when there is no tension throughout the body. In general, people who are well relaxed uniformly report later that they had no conscious awareness at all, including emotional feelings. Objective determination of the lack of tension is measured electromyographically.

To emphasize how emotionality can diminish, we know that the reflexes of the body are exaggerated when one is excessively tense. Chronic tonus of the striated muscles increases the amplitude of reflexes and decreases their latency. Conversely, reflexes diminish in amplitude and increase in latency when one learns to relax. For example, decreased tonus of the quadriceps femoris decreases the amplitude of the knee jerk while its latency increases; as there is diminution of tone in the arm muscles, the same thing happens to the flexion reflex; as there is diminution of general skeletal muscle tone, there is a decrease in involuntary startle reflex (Jacobson, 1938; Jacobson & Carlson, 1925). Sherrington (1909) also made this point when his research established that it is not possible to evoke the patellar tendon reflex in an absolutely toneless muscle. Sherrington concluded that the appearance of reflexes depends on the presence of tone in the muscles that constitute part of the reflex arc. The point is that as one learns to control the striated musculature in *both* its tonic and phasic activity, there is diminution of reflexes that accompany undesired emotions, such as proneness to anger, resentment, disgust, and embarrassment. Conversely, as general tension increases, the proprioceptive impulses thereby generated *increase* emotionality by activating neuromuscular circuits that reverberate to excite the central nervous system and the autonomic system. Thus, the degree to which one is in an emotional state can be objectively measured by the amplitude and latency of one's reflexes. The point is illustrated by everyday examples, such as when a saucer is accidentally dropped at a tea party. The excessively tense guest will emit an exaggerated startle reflex, perhaps with an emotional yelp, while the well-relaxed person, in an unemotional state, may not even blink or interrupt ongoing conversation. Toward the conclusion of my stress management classes I typically drop a large book onto the floor while my students are well into their relaxation period. Seldom can I ever observe even the blink of an eye, for the startle reflex is not overtly evoked as long as the students are in that relaxed condition.

Establishing the Meaning of Tension

The unique covert localized tension response patterns throughout the body during mental processes are especially important to study clinically. It is a basic principle of progressive relaxation that *every tension has a purpose—that every tension means something.* (I suspect that this principle derives from Titchener's [1909] context theory of meaning.) This point is obvious when the hand is vertically raised at the wrist, as in the first arm practice position (Figure 2). The learner detects the tension in the upper surface of the forearm, and it is readily apparent that the purpose of that tension was simply to raise the hand at the wrist. Similarly, if you walk out the door, the reason that you are tensing the muscles of your legs, the purpose and meaning of that tension, is simply to walk out the door.

What is not so obvious, and in fact clinically is quite subtle, is the interpretation of tensions present during various kinds of psychiatric difficulties. After careful training in detecting subtle tensions throughout the body and after careful training in developing the ability to report on the details of one's mental activity, the patient identifies subtle tensions, often in unexpected places of the body. The question then to be answered by both clinician and patient working together is why those tensions occur during a given kind of mental activity. By establishing the meaning of selected tensions, control can better be gained over the patient's difficulties. For instance, a patient who had difficulty in sitting quietly, with slight dizzy spells during excitement, eventually came to sit stiffly and formally. The question was *why* did she develop the tensions of sitting stiffly and formally. The interpretation was that the tensions *meant* that she was determined to maintain posture in her back because of a fear of developing a habit of faulty posture. That is, the purpose served by maintaining a stiff and formal posture was to fear having an everyday posture that was incorrect. Maintaining an incorrect posture in her daily life probably had some important interpersonal meaning for her, such as that women with incorrect posture were not ladies.

There are two ways to deal with such tensions: first, on a *meaning* level, by understanding the reasons *why* she held herself stiffly, and second, on a *tension* level, by directly relaxing the relevant controlling muscles.

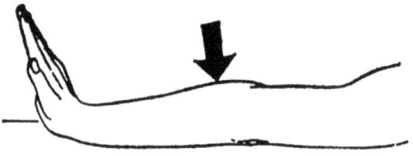

Figure 2. A preliminary position for learning tension control. The learner detects the muscular control signal of tension in the dorsal surface of the forearm as the hand is raised vertically at the wrist.

As another example, in anxiety, a fearful condition is represented in the skeletal musculature. Once the meaning of the striated muscle representation is ascertained, it is possible to then relax those critical tensions and thereupon diminish or eliminate the anxiety. In clinical work it may be a lengthy process to identify tensions characteristic of the neurotic condition of the patient, to interpret those tensions, and to deal effectively with them. But the history of clinical progressive relaxation is one of considerable success in developing self-control following this paradigm (Jacobson, 1938). Progressive relaxation has paved the way for much of the recent interest in the field of self-control, referred to by such terms as *stress management*, as indicated by a synonym developed by Jacobson (1964), known as *self-operations control*.

References

Chase, W. G. (Ed.). (1973). *Visual information processing*. New York: Academic Press.
Delafresnaye, J. F. (1954). *Brain mechanisms and consciousness*. Oxford: Blackwell Scientific.
Eccles, J. C. (1966). *Brain and conscious experience*. New York: Springer-Verlag.
Grings, W. W. (1973). Cognitive factors in electrodermal conditioning. *Psychological Bulletin, 79*, 200–210.
Hebb, D. O. (1968). The semiautonomous process: Its nature and nurture. *American Psychologist, 18*, 16–27.
Jacobson, E. (1925). Voluntary relaxation of the esophagus. *American Journal of Physiology, 72*, 387–394.
Jacobson, E. (1934). *You must relax*. New York: McGraw-Hill.
Jacobson, E. (1938). *Progressive relaxation* (rev. ed.). Chicago: University of Chicago Press. (Original work published 1929)
Jacobson, E. (1964). *Self-operations control*. Philadelphia: Lippincott.
Jacobson, E., & Carlson, A. J. (1925). The influence of relaxation upon the knee-jerk. *American Journal of Physiology, 73*, 324–328.
Lacey, B. C., & Lacey, J. I. (1974). Studies of heart rate and other bodily processes in sensorimotor behavior. In P. A. Obrist, A. H. Black, J. Brener, & L. V. DiCara (Eds.), *Cardiovascular psychophysiology: Current issues in response mechanisms, biofeedback, and methodology*. Chicago: Aldine-Atherton.
McGuigan, F. J. (1966). Covert oral behavior and auditory hallucinations *Psychophysiology, 3*, 73–80.
McGuigan, F. J. (1978). *Cognitive psychophysiology*. Hillsdale, NJ: Erlbaum.
McGuigan, F. J. (1981). *Calm-Down—A guide for stress and tension control*. San Diego: Institute for Stress Management, U.S. International University.
McGuigan, F. J. (1984). How is linguistic memory accessed?—A psychophysiological approach. *Pavlovian Journal of Biological Science, 19*, 119–136.
McGuigan, F. J. (1989). Patterns of covert speech behavior and phonetic coding. *Pavlovian Journal of Biological Science, 24*, 19–26.
Sherrington, C. S. (1909). On plastic tonus and proprioceptive reflexes. *Quarterly Journal of Experimental Physiology, 2*, 109–156.

Titchener, E. B. (1909). *Lectures on the experimental psychology of the thought-processes.* New York: Macmillan.

Wolpe, J. (1975). Relaxation as an instrument for breaking adverse emotional habits. In F. J. McGuigan (Ed.), *Tension control.* Blackburg, VA: University Publications.

Young, R. M. (1970). *Mind brain and adaptation in the nineteenth century.* New York: Oxford University Press.

CHAPTER 7

Control of Convulsions by Inhibitory and Excitatory Neurotransmitter Receptor Regulators in Epileptic El Mice and Neuromuscular Junction-Blocked Rats

Akitane Mori, Isao Yokoi, Hideaki Kabuto, Midori Hiramatsu, Michael J. Kwon, Masakatsu Shimada, and Kenji Akiyama

Currently there is considerable interest in the involvement of excitatory and inhibitory neurotransmitters in seizure mechanisms. Table 1 lists the substances that are known to participate in neuronal excitation and inhibition. There is ample information in the literature about these neurotransmitters and concerning their possible relationship to the etiology of seizures (Bradford & Peterson, 1987; Burley & Ferrendelli, 1984; Craig, 1984; Dragunow, 1986; Jobe, 1984; Laird, Dailey, & Jobe, 1984; McNamara, 1984; Meldrum, 1987; Ogawa & Mori, 1984; Sherwin & van Gelder, 1986). This chapter will focus on two of these neurotransmitters, namely, glutamic acid and γ-aminobutyric acid (GABA). These are the major neurotransmitters that have been implicated in seizure mechanisms. There is much evidence that excess excitatory glutamatergic

---

Akitane Mori, Isao Yokoi, Hideaki Kabuto, Midori Hiramatsu, Michael J. Kwon, Masakatsu Shimada, and Kenji Akiyama • Institute for Neurobiology, Okayama University Medical School, Okayama 700, Japan.

Table 1. Neurotransmitters Implicated in Seizure Mechanisms

1. Monoamines
    dopamine (inhibitory, excitatory)
    noradrenaline (inhibitory)
    serotonin (inhibitory)
    acetylcholine (excitatory, inhibitory)
2. Amino acids
    γ-aminobutyric acid (inhibitory)
    glutamic acid (excitatory)
    aspartic acid (excitatory)
    cysteine sulphinic acid (excitatory)
    cysteic acid (excitatory)
    homocysteic acid (excitatory)
    glycine (inhibitory)
    β-alanine (inhibitory)
    taurine (inhibitory)
    hypotaurine (inhibitory)
3. Neuropeptides
    somatostatin (excitatory?)
    methionine-enkephaline (excitatory?)
    leucine-enkephaline (excitatory?)
    thyrotropine-releasing hormone (inhibitory?)
4. Others
    β-carboline (excitatory)
    adenosine (inhibitory)
    inosine (inhibitory)
    prostaglandins (inhibitory)

nerve activity and/or the loss of inhibitory GABA-ergic nerve activity may lead to epilepsy (Bradford & Peterson, 1987; Jobe, 1984; Laird et al., 1984; McNamara, 1984).

In this chapter, we will discuss first the control of El mouse convulsions by antagonists of glutamate and aspartate receptors. Second, the control of El mouse convulsions by GABA receptor agonists or modulators will be described. Finally, the effect of baclofen, a $GABA_B$ receptor agonist, on the central nerve activity in the neuromuscular-junction-blocked rats will be discussed.

Materials and Methods

El mice (Imaizumi, Ito, Kutsukake, Takizawa, Fujiwara, & Tutikawa, 1959; Imaizumi & Nakano, 1964) are an inbred mutant strain that developed from ddY mice, and they are susceptible to convulsive seizures.

Although spontaneous seizures are sometimes observed, frequently the convulsions are induced by repeating a convenient "throwing" stimulation. The mice are thrown up in the air, approximately 10 cm from a tray held by hand, until the onset of convulsions. These are induced in all mice by this procedure usually within 80 "throws." The convulsions occur at about 7 weeks of age after such stimulation has been given once a week beginning at 4 weeks of age. We refer to stimulated El mice as El(+) and nonstimulated El mice as El(−).

A typical seizure begins with a prodrome such as a squeak and catatonic posture with tail erect for a few seconds. Then, suddenly, postural control is lost, clonic convulsions start in the hind limbs, and generalized tonic-clonic convulsions occur for a very short duration, followed by generalized tonic convulsions with ventroflexion of the neck and generalized tonic convulsions with dorsoflexion of the neck. Massive salivation, and urinary and fecal incontinence occur during this stage. After the convulsive stage, inertia and stupor are observed generally. The entire seizure process occurs within about 50 seconds. Sporadic spike and multiple polyspikes during the interictal period, and paroxysmal discharges during convulsions, have been recorded electroencephalographically (Sugiu, 1963; Suzuki, 1976).

Five El mice were used for each of the behavioral and biochemical experiments. For the biochemical determinations, El(+) about 3 to 4 months old and weighing about 30 g were decapitated 1 hour after the injection of the respective drug.

Sprague Dawley rats weighing 250 to 300 g were used for studying the effect of baclofen on the central nerve activity.

Drugs. DL-2-amino-3-phosphonopropionate (AP3), DL-2-amino-4-phosphonobutyrate (AP4), DL-2-amino-5-phosphonovalerate (AP5), DL-2-amino-6-phosphonohexanoate (AP6), and DL-2-amino-7-phosphonoheptanoate (AP7) were purchased from Sigma Chemical Co. They were dissolved in 0.6 mM phosphate buffer (pH 7.35), and the solutions were adjusted to pH 7.0 with 1M NaOH. Two µl (various concentrations) of each solution were injected intraventricularly into El mice, which were locally anesthetized with 1% lidocaine, exactly 1 hour before the convulsion test. The controls received injections of 2 µl of phosphate buffer in the same manner. γ-vinyl GABA, diazepam, progabide, and baclofen were kindly donated by Prof. H. F. Bradford, Imperial College of Science and Technology, London; Takeda Pharmaceutical Co. Ltd., Osaka; Fujisawa Pharmaceutical Co. Ltd., Osaka; and CIBA-Geigy Ltd., Takarazuka, Japan. Muscimol was purchased from Sigma Co. All drugs were dissolved in saline, except for diazepam, and were injected i.p.

into El mice, exactly 1 hour before the convulsion test. Diazepam was dissolved in dimethylsulfoxide (DMSO) and water (1:3). The dose was as follows: γ-vinyl GABA 1500 mg/kg (Jung, Lippert, Metcalf, Böhlen, & Schechter, 1977), muscimol 3 mg/kg (Guidotti & Ferrero, 1985), progabide 100 mg/kg (Bartholini et al., 1985), diazepam 32 mg/kg (Pratt, Jenner, & Marsden, 1985), and baclofen 20 mg/kg (Micheletti, Marescaux, Vergnes, Rumback, & Warter, 1985). Controls received injections of each vehicle. Baclofen (10 mg/kg) was injected i.p. into rats for EEG studies. Succinylcholine chloride (Katayama Chemicals, Osaka, 50 mg/kg), and Pancronium bromide (Myoblock, Sankyo Co. Ltd., Tokyo, 1 mg/kg) were used for immobilizing the rats.

Amino Acid Analyses. Amino acid levels in the cerebral cortex were analyzed in the following manner. The tissue was homogenized with 1% picric acid and centrifuged at 3000 rpm for 10 minutes. Picric acid in the resultant supernatant was absorbed onto Dowex 2X8. The remaining solution was evaporated, and the dried sample was dissolved in 0.01 N HCl (pH2.2). Taurine (Tau), glutamic acid (Glu), glutamine (Gln), aspartic acid (Asp), GABA, glycine (Gly), and alanine (Ala) levels were determined with an amino acid analyzer (A-5500E, Irika Kohgyo, Tokyo).

EEG Recording. EEGs were recorded with a model ME-95D electroencephalograph (Nihon Koden) from four unipolar leads: left frontal (LF)-indifferent electrode (E), left occipital (LO)-E, right frontal (RF)-E, and right occipital (RO)-E. Electrocardiograms (ECG) and electromyograms (EMG) were also recorded simultaneously.

Statistical analyses were carried out using Student's t test.

Results

Inhibitory Effects of ω-phosphono-α-aminocarboxylic Acid on El Mouse Seizures. Table 2 shows the effect of a series of ω-phosphono-α-aminocarboxylic acid. AP3 injected intraventricularly at a dose of 1.04 μmol had a marked anticonvulsant action, but at a lower dose it induced running fits. AP4 induced transitory excitation, followed by sedation. AP5 induced marked behavioral sedation. AP6 induced tonic-clonic convulsions and epileptic discharges in electroencephalograms. AP7 showed a strong anticonvulsant action at a dose of 1.27 μmol, though it induced myoclonic seizures at a lower dose.

Figure 1a shows the effect of AP5 on amino acid levels in El mouse brain. A significantly decreased level of glutamic acid was observed 1 hour after the injection of 1.8 μmol of AP5.

Table 2. Inhibitory Effects of ω-phosphono-α-aminocarboxylic Acid on E1 Mouse Seizures

Drug	Dose (mol)	Anticonvulsant effect	Remarks
AP3	1.04	++	
	0.1	−	Running fits
AP4	1.02	+	Excitation
AP5	1.8	+++	
AP6	0.8	−	Epileptic discharges
AP7	1.27	+++	
	0.02		Myoclonus

Inhibitory Effects of GABA Receptor Modulators on E1 Mouse Seizures and Amino Acid Levels in the Brain. GABA receptor modulators, γ-vinyl GABA, muscimol, progabide, diazepam, and baclofen showed very potent anticonvulsant effects.

Figure 1b illustrates the effects of GABA receptor modulators on amino acid levels in E1 mouse brain. γ-vinyl GABA markedly increased GABA level. Muscimol significantly increased glutamine level. Progabide did not effect amino acid levels in the brain; diazepam significantly increased glutamine level; and baclofen significantly decreased levels of GABA, glutamate and alanine.

Effect of Baclofen on the Central Nerve Activity in the Neuromuscular-Junction-Blocked Rats. We administered baclofen to freely moving rats and to rats immobilized by neuromuscular junction blockers and muscle relaxants, i.e., succinylcholine chloride or pancronium bromide.

The EEG in the left column of Figure 2 was recorded before 10 mg/kg baclofen injection intraperitoneally. The EEG in the right column was recorded 3 hours after baclofen injection. In each set of EEGs, four unipolar lead recordings from four epidural electrodes set on the left frontal, left occipital, right frontal, and right occipital cortex are shown from the top line to the fourth line. The following two lines show ECG and EMG recordings, respectively. In the first set, EEG recording from a freely moving rat, given neither anesthesia nor muscle relaxant, is shown. About 10 minutes after baclofen injection, motor activity of the rat began to depress and the rat seemed to fall asleep. In the EEG, fast wave activity was suppressed and high-voltage slow waves appeared. Three hours after baclofen injection, low activity of movement still continued and high voltage slow waves were dominant, as shown in the right upper EEG. When the rat was immobilized with succinylcholine

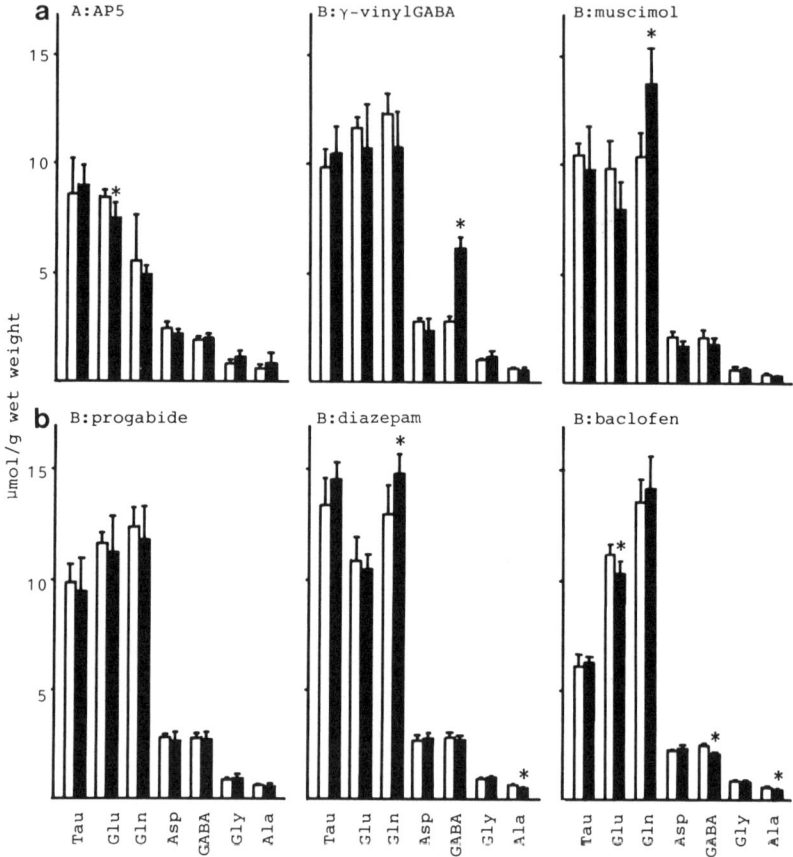

Figure 1. Effect of excitatory (a) and inhibitory (b) amino acid receptor modulators on amino acid levels in El mouse brain. Each bar represents amino acid levels (μmol/g tissue, means ± SD, $N = 5$). * = Significantly different from the corresponding control (Student's t test). (a) AP5 (0.8 μmol, i.p. inj.), (b) γ-vinyl GABA (1500 mg/kg, i.p. inj.), muscimol (3 mg/kg, i.p. inj.), progabide (100 mg/kg, i.p. inj.), diazepam (32 mg/kg, i.p. inj.), and baclofen (20 mg/kg, i.p. inj.). Amino acids were analyzed 60 minutes after drug administration.

chloride, as shown in the middle section, or with pancronium bromide, as shown at the bottom, under artificial ventilation, baclofen markedly suppressed the EEG activity. In the right middle and right bottom EEG, fast waves completely disappeared and low- or high-voltage very slow waves became dominant. High-voltage sharp or spike waves were seen sporadically.

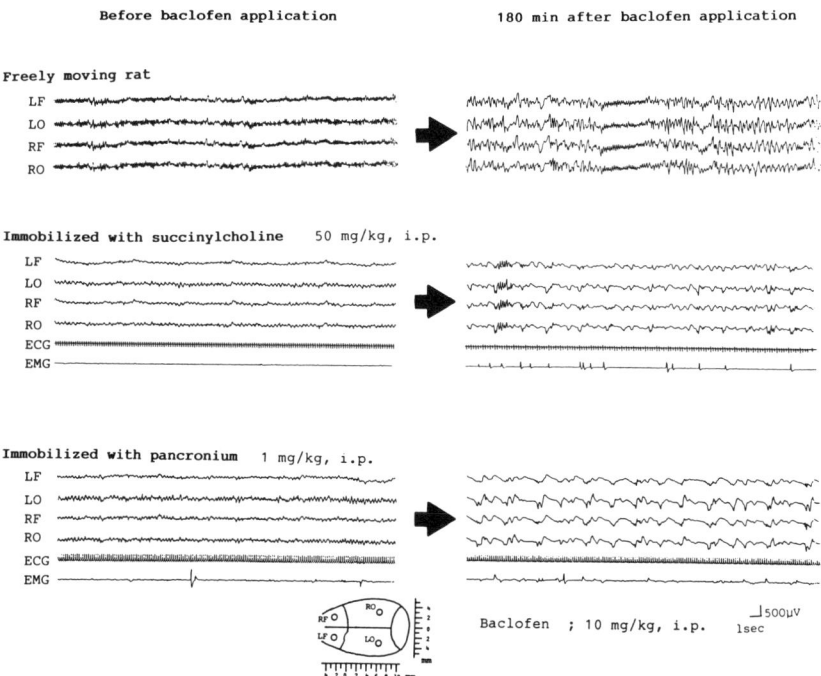

Figure 2. Effect of baclofen (10 mg/kg, i.p.) on rat EEG. Left column: Before baclofen application. Right column: 180 minutes after baclofen application. Upper: The EEGs were obtained from freely moving rat. Baclofen suppressed EEG activity slightly. Middle: The rat was immobilized with succinylcholine (50 mg/kg, i.p.). EEG was suppressed and high-voltage sharp waves and middle-voltage slow waves were observed 180 minutes after baclofen application. Lower: The rat was immobilized with pancronium (1 mg/kg, i.p.). High-voltage slow waves were observed 180 minutes after baclofen application. EEGs were recorded unipolarly from four epidural electrodes (see text).

Discussion

Excitatory amino acid receptors are classified into three types depending on their agonists—namely, N-methyl-D-aspartate (NMDA) receptor, kainate receptor, and quisqualate receptor. The ω-phosphono derivatives of α-aminocarboxylic acid (e.g., AP5 and AP7) are known to act as potent and selective antagonists at the NMDA receptors *in vivo* and *in vitro* (Fagg, Foster, Mena, & Cotman, 1982; Olverman, Jones, & Watkins, 1984; Watkins, 1984). They also have a pronounced anticonvulsant action on chemically induced seizures (Croucher, Collins, & Meldrum, 1982; Czuczwar, Frey, & Löscher, 1985; Czuczwar & Meldrum,

1982), on maximal electroconvulsions of rodents (Czuczwar et al., 1985), on audiogenic seizures of DBA/2 mice, and on the kindled amygdala model of epilepsy in rats (Peterson, Collins, & Bradford, 1983).

The brain levels of glutamic acid and aspartic acid are known to be significantly lower in stimulated El mice (i.e., El(+)) than in nonstimulated El mice (i.e., El(−)) (Suzuki, 1987). Other studies show both glutamic acid and aspartic acid levels in the El mouse brain to be lower than the levels of these amino acids in other strains of mice (dd, gpc, and BL-57) (Kurokawa, Machiyama, & Kato, 1963). These findings suggest that glutamic acid and aspartic acid may be involved in the trigger mechanism of El mouse seizures. We find AP5 to be an excellent anticonvulsant for El mouse seizures, though the effects of ω-phosphono-α-aminocarboxylic acid in the El mice are multiple and complicated depending on its carbon chain length.

We observed significantly decreased levels of glutamic acid, a potent excitatory neurotransmitter, 1 hour after the injection of 1.8 μmol of AP5. There was no change in the levels of other amino acids. This finding suggests that AP5 may occupy NMDA receptor sites in excess amounts, thus acting as an antagonist of the excitatory receptor sites while simultaneously decreasing the Glu level in the presynaptic neurons by down-regulation.

GABA is one of the important inhibitory neurotransmitters in the central nervous system, and it is known to relate closely to epileptic seizure mechanism (Löscher, 1982; Ribak, Harris, Vaughn, & Roberts, 1979; van Gelder, Sherwin, & Rasmussen, 1972; Wood, Hare, Glaeser, Ballenger, & Post, 1979). We studied the action of various GABA receptor modulators in El mice and found the El mouse seizures to be completely inhibited by γ-vinyl GABA, muscimol, progabide, diazepam, and baclofen.

With respect to the results of amino acid analyses, γ-vinyl GABA markedly increased GABA levels in the brain. This increased GABA may reflect an inhibited activity of GABA-transaminase, a GABA degrading enzyme, in the brain (Jung et al., 1977; Metcalf, 1979). Muscimol was found to significantly increase glutamine level. In this case, glutamate level was decreased but not significantly. Muscimol is a specific $GABA_A$ receptor agonist acting directly on GABA binding site (Bartholini et al., 1985; Krogsgaad-Larsen, Johnston, Lodge, & Curtis, 1977). The increase of glutamine may depend on other side effects of muscimol. No change in amino acid levels in the brain was observed by progabide. Progabide is known to act directly on $GABA_A$ binding site as an GABA agonist (Bartholini et al., 1985). Diazepam increases glutamine level in the brain.

Diazepam reinforces GABA receptor binding through benzodiazepine receptor (Costa, 1980). The increase in glutamine level in the brain by diazepam may depend on other pharmacological actions of this drug. Baclofen is thought to be a specific $GABA_B$ receptor agonist (Bowery, Hill, & Huxson, 1982). GABA receptors are classified as $GABA_A$ receptor and $GABA_B$ receptor. The $GABA_A$ receptors, located on the postsynaptic membrane, are linked to chloride channels. Consequently receptor activation by GABA levels leads mostly to an inward movement of Cl^- results in hyperpolarization, i.e., an inhibition of the postsynaptic cell. Bicuculline antagonizes this action of GABA, whereas muscimol mimics it. Baclofen has no effect on $GABA_A$ receptors. On the other hand, $GABA_B$ receptors are activated by baclofen and GABA, and are not blocked by bicuculline. Activation of $GABA_B$ receptors located on presynaptic excitatory terminal is thought to lead to a reduction of evoked excitatory neurotransmitter release, thereby resulting in decreased excitation of the postsynaptic cell. This effect is probably due to a blocked inward flux of Ca^{2+} and a decreased Ca^{2+}-dependent vesicular release process. In addition to these presynaptic $GABA_B$ receptor effects, a postsynaptic action has been reported. Baclofen acts postsynaptically by increasing membrane potassium conductance, resulting in hyperpolarization (Peet & McLennan, 1986). Activation of $GABA_B$ sites located on inhibitory interneurons could then result in disinhibition—in other words, excitation (Van Rijn, Berlo, Feenstra, Schoots, & Hommes, 1987). Our results demonstrate that baclofen decreased the levels of GABA, glutamate, and alanine in the brain. These changes in amino acid levels by baclofen may indicate an as yet unknown effect of this drug on the brain.

When baclofen was administered to freely moving rats and to rats immobilized by succinylcholine chloride or pancronium bromide, which are depolarizing and nondepolarizing type, respectively, the EEG activity was suppressed markedly. This suppressive effect seemed to be enhanced by both types of muscle relaxant. These observations suggest that electrical activity of muscle may have been completely suppressed under immobilization. Some afferent impulses from muscle movement, therefore, would not come to the central nervous system, thus failing to activate the brain function. Some sharp wave or spike activity may reflect postsynaptic effects, such as disinhibition, of $GABA_B$ receptor by baclofen.

In conclusion, we have shown that El mouse convulsions can be controlled by modulating the function of their major excitatory (glutamic acid) and inhibitory (GABA) neurotransmitter receptors. We have also demonstrated the effect of afferent inputs from muscles on the activity of the central nervous system using the neuromuscular-junction-blocked rats.

References

Bartholini, G., Scatton, B., Zivkovic, B., Lloyd, K. G., Deportere, H., Langer, S. Z., & Morselli, P. L. (1985). GABA receptor agonists as a new therapeutic class. In G. Bartholini, L. Bossi, K. G. Lloyd, & R. L. Morselli (Eds.), *Epilepsy and GABA receptor agonist* (L.E.R.S. Vol. 3, pp. 1–30). New York: Raven Press.

Bowery, N. K., Hill, D. R., & Huxson, A. (1982). Bicuculline-insensitive GABA receptors in mammalian brain: Specific binding of ^{3}H-baclofen. In Y. Okada & E. Roberts (Eds.), *Problems in GABA research* (pp. 302–310). Amsterdam: Excerpta Medica.

Bradford, H. F., & Peterson, D. W. (1987). Current views of the pathobiochemistry of epilepsy. *Molecular Aspects of Medicine, 9*, 119–172.

Burley, E. S., & Ferrendelli, J. A. (1984). Regulatory effects of neurotransmitters on electroshock and pentylenetetrazol seizures. *Federation Proceedings, 43*, 2521–2524.

Costa, E. (1980). Benzodiazepines and neurotransmitters. *Arzneimittel-Forschung, 30*, 858–860.

Craig, C. R. (1984). Evidence for a role of neurotransmitters in the mechanism of topical convulsant models. *Federation Proceedings, 43*, 2225–2528.

Croucher, M. J., Collins, J. F., & Meldrum, B. S. (1982). Anticonvulsant action of excitatory amino acid antagonists. *Science, 216*, 899–901.

Czuczwar, S. J., & Meldrum, B. (1982). Protection against chemically induced seizures by 2-amino-phosphonoheptanoic acid. *European Journal of Pharmacology, 83*, 335–338.

Czuczwar, S. J., Cavlheiro, E. A., Turski, L., Turski, W. A., & Kleinrock, Z. (1985a). Phosphonic analogues of excitatory amino acids raise the threshold for maximal electroconvulsions in mice, *Neurosciences Research, 3*, 86–90.

Czuczwar, S. J., Frey, H-H., & Löscher, W. (1985b). Antagonism of N-methyl-D, L-aspartic acid-induced convulsions by antiepileptic drugs and other agents. *European Journal of Pharmacology, 108*, 273–280.

Dragunow, M. (1986). Endogenous anticonvulsant substances. *Neuroscience and Biobehavioral Review, 10*, 229–244.

Fagg, G. E., Foster, A. C., Mena, E. E., & Cotman, C. W. (1982). Chloride and calcium ion reveal a pharmacologically distinct population of L-glutamate binding sites in synaptic membranes: Correspondence between biochemical and electrophysiological data. *Journal of Neuroscience, 2*, 958–965.

Guidotti, A., & Ferrero, P. (1985). Ex vivo binding of ^{3}H-muscimol to GABA$_A$ recognition sites: A tool to characterize GABA receptor agonist. In G. Bartholini, L. Bossi, K. G. Lloyd, & P. L. Morselli (Eds.), *Epilepsy and GABA receptor agonists* (L.E.R.S. Vol. 3, pp. 33–41). New York: Raven Press.

Imaizumi, K., & Nakano, T. (1964). Mutant stocks, strain. El. *Mouse News Letter, 31*, 57.

Imaizumi, K., Ito, S., Kutsukake, G., Takizawa, T., Fujiwara, K., & Tutikawa, K. (1959). Epilepsy like anomaly of mice. *Jikken Dobutsu (Bulletin of the Experimental Animal), 8*, 6–10.

Jobe, P. C. (1984). Neurotransmitters and epilepsy: An overview. *Federation Proceedings, 43*, 2503–2504.

Jung, M. J., Lippert, B., Metcalf, B. W., Böhlen, P., & Schechter, P. J. (1977). γ-vinyl GABA

(4-amino-hex-5-enoic acid), a new selective inhibitor of GABA-T: Effect on brain GABA metabolism in mice. *Journal of Neurochemistry, 29,* 797–802.
Krogsgaad-Larsen, P., Johnston, G. A. R., Lodge, D., & Curtis, D. R. (1977). A new class of GABA agonists. *Nature, 268,* 53–55.
Kurokawa, M., Machiyama, Y., & Kato, M. (1963). Distribution of acetylcholine in the brain during various states of activity. *Journal of Neurochemistry, 10,* 341–348.
Laird, H. E., II, Dailey, J. W., & Jobe, P. C. (1984). Neurotransmitter abnormalities. *Federation Proceedings, 43,* 2505–2509.
Löscher, W. (1982). Relationship between GABA concentrations in cerebrospinal fluid and seizure excitability. *Journal of Neurochemistry, 38,* 293–295.
McNamara, J. O. (1984). Role of neurotransmitters in seizure mechanisms in the kindling model of epilepsy. *Federation Proceedings, 43,* 2416–2520.
Meldrum, B. (1987). Neurotransmitter amino acids in epilepsy. *Electroencephalography and Clinical Neurophysiology, 39,* (Suppl.) 191–199.
Metcalf, B. W. (1979). Inhibitors of GABA metabolism. *Biochemical Pharmacology, 28,* 1705–1712.
Micheletti, G., Marescaux, C., Vergnes, M., Rumback, L., & Warter, J. M. (1985). Effects of GABA mimetics and GABA antagonists on spontaneous nonconvulsive seizures in Wistar rat. In G. Bartholini, L. Bossi, K. G. Lloyd, & P. L. Morselli (Eds.), *Epilepsy and GABA receptor agonists* (L.E.R.S. Vol. 3, pp. 129–137). New York: Raven Press.
Ogawa, N., & Mori, A. (1984). β-carbolines: Endogenous ligands for the benzodiazepine receptor. *Folia Psychiatrica et Neurologica Japonica, 38,* 207–211.
Olverman, H. J., Jones, A. W., & Watkins, J. C. (1984). L-glutamate has higher affinity than other amino acids for [^{3}H]D-AP5 binding sites in rat brain membranes. *Nature, 307,* 460–462.
Peet, M. J., & McLennan, H. (1986). Pre- and postsynaptic actions of baclofen: Blockade of the late synaptically-evoked hyperpolarization of CA1 hippocampal neurons. *Experimental Brain Research, 61,* 567–574.
Peterson, D. W., Collins, J. F., & Bradford, H. F. (1983). The kindled amygdala model of epilepsy; anticonvulsant action of amino acid antagonists. *Brain Research, 275,* 169–172.
Pratt, J. A., Jenner, P., & Marsden, C. D. (1985). Comparison of the effects of benzodiazepines and other anticonvulsant drugs on synthesis and utilizations of 5-HT in mouse brain. *Neuropharmacology, 24,* 59–68.
Ribak, C. E., Harris, A. B., Vaughn, J. E., & Roberts, E. (1979). Inhibitory, GABAergic terminals decrease at sites of focal epilepsy. *Science, 205,* 211–214.
Sherwin, A. L., & van Gelder, N. M. (1986). Amino acid and catecholamine markers of metabolic abnormalities in human focal epilepsy. *Advances in Neurology, 44,* 1011–1032.
Sugiu, R. (1963). Pathophysiological study of ep-mouse. *Okayama Igakkai-Zasshi, 75,* 145–188. (in Japanese)
Suzuki, J. (1976). Paroxysmal discharges in the electroencephalogram of the El mouse. *Experientia, 32,* 336–338.
Suzuki, S. (1987). Regional changes in amino acid levels in the brain of El mice due to convulsive disposition and seizures. *Okayama Igakkai Zasshi, 99,* 1517.
Takeuchi, N. (1968). Studies on alterations of cerebral free amino acids and related compounds in the convulsive disposition and during seizures of El mouse. *Osaka Igakkai-Zasshi, 20,* 387–398. (in Japanese)
van Gelder, N. M., Sherwin, A. L., & Rasmussen, R. (1972). Amino acid content of epileptic human brain: Focal versus surrounding regions. *Brain Research, 40,* 385–393.
Van Rijn, C. M., Berlo, M. J., Feenstra, M. G. P., Schoots, M. L. F., & Hommes, O. R.

(1987). R(−)-baclofen: Focal epilepsy after intracortical administration in the rat. *Epilepsy Research, 1,* 321–327.

Watkins, J. C. (1984). Excitatory amino acids and central synaptic transmissions. *Trends in Pharmacological Science, 5,* 373–376.

Wood, J. H., Hare, T. A., Glaeser, B. S., Ballenger, J. C., & Post, R. M. (1979). Low cerebrospinal fluid γ-aminobutyric acid content in seizure patients. *Neurology, 29,* 1203–1208.

CHAPTER 8

Fluency Enhancement in Stutterers
Advances in Self-Regulation through Sensory Augmentation

Ronald L. Webster

Stuttering is a uniquely human communications disorder that occurs in about 1% of the general population (Bloodstein, 1981). It is found approximately four times more often in males than in females (Andrews & Harris, 1964; Bloodstein, 1981). The median age of stuttering onset is 4 years, and approximately 95% of those who stutter will do so by the age of 7 years (Andrews & Harris, 1964). Most children who stutter (in the vicinity of 75%) "outgrow" the problem by the onset of puberty (Andrews & Harris, 1964; Bloodstein, 1981). Stuttering tends to run in families, with first-degree relatives of stutterers being over three times more likely to stutter than persons in the general population (Andrews, Craig, Feyer, Hoddinot, and Neilson, 1983). Observed familial patterns of stuttering can be accounted for by single major locus and multifactorial genetic models (Kidd, 1980). There is no evidence from the controlled study of unselected populations that stutterers are different from nonstutterers on measures of anxiety or neuroticism (Andrews *et al.*, 1983). Some evidence exists suggesting that stutterers exhibit more problems with social adjustment than nonstutterers (Andrews *et al.*, 1983); however, it seems likely that these results can best be explained by viewing stuttering as the antecedent factor (Prins, 1972).

Ronald L. Webster • Department of Psychology, Hollins College, Roanoke, Virginia 24020, USA.

Definition and Measurement of Stuttering

Stuttered speech has a number of perceptually salient features. Among them are (1) repetitions of sounds, syllables, and words, (2) prolongations of syllable initial sounds, and (3) hesitations associated with voice blockage (Van Riper, 1971; Webster, 1974). In addition, accessory behaviors may be noticed during attempts to speak. Such behaviors can include introjections of sounds or words unrelated to the message to be delivered; starter words or sounds that occur just prior to attempts to deliver a specific message; and facial grimaces, distorted breathing, and autonomic arousal (Webster, 1978). The usual defining features of stuttering—repetitions, prolongations, and voice blockage—occur at the level of simple, unaided observation. While it seems obvious that distortions in speech muscle movements yield the events recognized as stuttering, much remains to be learned about specific physical details that differentiate the speech of stutterers from that of normally fluent persons. A number of studies are summarized below that indicate the nature of current research efforts directed toward the improved definition and measurement of stuttered speech.

Freeman and Ushijima (1978) used hooked wire electrodes to record EMG levels from oral and intrinsic laryngeal muscles in stutterers during instances of stuttered and fluent speech. Higher levels of EMG activity were observed during stuttered speech compared with fluent speech. In the stutterers under fluency-enhancing conditions that included delayed auditory feedback, speaking under white noise masking, speech pacing with a metronome, and speaking in chorus with others, it was found that both oral and laryngeal muscles showed lower levels of activity than during stuttering. Freeman and Ushijima also reported that the normal reciprocity between laryngeal adductors and abductors did not occur during the moments of stuttering. Specifically, adductors and abductors were activated simultaneously. Similar findings regarding loss of reciprocity during stuttering were reported by Shapiro (1980). Both Shapiro and Freeman and Ushijima noted that abnormal muscle activity also occurred within perceptually fluent utterances. Freeman (1984) suggested that stutterers may experience many instances of speech muscle coordination that do not yield the perception of stuttering.

Conture, McCall, and Brewer (1977) conducted frame-by-frame analyses of videotapes made via a fiberscope of laryngeal activity during stuttering. These investigators reported that during instances of stuttering the larynx was inappropriately open on some occasions and inappropriately closed on others. Conture (1984) also noted that different patterns of laryngeal closure were associated with repetitions when contrasted with prolongations. The larynx was observed to lower during repetitions when compared with its height during fluent utterances of vowels. Sound prolongations were frequently associated with tight adduction of the vocal folds on voiced sounds and excessive abduction of the vocal folds on voiceless sounds.

Acoustic analyses of voice onsets (Webster, Morgan, & Cannon, 1987) have shown that fluent one-syllable words initiated with vowels have significantly more abrupt beginnings in stutterers than in fluent speakers. Initial acoustic pulses in voiced one-syllable utterances were also found to be significantly reduced in stutterers who experienced white noise masking compared with a "no-noise" condition (McClure, 1983). The reports of Freeman and Ushijima (1978), Conture et al. (1977), and Webster et al. (1987) have demonstrated through a variety of measurement techniques that abnormal vocal gestures are associated with stuttered speech and with the fluent speech of stutterers.

Articulatory gestures—the movements of tongue, lips, soft palate, and jaw that shape speech sounds—have also been shown to be aberrant in stutterers. Zimmerman (1980) used high-speed cineradiography to describe the temporal and spatial properties of perceptually fluent speech in stutterers and normal speakers. Standardized consonant-vowel-consonant syllables were spoken and movements of the jaw and lower lip were analyzed. When compared with fluent speakers, stutterers were found to display longer transition times for the downward movement of the lip and jaw, longer intervals between movement onset and peak velocity in the gesture moving from the initial consonant to the vowel, and somewhat longer steady-state positions of the jaw and lip during utterance of the vowel element in the syllable.

In a study of stutterers' articulatory movements using acoustic analyses of vowel-consonant-vowel syllables, Pindzola (1987) reported that stutterers spent longer times in static articulatory positions than nonstutterers. This was true even though total vowel durations were not significantly different for the two groups. Transitions from the initial vowel to the consonant were significantly shorter in stutterers than in nonstutterers.

Multiple measures of upper lip, lower lip, and jaw kinematics in the fluent speech of stutterers and normal speakers were made on standard speech tasks by Caruso, Abbs, and Gracco (1988). In general, stutterers did not show difficulties in the coordination of speech movements. However, stutterers were significantly different from normals in subtle measures of the sequencing in the initiation of articulatory movements and in the velocity peaks of these movements.

Speech sounds result from the action of voicing and articulation upon the expelled air stream. Muscle systems involved in management of the air stream of stutterers also show deviant activity. Peters and Boves (1987) conducted an extensive study of subglottal air pressure buildups and phonation in stutterers and normal speakers. These investigators found that seven patterns of air pressure buildup were definable. Three types of pressure buildup were determined to be normal and four were judged to be deviant. Deviant patterns of pressure buildup occurred significantly more often in fluent utterances of stutterers than in those of normal speakers. The three major deviant patterns of subglottal air pressure buildup involved rapid, excessive increases in air pressure prior to phonation or nonmonotonic increases in air pressure in advance of phonation. Again, the major finding was that subtle distortions were found in the behaviors used by stutterers even when speech was judged to be perceptually fluent.

These beginning efforts to describe stuttering have typically used small numbers of subjects and speech tasks that are not directly comparable, and have tended to measure a restricted number of responses. Nonetheless, they do suggest the merit in moving beyond simple, perceptual judgments of stuttered speech through improved resolution of observation via instrumental analysis. Clearly, a number of subtle and potentially important phenomena are starting to be recognized that differentiate stutterers from normally fluent speakers through measurement of movement characteristics in muscle systems involved with respiration, phonation, and articulation. There is much to be gained through these efforts, both in terms of improving basic understandings of stuttering and in creating improved methods for treating stuttering, by the continuation of research that emphasizes the measurement and objectification of phenomena in stuttering.

Fluency-Enhancing Conditions

A number of variables have strong, immediate fluency enhancing effects on stutterers. Among them are (1) delayed auditory feedback (DAF), a condition in which speech is returned electronically to the ears of a speaker a fraction of a second after he talks; (2) white noise masking, a condition in which high levels of white noise are presented through headphones while the stutterer is speaking; (3) rhythmic stimulation, a condition in which the stutterer is instructed to release syllables in time with an external rhythmic cue such as the tick of a metronome; (4) whispering, a condition of speech in which the vocal folds are not approximated and speech is produced via the excitation of the vocal tract resonance through the turbulence of air passing through the tract; (5) adaptation, a condition in which the stutterer reads a short paragraph a number of times aloud with an observed decrease in stuttering; (6) singing; (7) choral reading; (8) deafness; and (9) therapy.

DAF represents a curious stimulus condition inasmuch as it reduces dysfluencies in stutterers and markedly increases dysfluencies in normal speakers (Lechner, 1979; Stark & Pierce, 1970; Stephen & Haggard, 1980; Webster, Lubker, & Schumacher, 1970). The delay interval that produces maximum disruption in fluent speakers is about the duration of a normal syllable (180 msec). Shorter delay intervals are usually effective in improving the fluency of stutterers (Webster et al., 1970).

White noise masking also differentially influences the speech of stutterers and normally fluent speakers. Stutterers speak with improved fluency under high-amplitude masking (Adams & Hutchinson, 1974; Adams & Moore, 1972; Garber & Martin, 1977; Webster & Dorman, 1970). Both stutterers and normally fluent speakers generally increase vocal intensity and extend syllable durations when experiencing white noise (Adams & Hutchinson, 1974). When vocal intensity levels are controlled in stutterers, white noise masking is still effective in reducing or eliminating dysfluencies (Garber & Martin, 1977). Speech contingent and noncontingent white noise masking improved fluency to the same extent in stutterers (Webster & Dorman, 1970).

It has also been demonstrated that stutterers improve their fluency when speech is released in synchronization with a regular, repetitive external stimulus, such as the tick of the metronome or the blink of a light (Brady, 1971; Brayton & Conture, 1978; Silverman & Trotter, 1973).

A number of altered speaking conditions have been demonstrated to have fluency-enhancing effects with stutterers: whispering (Bruce & Adams, 1978; Cherry & Sayers, 1956) choral reading (Adams & Ramig, 1980; Andrews, Howie, Dozsa, & Guitar, 1982), singing (Andrews et al., 1983) and adaptation (Bruce & Adams, 1978; Johnson & Knott, 1937; Webster & Dorman, 1971). The reliability of fluency enhancement under these circumstances is very good, with almost all stutterers showing speech improvement.

Studies of the congenitally deaf (Backus, 1938; Harmes & Malone, 1939) indicate that stuttering occurs rarely, if at all. Most of the research reported on deafness and stuttering has involved questionnaire surveys of institutions for the deaf. Even though various interpretations of what might constitute stuttering have been used by those who respond to the questionnaires, the incidence of stuttering reported is virtually nil.

An interesting and important issue involves how the fluency-enhancing effects noted can be explained. One approach to interpretation that appears to have merit is to attempt to define a locus of action for each condition. It would appear that there are two clear-cut loci upon which these fluency-enhancing conditions have effects. First, the auditory feedback system of the stutterer is clearly influenced by the conditions of delayed auditory feedback, masking and deafness. In addition, Webster and Dorman (1971) showed that adaptation effects could be accounted for by temporary decreases in the speaker's reliance upon auditory feedback cues. Therefore, it would appear that adaptation is properly associated with the auditory locus. The auditory modality appears to be involved again with whispering. However, as will be seen below, whispering could act upon another locus.

The second major locus of action appears to be in the area of laryngeal activity. Whispering clearly involves a cessation of voicing. The powerful vibrations that constitute voice are simply not present because they are not generated through the act of whispering. Some of the internal sensory feedback associated with normal speech is necessarily absent during whispering. Specifically, the vibrations of voice that are normally transmitted from the larynx through the tissues and bones of the body to the ear are absent. In singing, the voiced segments of speech are increased in duration and also may be altered in terms of onset characteristics. Under conditions of choral reading, syllable durations are altered. Rhythmic stimuli may be important because they provide timing cues to guide the release of syllables and to anchor the initiation of voicing on a temporal basis. Finally, therapy (Webster, 1975, 1980) provides specific training that alters parameters of speech muscle movements in terms of position, force, acceleration, and timing.

Considerations Regarding Sensory Feedback

While it is possible to discuss speech in terms of mechanics of respiration, phonation, and articulation, the act of speaking involves a set of complex sensory, neural, and motor systems. One of the early models proposed to conceptualize the working of the speech system was presented by Fairbanks (1954). In this model, speech is considered as a servosystem (Figure 1). Control signals that activate muscles are originated in the brain and are converted to neuromuscular commands that result in movements of the speech musculature. Sensory feedback is generated during the act of speaking and is returned through various channels to the brain, where it is presumed to be evaluated and com-

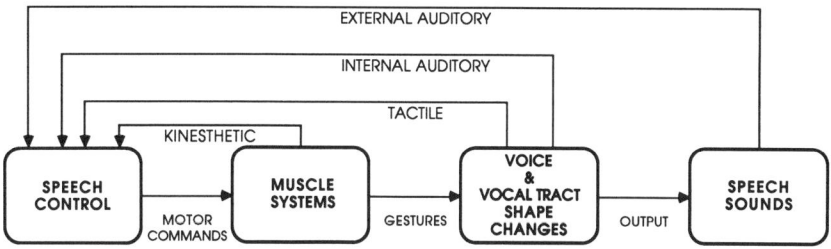

Figure 1. Schematic representation of speech production with a servomechanistic model.

pared with the intended movements, and then rapid adjustments are made to cause output of the system to conform with the intended values. In this model, the closed-loop feedback system permits ongoing, continuous control of speech production (Sussman, 1972). Webster and Lubker (1968) indicated that a flaw in the return of sensory information could result in the disruption of feedback information, which in turn could lead to the disturbance in efforts to produce ongoing muscle movements of speech reduction.

Therapies at Two Fluency-Inducing Loci

It appears reasonable to speculate that therapeutic efforts with stutterers could be effective at either the motor control locus or the auditory feedback locus. Indeed, there is evidence to support this conjecture. Webster (1975, 1980) described the Precision Fluency Shaping Program, a comprehensive behavior therapy program for stutterers that is based on the systematic establishment of specific motor patterns that generate fluent speech. The emphasis in this therapy is upon the reconstruction of fine-grain topographic details of responses involving respiration, articulation, and phonation. A series of fluency-propagating targets have been identified and instructional sequences developed that appear to be relevant to the treatment of stuttering. A special-purpose instrument, the Voice Monitor, has also been created to provide clients in treatment with ongoing, immediate feedback about voice-onset properties. This instrument is used as a standard training aid in administration of the Precision Fluency Shaping Program. Approximately 2600 stutterers have been treated at our center with this program. With the Precision Fluency Shaping Program, approximately 90 to 95% of treated cases attain normal levels of fluency (dysfluency rates at or below 3%) at the end of a 3-week treatment program and display normal reactions to daily speaking situations. Follow-up studies at 1 year and 2 years posttreatment indicate that approximately 70 to 75% of the treated cases retain normal fluency and normal reactions to everyday speaking situations.

Treatment efforts have also been directed toward the auditory locus. For example, Goldiamond (1965), Ryan and Van Kirk (1974), and Lee, McGough, and Peins (1973) attempted the employment of DAF in stuttering therapy. While the presence of DAF conditions was reliably associated with fluent speech, in general there was little evidence that fluency transferred well to extraclinic environments or was well retained after the cessation of treatment (Ingham, 1984). Portable DAF devices are available in the marketplace for those stutterers who wish to use them. White noise masking has also been used in an effort to reduce stuttering in daily life. Dewar, Dewar, and Anthony (1976) and Dewar, Dewar, Austin, and Brash (1979) reported improvements in fluency with stutterers who used a portable, voice-operated masking device, the Edinburgh Masker. Ingham (1984) noted that the Dewar *et al.* (1979) study was not based on objective data and failed to provide details on how subject responsiveness to the instrument was evaluated. The Edinburgh Masker may also be purchased for use by individual stutterers. Metronomes have been developed for use by stutterers in everyday life. Brady (1968, 1971) reported on a metronome-based form of behavior therapy for stutterers. Some reservations about the efficacy of the metronome program were expressed by Ingham (1984) because of the lack of information on measurement reliability, speech rate, and extraclinic consequences of metronome use.

The devices mentioned above, DAF, masking, and metronome systems, have a number of practical negative consequences associated with their use. Both the DAF and masking units are relatively large, must be attached to the body with unwieldy straps, and do not appear to be well adapted for daily wear. The metronome, while relatively small and easy to mount on the body, occludes the ear canal in which the unit is used, thereby reducing audition in the selected ear. Numerous stutterers who have attended our clinic have reported that these devices are simply not practical for use on an everyday basis. All three of the devices were judged to become nuisances when used every day. For example, the constant ticking of the metronome, the spurious, nonspeech activation of the masker, and the delay of all sounds to the ear with the DAF device soon annoyed many users of these devices.

A Development in Vocal Enhancement for Stutterers

Our past work with the auditory locus involved tests of DAF and masking (Webster et al., 1970; Webster & Dorman, 1970). As we recently considered the sensory channel employed by masking and DAF, we became aware of the fact that speech signals (those sounds that emanate from the oral cavity) were processed by these devices. However, the voice signal, the buzz originating at the vocal folds, was not directly manipulated by DAF and was possibly only marginally affected by masking.

We speculated about the merit of transmitting the vocal buzz directly to the ear. Our first efforts were conducted with a miniature stethoscope. The head of the stethoscope was mounted on the throat, and the earpieces were placed in the user's ears. About one-third of the stutterers tested with this device spoke with improved fluency. The remainder showed only slight gains or no gains in fluency. An electronic system was also tested that used a small throat microphone, an amplifier, and earphones, but it seemed to be even less effective than the relatively primitive stethoscope system. We eventually recognized that the sound quality in the ear was substantially different when we subjectively compared the stethoscope and the first electronic system.

Our next step was to attempt an electronic system that delivered sound directly into the occluded ear canal. We noticed that the apparent resonance of the vocal buzz was enhanced when we compared the new system with the previous one that used headphones. We also observed that about one-third of the stutterers showed improvements in their fluency with this system. We then prepared in consultation with a hearing aid manufacturer a miniaturized version of the amplifier-speaker system that could be placed within the external ear canal of the user and developed a smaller and more effective throat microphone. The sound quality of the instrument was good; that is, the vocal buzz was heard with strong resonance in the ear canal during speech. A U.S. Patent application was filed on the device. As this chapter is being prepared, notice has been received that the claims made in the patent application have been allowed by the Patent Office.

The fluency-generating efficacy of the new device was evaluated at Hollins College with 21 stutterers. The most recent 100 stutterers who applied for and were on the waiting list for the Precision Fluency Shaping Program were sent letters that described the proposed evaluation of the new fluency device and asked for volunteers. Stutterers were selected who represented different ages, education levels, and places of residence. The participants were 20 males and 1 female. They ranged in age from 23 to 57 years, with a mean age of 35.5 years. Levels of stuttering severity extended from mild to severe. Subjective clinical ratings by experienced clinicians placed 9 in the mild category, 3 in the moderate category, and 9 in the severe category. Each participant was permitted to retain the prototype fluency device that was used in the tests.

Speech samples were collected from the participants during standardized oral reading and conversational tasks. Videotape recordings were made of all speech samples. Three double-spaced typed reading passages were used. The total number of words in each of two passages was 398 and for the third passage, 397. Conversational speech samples were collected as participants responded to one of the three standardized lists of questions. Reading passages and conversational question lists were randomly assigned to the three different test conditions. Approximately 500 words of conversation were collected from each participant.

After the initial conversational and reading samples were recorded, each participant was fitted with a fluency device that was molded specifically for his right ear. A thin wire extended from the earpiece, behind the ear, and along the neck to a small contact microphone that was held in place approximately 2 centimeters above the sternal notch by a thin elastic neck band. After being fitted with the device and being instructed how to adjust the volume of vocal sound heard in the ear to a relatively loud, but comfortable level, the participants were placed together in pairs and were instructed to converse with each other for a period of 20 to 30 minutes. The signal level in the subjects' ears was set so a slightly audible buzz could be heard by an observer standing approximately ½ meter from the user as he talked.

A second testing session followed the initial habituation to the device. Again, standard reading and conversational speech samples were collected on videotape.

During the next phase of the investigation all participants were given small group instruction in the control of respiration and gentle initiation of voicing. An experienced clinician explained how diaphragmatic breathing and the gentle initiation of voicing were to be produced. Participants practiced these skills in pairs for 1 hour while their voice onsets were electronically evaluated by a special-purpose computer. Clinicians provided additional instruction with any cases that had difficulty in attaining the fluency skills. Following completion of the paired practice exercises, participants were placed in small groups of four or five members and practiced their fluency skills while wearing the fluency devices. Participants were instructed to wear and use their fluency devices in all conversations for one evening and one morning. Final evaluations of speech for all participants were conducted approximately 24 hours after the devices were fitted. Again, standard reading and conversational tasks were used and speech samples were videotaped.

Results of Clinical Trials

Analyses of percent dysfluent word measures in reading and conversation were conducted with paired t tests (two-tailed). Table 1 shows the mean percent dysfluent word scores for all participants under all conditions of the study.

Mean reading dysfluency scores decreased significantly from the first session to the second, $t(20) = 3.33$, $p < .001$, indicating that the fluency device alone was having a positive effect. A significant decrease in dysfluencies was also found, $t(20) = 3.04$, $p < .01$, when the second session was compared with the third session. Training in respiration and gentle voice onsets appeared to further strengthen the fluency-enhancing effects of the device. Mean word-per-minute rates were also calculated and analyzed for the reading condition. The mean word-per-minute rate for session one was 106.43; for session two, 118.0; and for session three, 105.67. Only the difference between session one and session two was significant, $t(20) = 2.72$, $p < .05$. Thus, the device alone both reduced dysfluencies and increased word-per-minute rates.

Mean percent dysfluencies did not decrease significantly when the conversational measures for session one and session two were compared, $t(20) = 1.58$, $p > .05$. However, there were significant drops in dysfluencies during conversation when session one was compared with session three, $t(20) = 2.54$, $p < .05$, and when session two was compared with session three, $t(20) = 3.90$, $p < .001$. Word-per-minute rates were not calculated for the conversational samples. Clinicians noted that the dysfluencies occurring during both reading and conversation with the device in place were shorter and less intense.

Table 1. Mean Percent Dysfluent Words in Reading and Conversation

	Session 1	Session 2	Session 3
Reading	17.44	11.86	5.07
Conversation	20.72	18.11	12.87

Inspection of the raw scores indicated that 17 stutterers had dysfluencies on the initial reading task that were outside the range usually considered fluent in normal speakers (i.e., dysfluency rates over 3%). When compared with the first session, 14 showed reductions in dysfluencies in the second session and 15 showed reductions in the third session. A total of 12 stutterers showed reductions in dysfluencies between sessions two and three.

Inspection of raw scores for the conversational task showed that all participants had dysfluency rates over 3% in session one. When compared with the first session, 13 cases decreased dysfluencies on the second session and 20 showed decreases in the third session. From the second to the third session 14 cases showed reductions in dysfluencies.

Participants were permitted to keep their ear devices for daily use. In preliminary follow-ups, participants indicated that the devices were useful in reducing dysfluencies. During the first month at home, 17 of the 21 cases used their devices every day. There were few reports of difficulty with operation or comfort of the devices. Most users indicated that they experienced a greater willingness to venture into situations that they had previously avoided because of their stuttering problem. About half of the users indicated that they were experiencing noticeable carryover of fluency into times when they were not wearing their ear devices.

Conclusions

The new device was a more effective fluency enhancer in reading than in conversation. This was true with the device alone as well as when the device and training were combined. It appears that users of the device benefited most when they actively listened to the details of their voices as they talked. The burden of concentration imposed by conversation may have reduced the users' attention to their voices. Another suggestion is that the effectiveness of the device is strengthened with use. This would be especially true with those stutterers who become aware of the need to exert some initial level of control during the initiation of voicing. It appears as if awareness of specific behavioral details involved with the onset of voicing would benefit the user.

Rather large improvements in fluency were associated with the device plus training, even though the training in diaphragmatic breathing and gentle voice onsets was minimal. This result was rather surprising since training in these fluency skills without voice feedback augmentation usually requires a great deal of time and the effort of a skilled clinician. It should be noted that the emphasis here is upon voice feedback and not speech feedback. Other observations in our laboratory have indicated that augmentation of speech feedback does not produce fluency enhancement. The role of the vocal feedback system in speech guidance merits further careful study.

The devices tested in this study were early prototypes. It seems likely that we shall be able to define and improve detection and presentation of the acoustic signal in the ear canal of the stutterer. A number of engineering changes in circuit components, microphones, amplifiers, filters, phase shifters, and speakers may strengthen the fluency-generating capabilities of the device. It is also possible that exploration of ear mold materials and shapes may yield improved operation of the device.

The results of the study were quite promising. However, it seems clear that additional research focusing on the role of sensory feedback in stutterers is needed. We are just beginning to recognize the potentially important role that bone-conducted auditory feedback may have in stutterers. And it seems fair to suggest that stutterers are just beginning to benefit from the practical application of knowledge about their sensory feedback systems.

References

Adams, M. R., & Hutchinson, J. (1974). The effects of three levels of auditory masking on selected vocal characteristics and the frequency of dysfluency of adult stutterers. *Journal of Speech and Hearing Research, 17*, 682–688.

Adams, M. R., & Moore, W. H., Jr. (1972). The effects of auditory masking on the anxiety level, frequency of dysfluency, and selected vocal characteristics of stutterers. *Journal of Speech and Hearing Research, 15*, 572–578.

Adams, M. R., & Ramig, P. (1980). Vocal characteristics of normal speakers and stutterers during choral reading. *Journal of Speech and Hearing Research, 23*, 257–469.

Andrews, G., & Harris, M. (1964). *The syndrome of stuttering* (Clinics in Developmental Medicine no. 17). London: Heinemann.

Andrews, G., Howie, P. M., Dozsa, M., & Guitar, B. E. (1982). Stuttering: Speech pattern characteristics under fluency-inducing conditions. *Journal of Speech and Hearing Research, 25*, 208–216.

Andrews, G., Craig, A., Feyer, A., Hoddinott, S., Howie, P., & Neilson, M. (1983). Stuttering: A review of research findings and theories. Circa, 1982. *Journal of Speech and Hearing Disorders, 48*, 226–246.

Backus, O. (1938). Incidence of stuttering among the deaf. *Annals of Otolaryngology, Rhinology, and Laryngology, 47*, 632–635.

Bloodstein, O. (1981). *A handbook on stuttering* (3rd ed.). Chicago: National Easter Seal Society.

Brady, J. P. (1968). A behavioral approach to the treatment of stuttering. *American Journal of Psychiatry, 125*, 843–848.

Brady, J. P. (1971). Metronome-conditioned speech retraining for stuttering. *Behavior Therapy, 2,* 129–150.

Brayton, E. R., & Conture, E. G. (1978). Effects of noise and rhythmic stimulation on the speech of stutterers. *Journal of Speech and Hearing Research, 21,* 285–294.

Bruce, M. C., & Adams, M. R. (1978). Effects of two types of motor practice on stuttering adaptation. *Journal of Speech and Hearing Research, 21,* 421–428.

Caruso, A. J., Abbs, J. H., & Gracco, V. L. (1988). Kinematic analysis of multiple movement coordination during speech in stutterers. *Brain, 111,* 439–455.

Cherry, C., & Sayers, B. McA. (1956). Experiments upon the total inhibition of stammering by external control and some clinical results. *Journal of Psychosomatic Research, 1,* 233–246.

Conture, E. G. (1984). Observing laryngeal movements of stutterers. In R. F. Curlee & W. H. Perkins (Eds.), *Nature and Treatment of stuttering: New directions.* San Diego: College Hill Press.

Conture, E., McCall, G., & Brewer, D. (1977). Laryngeal behavior during stuttering. *Journal of Speech and Hearing Research, 20,* 661–668.

Dewar, A., Dewar, A. D., & Anthony, J. F. K. (1976). The effect of auditory feedback masking concomitant movements of stammering. *British Journal of Disorders of Communication, 11,* 95–102.

Dewar, A., Dewar, A. D., Austin, W. T. S., & Brash, H. M. (1979). The long term use of an automatically triggered auditory feedback masking device in the treatment of stammering. *British Journal of Disorders of Communication, 14,* 219–229.

Fairbanks, G. (1954). Systematic research in experimental phonetics: I. A theory of the speech mechanism as a servosystem. *Journal of Speech and Hearing Disorders, 19,* 133–139.

Freeman, F. J. (1984). Laryngeal muscle activity of stutterers. In R. F. Curlee & W. H. Perkins (Eds.), *Nature and treatment of stuttering: New directions.* San Diego: College Hill Press.

Freeman, F., & Ushijima, T. (1978). Laryngeal muscle activity during stuttering. *Journal of Speech and Hearing Research, 21,* 538–562.

Garber, S. F., & Martin, R. R. (1977). Effects of noise and increased vocal intensity on stuttering. *Journal of Speech and Hearing Research, 20,* 233–240.

Goldiamond, I. (1965). Stuttering and fluency as manipulatable operant response classes. In L. Krasner & L. P. Ullman (Eds.), *Research and behavior modification.* New York: Holt, Rinehart & Winston.

Harmes, M. A., & Malone, J. Y. (1939). The relationship of hearing acuity to stammering. *Journal of Speech Disorders, 4,* 363–370.

Ingham, R. J. (1984). *Stuttering and behavior therapy: Current status and experimental foundations.* San Diego: College Hill Press.

Johnson, W., & Knott, J. R. (1937). Studies in the psychology of stuttering: I. The distribution of moments of stuttering in successive readings of the same material. *Journal of Speech Disorders, 2,* 17–19.

Kidd, K. K. (1980). Genetic models of stuttering. *Journal of Fluency Disorders, 5,* 187–201.

Lechner, B. K. (1979). The effects of delayed auditory feedback and masking on the fundamental frequency of stutterers and nonstutterers. *Journal of Speech and Hearing Research, 22,* 343–353.

Lee, B. S., McGough, W. E., & Peins, M. M. (1973). A new method for stutter therapy. *Folia Phoniatrica, 25,* 186–195.

McClure, J. T. (1983). *Voice onset abruptness of stutterers and normal speakers as a function of white noise masking.* Unpublished master's thesis, Hollins College, Roanoke, VA.

Peters, H. F. M., & Boves, L. (1987). Aerodynamic functions in fluent speech utterances of stutterers and nonstutterers in different speech conditions. In H. F. M. Peters & W. Hulstijn (Eds.), *Speech motor dynamics in stuttering*. New York: Springer-Verlag.

Pindzola, R. H. (1987). Durational characteristics of the fluent speech of stutterers and nonstutterers. *Folia Phoniatrica, 39*, 90–97.

Prins, D. (1972). Personality, stuttering severity and age. *Journal of Speech and Hearing Research, 15*, 148–154.

Ryan, B. P., Van Kirk, B. (1974). The establishment, transfer, and maintenance of fluent speech in 50 stutterers using delayed auditory feedback and operant procedures. *Journal of Speech and Hearing Disorders, 39*, 3–10.

Shapiro, A. I. (1980). An electromyographic analysis of the fluent and dysfluent utterances of several types of stutterers. *Journal of Fluency Disorders, 5*, 203–232.

Silverman, H., & Trotter, D. (1973). Impact of pacing speech with a miniature electronic metronome upon the manner in which a stutterer is perceived. *Behavior Therapy, 4*, 414–419.

Stark, R. E., & Pierce, B. R. (1970). The effects of delayed auditory feedback on a speech related task in stutterers. *Journal of Speech and Hearing Research, 13*, 245–253.

Stephen, S. C. G., & Haggard, M. P. (1980). Acoustic properties of masking/delayed feedback and the fluency of stutterers and controls. *Journals of Speech and Hearing Research, 23*, 527–538.

Sussman, H. M. (1972). What the tongue tells the brain. *Psychological Bulletin, 77*, 262–272.

Van Riper, H. (1971). *The nature of stuttering*. Englewood Cliffs, NJ: Prentice-Hall.

Webster, R. L. (1974). A behavioral analysis of stuttering: Treatment and theory. In K. S. Calhoun, H. L. Adams, & K. M. Mitchell (Eds.), *Innovative treatment methods in psychopathology*. New York: Wiley.

Webster, R. L. (1975). *The precision fluency shaping program: Speech reconstruction for stutterers* (Vol. 1 & 2). Roanoke, VA: Communications Development Corporation.

Webster, R. L. (1978). Empirical considerations regarding controversies in stuttering therapy. In H. Gregory (Ed.), *Controversies in stuttering therapy*. Baltimore: University Park Press.

Webster, R. L. (1980). Evaluation of a target based stuttering therapy. *Journal of Fluency Disorders, 5*, 303–320.

Webster, R. L., & Dorman, M. F. (1970). Decreases in stuttering frequency as a function of continuous and contingent forms of auditory masking. *Journal of Speech and Hearing Research, 13*, 82–86.

Webster, R. L., & Dorman, M. F. (1971). Changes in reliance on auditory feedback cues as a function of oral practice. *Journal of Speech and Hearing Research, 14*, 307–311.

Webster, R. L., & Lubker, B. B. (1968). Interrelationships among fluency producing variables in stuttered speech. *Journal of Speech and Hearing Research, 11*, 754–766.

Webster, R. L., Lubker, B. B., & Schumacher, S. J. (1970). Changes in stuttering frequency as a function of various intervals of delayed auditory feedback. *Journal of Abnormal Psychology, 75*, 45–49.

Webster, R. L., Morgan, B. T., & Cannon, M. W. (1987). Voice onset abruptness in stutterers before and after therapy. In H. F. M. Peters & W. Hulstijn (Eds.), *Speech motor dynamics in stuttering*. New York: Springer-Verlag.

Zimmerman, G. N. (1980). Articulatory dynamics of simple, "fluent" utterances of stutterers and nonstutterers. *Journal of Speech and Hearing Research, 23*, 95–107.

PART III

Psychoneuroimmunology

In the psychoneuroimmunology section, three strong chapters argue for the role of behavioral processes in immune functions. Robert Ader summarizes the impact of conditioning of lowered immunity on mice, Nicholas R. S. Hall and Robert Kvarnes provide us with an overview of potential mechanisms and difficulties in this area, and Maurice G. King and Alan J. Husband deal specifically with some of the mechanisms of conditioned immunity that Hall and Kvarnes suggest are so badly in need of articulation.

In Chapter 9, Ader argues that the strongest data for the role of behavioral processes in immunity derive from studies of conditioned changes in immune processes in his laboratory and others. These studies suggest that immune functions generate stimuli that are detectable to animals and that animals somehow act on the information in these signals. On the basis of other data, Ader maintains that for some genetic strains of mice the importance of certain immune agents for survival through conditioned immunity is a factor in determining effectiveness in producing a conditioned aversion response. Ader's careful attention to proper controls and willingness to admit the limitations of his methods lend even greater credibility to his conjectures regarding the conditioning of immune functions.

In Chapter 10, Hall and Kvarnes argue that individual, physician, environmental, and cultural factors must be taken into account in evaluating treatment outcomes. The central nervous system is probably involved in the transduction of emotional states into an immunomodulatory signal via direct pathways in behaviorally based interventions, placebo effects, and other phenomena. Although there is no direct evidence in man, the mechanism may include hormones. On the other hand, *in vitro* and animal models demonstrate clear connections between the brain and the immune system. Hall and Kvarnes provide a balanced approach to the problems of self-regulation of immune functions and an outline for numerous directions of research that will help to clarify the mechanisms of psychoneuroimmunology.

In Chapter 11, dealing with altered immune reactions, King and Husband explore the determinants of effective unconditional stimuli in the conditioned taste aversion procedure and the components of the unconditional response that renders it more readily conditionable. In addition, they summarize studies they have begun that so far support a central mediation process for the conditioning of sensory CSs to immunological reactions that involve neuropeptides. These fine studies have important theoretical implications for mechanisms of altered immunity through conditioning as well as clinical implications for combining immune agents with behavioral approaches.

CHAPTER 9

Behavior in Autoimmune Mice

Robert Ader

Introduction

Several lines of research suggest that the nervous system and the immune system interact at several levels to constitute an integrated mechanism of defense. For example, recent studies document that lymphoid tissue is innervated by the sympathetic nervous system (Felten, Felten, Bellinger, Carlson, Ackerman, Madden, Olschowka, & Livnat, 1987), and lesions or electrical stimulation of hypothalamic structures alter immunologic reactivity (Roszman, Jackson, Cross, Titus, Markesbery, & Brooks, 1985; Stein, Schleifer, & Keller, 1981). Conversely, activation of the immune system by injecting animals with antigen results in an increase in the firing rate of neurons within the ventromedial hypothalamus (Besedovsky, Sorkin, Keller, Felix, & Haas, 1977). The exogenous alteration of blood levels of a variety of hormones also influences immune responses, and, conversely, activation of the immune system elicits endocrine responses such as changes in adrenocortical steroid and catecholamine levels (Besedovsky, del Rey, Sorkin, DaPrada, Burri, & Honegger, 1983; Besedovsky, Sorkin, Keller, & Muller, 1975; Livnat, Felten, Carlson, Bellinger, & Felten, 1985; Shek & Sabiston, 1983). In this chapter, I propose to discuss some of the evidence for a similar reciprocal relationship between behavior and immune function based, presumably, on the existence of neural and endocrine pathways that provide a link between these adaptive systems.

Robert Ader • Department of Psychiatry, University of Rochester School of Medicine and Dentistry, Rochester, New York 14642, USA.

Effects of Stress on Immune Function

There are abundant data indicating that "stress" is capable of influencing immune responses in man as well as in subhuman animals (Ader, 1981). The results of such studies yield a complex pattern of effects, the interpretation and mechanisms of which are not yet fully understood. The effects of stress are not uniform but appear to depend upon the quality and quantity of environmental or stressful stimulation, the quality and quantity of immunogenic stimulation, the temporal relationship between stressful and immunogenic stimulation, the parameters of immune function chosen for study and the time(s) at which immune function is sampled, a variety of host factors (e.g., species, strain, sex, age), and the interaction among these variables. Nevertheless, direct evidence indicates that stressful stimulation is, indeed, capable of altering antibody- and cell-mediated immune responses.

Stress is also capable of influencing the susceptibility to and/or the progression of a variety of pathophysiological processes from which it is sometimes inferred that stress is influencing the immune system. With respect to cancer, for example, the link between immune function and neoplastic disease does not necessarily provide grounds for inferring a stress-induced change in immune function as the mediating mechanism. Even studies in which immunocompetence or, rather, some parameter of immune function is measured along with the development or progression of cancer provide, at best, correlational data. Few conclusions can be drawn about the relationship between these events unless one is measuring a parameter of immune function that is relevant to the development or metastatic spread of the particular neoplastic process under study. There are data, however, on the effects of psychosocial factors and stress on infectious disease (Plaut & Friedman, 1981) from which we may infer, with some justification, an action of stress on the immune system. And, conversely, there are data to indicate that behavior is altered by the induction or response to a variety of infectious diseases (Dolinsky, Hardy, Burright, & Donovick, 1985; Hotchin & Seegal, 1977; McFarland & Hotchin, 1983, 1984; McFarland, Sikora, & Hotchin, 1981). Bouchon and Will (1982a, 1982b), for example, have described behavioral differences between dwarf and control mice, including a deficit in the maze-learning performance of these immunologically compromised animals. Rats with experimentally induced immune complex disease show less resistance to extinction of an active avoidance response than healthy controls (Hoffman, Shucard, Harbeck, & Hoffman, 1978). Also, the viral infection of mice during early or fetal life can result in a variety of behavioral changes later in life (e.g., Hotchin, Benson & Gardner, 1970; McFarland et al., 1981).

Conditioned Changes in Immunologic Reactivity

From an experimental point of view, conditioned changes in immunologic reactivity are perhaps the most dramatic illustration of the effects of behavior on immune function. Ader and Cohen (1975) found that the single pairing of a novel taste stimulus, saccharin, the conditioned stimulus (CS), with an injection of the immunosuppressive drug cyclophosphamide (CY), the unconditioned stimulus (UCS), resulted in an attenuation of antibody production when conditioned animals were reexposed to the CS at the time of immunization with sheep erythrocytes. These observations have been replicated in other laboratories (Rogers, Reich, Strom, & Carpenter, 1976; Wayner, Flannery, & Singer, 1978) and extended by taste aversion studies measuring the suppression of plaque-forming cell (PFC) responses (Gorczynski, Macrae, & Kennedy, 1982; McCoy, Roszman, Miller, Kelly, & Titus, 1986) and arthritic inflammation (Klosterhalfen & Klosterhalfen, 1983), and attenuation of the PFC response or mitogen responsiveness to a CS previously paired with stressful stimulation (Lysle, Cunnick, Fowler, & Rabin, 1988; Sato, Flood, & Makinodan, 1984). Conditioned changes in cell-mediated immunity have also been observed. Bovbjerg, Ader, and Cohen (1982, 1984) described the acquisition and extinction of the conditioned suppression of a graft-versus-host response in rats, and Gorczynski, Macrae, & Kennedy, (1984) demonstrated the acquisition and extinction of a conditioned enhancement of one parameter of the response to allogenic skin grafting in mice. Other observations of conditioned changes of cell-mediated responses have involved conditioned enhancement of a delayed-type hypersensitivity response (Bovbjerg, Cohen, & Ader, 1987), the use of antilymphocyte serum, a biological rather than a pharmacologic immunosuppressant, as the UCS (Kusnecov, Sivyer, King, Husband, & Cripps, 1983), and the conditioned release of histamine in a discriminative conditioning paradigm (Peeke, Ellman, Dark, Salfi, & Reus, 1987; Russell, Dark, Cummins, Ellman, Calloway, & Peeke, 1984). Still other studies (O'Reilly & Exon, 1986; Solvason, Ghanta, & Hiramoto, 1988) have shown conditioned changes in natural killer cell activity.

Effects of Conditioning in the Pharmacotherapy of Autoimmune Disease

In an effort to assess the biological impact of conditioned immunosuppressive responses, Ader and Cohen (1982) examined the effects of conditioning in the context of a regimen of pharmacotherapy designed to influence the progression of autoimmune disease in New Zealand mice. The (NZBxNZW)F_1 female mouse develops systemic lupus erythematosus and a lethal glomerulonephritis at about 8 to 14 months of age. The development of autoimmune disease, however, can be delayed by weekly treatment with low doses of immunosuppressive drug. Over a 2-month period, (NZBxNZW)F_1 female mice were treated weekly with a low dose of CY (30 mg/kg). Each treatment was paired with the taste of saccharin; that is, these animals were treated under a continuous or 100% reinforcement schedule. A second conditioned group was treated under a 50% reinforcement schedule; that is, saccharin was followed by an injection of CY on only half the trials. A nonconditioned group received the same number of saccharin and CY treatments in a noncontingent manner, and a nontreated control group received saccharin and injections of saline in a noncontingent manner. As hypothesized, the onset of disease and mortality was delayed in conditioned mice treated under a 50% reinforcement schedule relative to nonconditioned animals treated with the same amount of saccharin and CY. Nonconditioned animals did not differ from untreated mice. Thus, by taking advantage of conditioned immunosuppressive responses, the progression of disease was delayed using a cumulative amount of drug that was ineffective by itself in influencing the progression of the autoimmune disease.

Conditioned Taste Aversion in Lupus-Prone (NZBxNZW)F_1 Mice

In the course of this "pharmacotherapy" study, conditioned mice were tested to determine if they would display an aversion to the saccharin solution that had been paired with CY on the previous three trials. Contrary to expectations, there was no evidence of a conditioned aversion to saccharin. Increasing the dose of CY from 30 to 60 and to 120 mg/kg resulted in only a modest decrease in the preference for saccharin relative to plain water in conditioned compared with nonconditioned mice.

The failure to observe a taste aversion to saccharin paired with CY in lupus-prone mice prompted an experiment to determine if the behavior of the (NZBxNZW)F_1 mice was specific to the use of CY as the UCS or reflected a deficit in the learning ability of animals with active autoimmune disease. In humans, 50% of patients with systemic lupus erythematosus have impairments of orientation and perception, show a loss of memory, and display functional symptoms of depression and anxiety (Hughes, 1982; Tan & Rothfield, 1978). Also, Nandy, Lal, Bennett, & Bennett (1983) noted that NZB mice are inferior to normal C57BL/6 mice in performing a conditioned response motivated by the active avoidance of electric shock stimulation. We assessed taste aversion behavior (preference for saccharin) 3 days after (NZBxNZW)F_1 and C57BL/6 mice were conditioned by pairing saccharin with either CY or LiCl. The results of this study (Figure 1) provided no evidence of a generalized learning deficit in the lupus-prone mice. The normal, C57BL/6 animals showed a conditioned aversion to saccharin after a single trial on which saccharin was paired with either CY or LiCl. The (NZBxNZW)F_1 mice showed relatively poor avoidance conditioning when saccharin was paired with CY, but they showed a conditioned aversion to saccharin that had previously been paired with LiCl. Thus, lupus-prone mice do not appear to have a deficit in learning ability, per se, even though they do not display much of an aversion to a distinctive gustatory stimulus associated with the effects of an immunosuppressive drug.

Effects of Immune Status on Behavior in Lupus-Prone Mice

In light of these preliminary observations, it was hypothesized that the avoidance learning behavior of (NZBxNZW)F_1 mice in a conditioned taste aversion paradigm when an immunosuppressive drug was used as the UCS reflected the animals' "recognition" of their immunologic dysregulation. That is, the lupus-prone animals did not acquire a taste aversion to saccharin paired with CY as well as normal mice—or as well

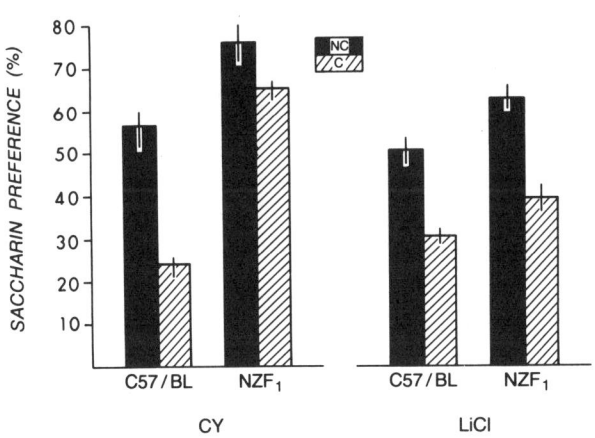

Figure 1. Mean (± SE) preference for saccharin in (NZBxNZW)F_1 and C57BL/6 mice following a single conditioning trial on which consumption of a 0.15% saccharin solution was paired with an ip injection of either CY (240 mg/kg) or LiCl (125 mg/kg). NC = nonconditioned mice. (Reprinted from Ader, Grota, & Cohen, 1987, with permission of the New York Academy of Sciences.)

as they acquired an aversion to saccharin paired with a nonimmunosuppressive drug—because CY, in suppressing the immune system, was acting to promote their ultimate survival. Such a hypothesis is entirely consistent with a large literature on the role of behavior in the regulation of physiological states. Behavioral processes are adopted to maintain body temperature within homeostatic limits (Alberts, 1978; Satinoff & Henderson, 1977) and to meet nutritional requirements (Davis & Levine, 1977; Peck, 1978). Protein-deficient rats, for example, prefer odors that have been associated with a balanced protein food (Booth & Simson, 1971). Hyperglycemic rats show an aversion to a normally preferred saccharin solution (Brookshire, 1974), and adrenalectomized animals choose to drink saline solutions containing corticosterone in preference to plain saline (Castonguay, Smith, & Stern, 1985). The role of learning in the regulation of homeostasis is also illustrated by the fact that salt- or water-loaded diabetes insipidus rats will differentially traverse a maze rewarded by an injection of antidiuretic hormone (Miller, DiCara, & Wolf, 1968), and distinctively flavored, nonpreferred drinking solutions become preferred solutions as a result of their association with recovery from illness or the reinstatement of homeostasis (Garcia, Hankins, & Rusiniak, 1974; Rozin & Kalat, 1971; Zahorik, Maier, & Pies, 1974). The potential role of learning in the regulation of physiological processes is further illustrated by data on the instrumental conditioning of autonomic and visceral responses (Miller, 1969) and the extensive literature on conditioned pharmacologic responses (Eikelboom & Stewart, 1982).

Miller et al. (1968) hypothesized that "at least in cases where homeostasis is mediated via the central nervous system, deviations in any direction, if large enough, can function as a drive and the prompt restoration to normal levels by any means can function as a reward" (p. 686). As these authors point out, sufficiently large deviations from homeostasis may occur only under abnormal circumstances. The dysregulation that characterizes the development of autoimmune disease (Smith, & Steinberg, 1983) may represent an abnormal circumstance under which there is a large deviation from homeostasis, and, considering the impact of conditioning in modulating immune responses (Ader & Cohen, 1985) and the development of autoimmune disease (Ader, 1985; Ader & Cohen, 1982), the development of autoimmune disease in lupus-prone animals may constitute a sensitive model in which to examine the role of learning in the maintenance of homeostasis.

It seemed reasonable, therefore, to hypothesize that the relatively poor aversive conditioning of the lupus-prone (NZBxNZW)F_1 mice to a taste stimulus that was associated with the effects of an immunosuppressive drug was an adaptive response to the immunorestorative effects of that drug in animals that spontaneously develop autoimmune disease. However, CY has noxious gastrointestinal consequences even in lupus-prone mice. Thus, the hypothesis that lupus-prone mice are "aware" of their immunologic dysregulation and are capable of "recognizing" the immunorestorative effects of CY would, operationally, translate into the hypothesis that there would be an interaction between the degree of immune dysfunction and the dose of CY that would determine the response to a distinctive taste stimulus that was paired with an immunosuppressive drug. That is, with advancing disease, it would require higher doses of immunosuppressive drug—or, for example, a larger number of conditioning trials at a constant dose of drug—to induce a taste aversion in lupus-prone mice than in a healthy control group. It follows, conversely, that, compared with healthy animals, mice with autoimmune disease would acquire a taste aversion more rapidly or at lower doses of drug when an immunoenhancing agent was used as the unconditional stimulus. Furthermore, if learning processes can be enlisted to correct immunologically based deviations from homeostasis, these predictions would be reversed in other animals for whom imunosuppressing and immunoenhancing drugs were acting to potentiate or attenuate, respectively, the homeostatic imbalance.

Differences in taste aversion learning were explored in the lupus-prone MRL strain of mice. These animals were derived from the LG (75%), AKR (12.6%), C3H (12.1%), and the C57BL/6 (0.3%) strains (Murphy & Roths, 1978). A spontaneous autosomal recessive mutation divided the MRL mice into two congenic inbred strains: one substrain, MRL-lpr/lpr, carries the lpr (lymphoproliferative) gene, and the other, MRL +/+ does not, but these strains share at least 89% of their genomes. In contrast to $(NZBxNZW)F_1$ animals, MRL-lpr/lpr mice develop symptoms of disease (lymphadenopathy and anti-DNA antibodies) relatively early in life (10–12 weeks), and there is a 50% mortality in males and females at approximately 5 to 6 months of age, with females developing disease only slightly more rapidly than males. MRL +/+ mice do not develop autoimmune disease until relatively late in life, and a 50% mortality is not reached until approximately 17 and 23 months of age in females and males, respectively. The reasons for studying MRL mice were based on the practical consideration that manifest symptoms of disease occurred relatively early in life and on the strategic advantages of having a healthy, congenic strain of control mice.

The experiments described below were designed to elaborate on the observations that there is a difference in taste aversion behavior of lupus-prone and normal mice when an immunosuppressive drug is used as the UCS. Thus, the learning performance of MRL-lpr/lpr and

MRL +/+ mice in response to CY, an immunosuppressive drug, and lithium chloride was assessed before as well as after the development of symptoms of autoimmune disease. Conditioning performance was also assessed in a situation involving the passive avoidance of electric shock. In addition, a preliminary study examined the voluntary consumption of a distinctively flavored drinking solution containing different concentrations of cyclophosphamide.

Taste Aversion Learning in MRL-lpr/lpr and MRL +/+ Mice

Six-week-old MRL-lpr/lpr and MRL +/+ mice were individually housed and maintained under a 12-hour light-dark cycle (light onset at 7:00 a.m.) in a temperature- and humidity-controlled colony room with food and water provided *ad libitum*. Experiments on animals with manifest symptoms of disease began when 80% of the MRL-lpr/lpr mice displayed a palpable lymphadenopathy (22 and 25 weeks of age for females and males, respectively). The animals were randomly assigned to treatment groups and gradually adapted to and then maintained on a 1-hour drinking period (between 9:00 and 11:00 a.m.) each day throughout the experiment. On the first conditioning trial, mice were provided with a single bottle containing chocolate milk (undiluted Sealtest chocolate homogenized whole milk), the conditioned stimulus (CS), in place of their usual plain tap water. Immediately thereafter, groups were injected intraperitoneally (ip) with vehicle (water) or 25, 50, 100, or 200 mg/kg CY. Nonconditioned mice were injected with drug at the same time, but they had been exposed to chocolate milk 1 week earlier.

Taste aversion performance was assessed at 2- to 3-day intervals after conditioning by providing mice with two drinking bottles, one of which contained plain water and the other chocolate milk. Following each test hour, the animals were again injected with vehicle or drug. Consumption was determined by weighing the bottles before and after the drinking period, and consumption of chocolate milk was recorded as a percentage of total fluid intake.

It should be noted, first, that there were no strain differences in the absolute amounts of chocolate milk consumed by conditioned and nonconditioned animals on their initial exposure to the flavored solution, and on the first, post-conditioning test trial, there were no differences in the preference scores of conditioned MRL-lpr/lpr and MRL +/+ mice. Thus, it becomes unlikely that any subsequent differences in avoidance behavior could be attributed to a differential, nonassociative effect of CY in these congenic substrains. Data from the initial test trial (Figure 2) also showed that there were no differences between conditioned and non-

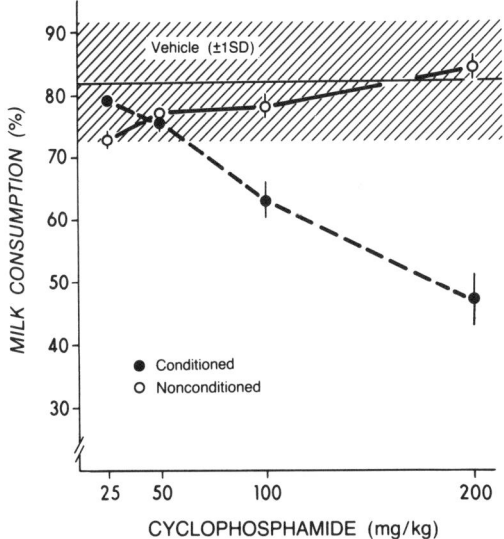

Figure 2. Consumption of chocolate milk (mean ± *SE* percentage of total fluid intake) following a single trial on which conditioned MRL-lpr/lpr and MRL +/+ mice (combined) received an ip injection of different doses of cyclophosphamide (CY) and nonconditioned groups (combined) received chocolate milk and CY in an unpaired manner (*N* = 27–32 conditioned and 12–15 unconditioned mice per group). (Reprinted from Grota, Ader, & Cohen, 1987, with permission of Academic Press.)

conditioned animals at doses of 25 and 50 mg/kg CY; at doses of 100 and 200 mg/kg CY, however, conditioned mice displayed a reduced preference for the CS solution compared with nonconditioned animals, indicating that the decreased consumption of chocolate milk was the result of its pairing with CY and not a direct effect of CY per se.

Figure 3 shows the number of animals that met a criterion for taste aversion learning (defined by the performance of MRL +/+ mice) within 10 trials. There were no differences between MRL-lpr/lpr and MRL +/+ mice at the two lowest doses of CY, which induced a taste aversion in less than half the animals, and there were no strain differences at the highest dose of CY, which induced a taste aversion in more than 90% of the animals. At 100 mg/kg CY, a dose that was effective in differentiating between MRL-lpr/lpr and MRL +/+ mice in previous experiments (Ader, Grota, & Cohen, 1987), fewer than 50% of the MRL-lpr/lpr mice reached the conditioning criterion, whereas 92% of the congenic control mice displayed a taste aversion to chocolate milk.

The actual number of trials required to achieve the acquisition crite-

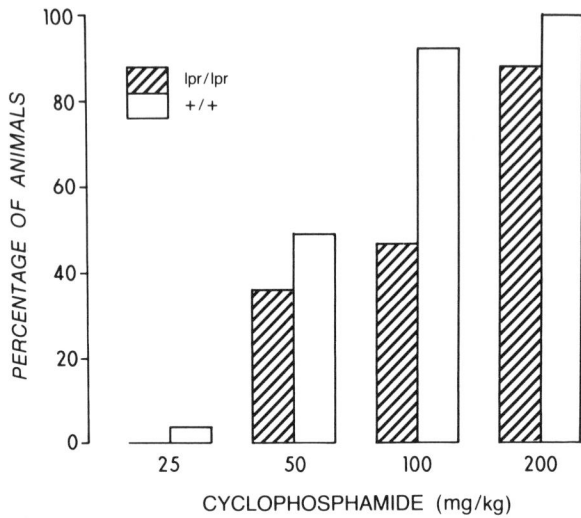

Figure 3. Percentage of MRL-lpr/lpr and MRL +/+ mice that attained the criterion for acquisition of a taste aversion within 10 conditioning trials ($N = 13$–17 per group). (Reprinted from Grota, Ader, & Cohen, 1987, with permission of Academic Press.)

rion did not prove adequate for comparing the performance of MRL-lpr/lpr and MRL +/+ mice; asymptotic performance occurred after only a few trials. However, all conditioned animals were exposed to chocolate milk followed by an injection of CY on the first three trials. Thus, a direct comparison of MRL-lpr/lpr and MRL +/+ mice, unconfounded by differences in the number of subsequent reinforced exposures to the CS, could be made for the first three preference tests. As predicted, there was an interaction between Strain and Dose of CY and, in this instance, Trials. Neither strain acquired a taste aversion at the low doses of CY, and both strains showed a conditioned aversion at the high dose of CY. However, as shown in Figure 4, MRL-lpr/lpr mice did not show an aversion to a taste stimulus paired with an intermediate dose of CY that was effective in inducing a taste aversion in MRL +/+ animals; that is, it evidently requires a higher dose of CY to induce an aversion to a distinctive taste stimulus in mice with manifest symptoms of autoimmune disease than in healthy, congenic control animals.

When the same experiment is conducted in animals that are 10 weeks of age—i.e., before the development of lymphadenopathy in MRL-lpr/lpr mice—the rate of development of conditioned taste aversions varies directly with the dose of CY, but there are no significant

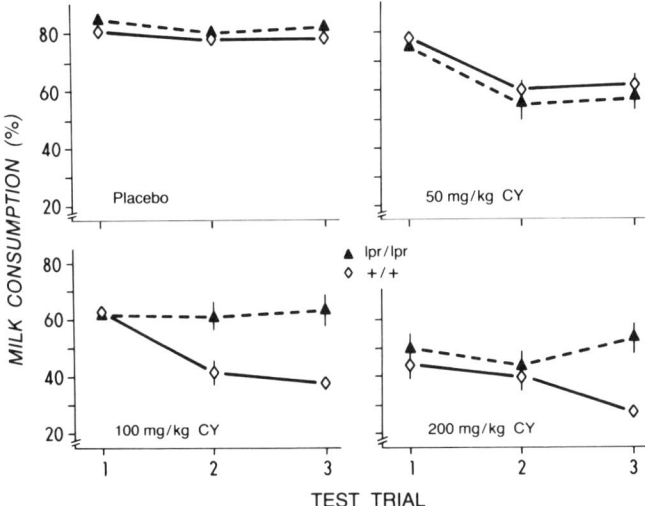

Figure 4. Taste aversion performance in mice conditioned after the development of lymphadenopathy in MRL-lpr/lpr mice; mean ± SE preference for chocolate milk in MRL-lpr/lpr and MRL +/+ mice following each of three conditioning trials on which chocolate milk consumption was paired with different doses of CY (N = 11–19 per group). (Reprinted from Grota, Ader, & Cohen, 1987, with permission of Academic Press.)

differences between the two strains (Figure 5). This finding, which, again, verifies preliminary observations (Ader et al., 1987), supports the hypothesis that the avoidance performance of lupus-prone mice in response to an immunosuppressive drug is related to the presence of active disease. As previously observed in New Zealand hybrid mice, lupus-prone MRL-lpr/lpr mice do not appear to have a deficit in learning ability, as such; there are no differences between 10- and 18-week-old male and female MRL-lpr/lpr and MRL +/+ mice in the acquisition of a taste aversion based on the pairing of chocolate milk with lithium chloride or in the acquisition of a passive avoidance response based on electric shock stimulation (Grota, Ader, & Cohen, 1987).

Voluntary Consumption of Cyclophosphamide by Lupus-Prone Mice

If, as hypothesized, the failure to display a taste aversion to a flavored solution paired with the noxious gastrointestinal effects of an immunosuppressive drug actually represents the animal's recognition of the effects of the drug in ameliorating symptoms of autoimmune dis-

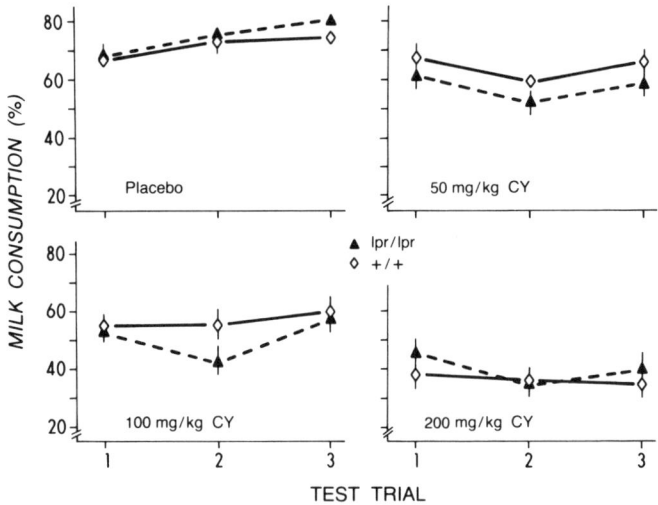

Figure 5. Taste aversion performance in mice conditioned before the development of lymphadenopathy; mean ± SE preference for chocolate milk in MRL-lpr/lpr and MRL +/+ mice following each of three conditioning trials on which chocolate milk consumption was paired with different doses of CY ($N = 20$ per group). (Reprinted from Grota, Ader, & Cohen, 1987, with permission of Academic Press.)

ease, animals with lupus might, under certain circumstances, be capable of learning to voluntarily consume cyclophosphamide if it was made sufficiently palatable. This possibility was examined after determining a range of concentrations of CY added to undiluted chocolate milk that mice would drink in a volume that was sufficient to suppress immunologic reactivity. Preliminary observations in male MRL-lpr/lpr mice suggest that this is, in fact, the case.

Five days each week, water-deprived MRL-lpr/lpr and MRL +/+ mice, 19 to 20 weeks of age (i.e., after lymphadenopathy had developed in the lpr animals), were provided with chocolate milk containing 0, 0.2, 0.4, or 0.8 mg/ml CY. The single drinking bottle containing chocolate milk was available for 1 hour; plain water was provided for 1 hour in the afternoon of that same day. Based on five to nine mice per group in each of two replications of this experiment, there was an inverse relationship between the amount of chocolate milk consumed and the concentration of CY. At the end of 1 week, there were no differences between MRL-lpr/lpr and MRL +/+ mice. However, after 2 or more weeks, MRL-lpr/lpr mice consumed significantly more chocolate milk containing 0.2 and 0.4 mg/ml CY than did MRL +/+ mice. The substrains did not differ in their consumption of plain chocolate milk, and they did not differ in their (significantly reduced) consumption of the most concentrated CY solution. Furthermore, the animals with lupus consumed sufficient volumes of the CY solution to reduce lymphadenopathy and anti-DNA antibody titer over the course of 4 weeks.

Thus far, we have been unable to discriminate between MRL-lpr/lpr and MRL +/+ mice that are given a choice between chocolate milk containing CY and either plain chocolate milk or plain water. Even when CY is diluted in chocolate milk, it is a solution that is avoided if an alternative is available. Therefore, a single bottle containing the CY solution was used to ensure exposure to the drug (a procedure that, in principle, may have to be introduced before preference testing would be possible). It is important to note that there were no differences in the consumption of unadulterated chocolate milk—or in the consumption of plain water later in the day—between MRL-lpr/lpr and MRL +/+ mice, and there were no substrain differences in the initial consumption of chocolate milk containing CY—i.e., during the first week of daily testing. These observations would be consistent with the interpretation that the subsequent differences between MRL-lpr/lpr and MRL +/+ animals were the result of learning on the part of the animals with lupus. The observation that animals with autoimmune disease would consume more of a chocolate milk solution containing an immunosuppressive drug than would healthy, congenic control animals is in keeping with the substrain differences in taste aversion conditioning described above and with the notion that the animal with lupus is capable of behaving in a manner that alleviates symptoms of an immunologic dysregulation.

Discussion

Since the immunosuppressive effects of CY act to correct the immunologic dysregulation of lupus-prone mice, (Shiraki, Fujiwara, & Tomura, 1984; Smith, Chused, & Steinberg, 1984) it was hypothesized that higher concentrations of CY would be required to induce a taste aversion in animals with autoimmune disease than in a normal control group. As predicted, lupus-prone MRL-lpr/lpr mice with manifest symptoms of autoimmune disease do not display an aversion to a taste stimulus that had previously been paired with the noxious and immunosuppressive effects of a dose of CY that is effective in inducing a conditional taste aversion in healthy, congenic MRL +/+ mice. These results confirm earlier observations (Ader et al., 1987) of differences in conditioning to an immunosuppressive UCS between autoimmune

(NZBxNZW)F_1 and healthy C57BL/6 mice. They also replicate previously reported differences between MRL-lpr/lpr and MRL +/+ mice. Since these are congenic substrains, the observed differences would not appear to be attributable to any genetic differences other than those related to the immunologic status of the animals. When conditioning performance is assessed before MRL-lpr/lpr mice show manifest symptoms of disease, there are no differences between the lpr and +/+ substrains, and when taste aversion conditioning is assessed in response to LiCl rather than CY or in the passive avoidance of electric shock stimulation, there are no differences between lpr and +/+ substrains. These observations lend further support to the interpretation that the differences in behavior between MRL-lpr/lpr and Mrl +/+ in response to an immunosuppressive drug are a reflection of differences in the immunologic status of these congenic strains.

One cannot completely eliminate the possibility that there are sensory threshold differences between MRL-lpr/lpr and MRL +/+ mice. It is not likely that the differences in learning can be attributed to substrain differences in taste thresholds because nonconditioned MRL-lpr/lpr mice displayed a slightly *lower* preference for chocolate milk than did similarly treated MRL +/+ mice. One cannot be sure, however, that the noxious gastrointestinal effects of CY are equally salient for animals with active autoimmune disease in comparison with healthy controls even though our (unpublished) data on pain thresholds to exteroceptive stimulation have failed thus far to discriminate between MRL-lpr/lpr and MRL +/+ mice. We are continuing to assess differences in the palatability of different CS solutions and gustatory as well as pain thresholds between male and female MRL-lpr/lpr and Mrl +/+ mice at different ages.

As noted above, other studies (e.g., Hoffman et al., 1978; Hotchin & Seegal, 1977; McFarland et al., 1981; McFarland & Hotchin, 1984) have documented differences in behavior between animals with autoimmune disease and healthy controls. Nandy et al. (1983) and Forster, Popper, Retz, and Lal (1987) found that lupus-prone strains of mice that show early-onset disease (including MRL-lpr/lpr mice) show poorer learning of an *active* avoidance response than age-matched normal (C57BL/6) or healthy, late-onset lupus-prone (MRL +/+) mice. Also, performance deficits among NZB mice were correlated with the early development of brain-reactive antibodies in these animals. In the *passive* avoidance paradigms used in our studies, however, we have been unable to detect differences in performance between (NZBxNZW)F_1 and C57BL/6 or between MRL-lpr/lpr and MRL +/+ mice except when an immunosuppressive drug was used as the unconditioned stimulus to induce a taste aversion.

The present data indicate that the performance of MRL-lpr/lpr and (NZBxNZW)F_1 mice in response to cyclophosphamide, and immunosuppressive drug, is related to their immunologic disorder. The results are consistent with the hypothesis that lupus-prone animals with manifest signs of autoimmune disease would not avoid a gustatory stimulus associated with doses of cyclophosphamide that are effective in inducing taste aversions in control mice because the effects of the drug, although noxious, act to correct the autoimmune disorder.

If behavior can reflect immunologic processes, one would infer that alterations in immune function generate signals that can be detected by the central nervous system (CNS). Consistent with the notion of the immune system acting as a sensory organ (Blalock, 1984), our preliminary data on the voluntary consumption of a drinking solution containing CY suggest, further, that the organism is capable of acting on the information being transmitted from the immune system to the brain. It is not yet clear, however, whether any such signals emanating from the immune system have a direct and/or an indirect effect on the nervous system and on behavior. Indirect or nonspecific signals might include fluctuations in the level of hormones and neurotransmitter substances. Several studies have shown that the response to antigenic stimulation includes neuroendocrine changes mediated by products of activated lymphocytes (e.g., Besedovsky et al., 1983). Indirect effects on the CNS might also include secondary signals derived from the peripheral lymphoid and nonlymphoid targets of immunologic dysregulations—e.g., changes in the lymph nodes or kidneys. The neuroendocrine concomitants of autoimmune disease might thus contribute to differences in the behavior of lupus-prone and normal mice. However, some additional mechanism needs to be postulated to account for the fact that, in our studies, behavioral differences did not occur in all learning situations but were confined to taste aversion learning situations in which CY, an immunosuppressive agent, was used as the unconditioned stimulus.

If the animal with lupus responds differently to the effects of immunosuppressive and nonimmunosuppressive stimuli, one may postulate that the drug-induced immunologic changes are capable of being detected by the CNS. If animals with autoimmune disease do not (except at high doses) avoid the noxious effects of CY because of its perceivable effects in restoring homeostasis, we would hypothesize that lupus-prone mice with active disease would acquire a taste aversion more rapidly (or at lower doses) than healthy controls in response to drugs that exacerbated their autoimmune disorder. Such a hypothesis is entirely consistent with a large literature on the role of behavior in regulating a variety of physiological states and, more specifically, with studies showing that taste stimuli associated with the restoration of homeostasis or the recovery from experimentally induced alterations of physiological function become preferred stimuli (e.g., Rozin & Kalat, 1971). The suggestion that animals with lupus voluntarily consume more of a drinking solution containing CY than do healthy, congenic control mice—and consume a volume sufficient to attenuate some of the symptoms of the autoimmune disease—is in keeping with the notion that sufficiently large deviations from homeostasis (even within the immune system) can motivate behaviors that are reinforced by the restoration of a physiologic balance (Miller et al., 1968). These preliminary observations also implicate instrumental learning processes in the regulation of immune function.

The source(s) and nature of the postulated signals emanating from the immune system and the reception of these signals within the CNS and/or by peripheral target organs need to be explored. Whatever these may be, these observations suggest that, as might be expected on the basis of the bidirectional influences of neural and immune function and endocrine and immune function, behavior is capable of modifying immune responses, and immune functioning has implications for behavior. Under some conditions, it appears that behavioral processes can serve an *in vivo* immunoregulatory mechanism to maintain or restore homeostasis. At the very least, these data provide additional evidence for CNS–immune system interactions and expand the role to behavior in the regulation of physiological processes.

ACKNOWLEDGMENTS. The research described in this chapter was supported by a Research Scientist Award (K3-MH6318) from the National Institute of Mental Health and by research grants from the National Institute for Neurological and Communicative Diseases and Stroke (NS22228) and from RJR Nabisco, Inc.

References

Ader, R. (Ed.). (1981). *Psychoneuroimmunology*. New York: Academic Press.
Ader, R. (1985). Conditioned immunopharmacologic effects in animals: Implications for a conditioning model of pharmacotherapy. In L. White, B. Tursky, & G. Schwartz (Eds.), *Placebo: Theory, research, and mechanisms*. New York: Guilford.
Ader, R., & Cohen, N. (1975). Behaviorally conditioned immunosuppression. *Psychosomatic Medicine, 37,* 333–340.
Ader, R., & Cohen, N. (1982). Behaviorally conditioned immunosuppression and murine systemic lupus erythematosus. *Science, 215,* 1534–1536.
Ader, R., & Cohen, N. (1985). CNS-immune system interactions: Conditioning phenomena. *Behavioral and Brain Science, 8,* 379–426.

Ader, R., Grota, L. J., & Cohen, N. (1987). Conditioning phenomena and immune function. *Annals of the New York Academy of Sciences, 496,* 532–544.
Alberts, J. R. (1978). Huddling by rat pups: Group behavioral mechanisms of temperature regulation and energy conservation. *Journal of Comparative and Physiological Psychology, 92,* 231–245.
Besedovsky, H. O., Sorkin, E., Keller, M., & Muller, J. (1975). Changes in blood hormone levels during the immune response. *Proceedings of the Society for Experimental Biology and Medicine, 150,* 446—470.
Besedovsky, H. O., Sorkin, E., Felix, R., & Haas, H. (1977). Hypothalamic changes during the immune response. *European Journal of Immunology, 7,* 325–328.
Besedovsky, H. O., del Rey, A. E., Sorkin, E., DaPrada, M., Burri, R., & Honegger, C. (1983). The immune response evokes changes in brain noradrenergic neurons. *Science, 221,* 564–566.
Blalock, J. E. (1984). The immune system as a sensory organ. *Journal of Immunology, 132,* 1067–1070.
Booth, D. A., & Simson, P. C. (1971). Food preferences acquired by association with variations in amino acid nutrition. *Quarterly Journal of Experimental Psychology, 23,* 135–145.
Bouchon, R., & Will, B. (1982a). Effects of early enriched and restricted environments on the exploratory and locomotor activity of dwarf mice. *Behavioral and Neural Biology, 35,* 174–186.
Bouchon, R., & Will, B. (1982b). Effets de condition d'élevage après le sevrage sur les performances d'apprentissage des souris "dwarf." *Physiology and Behavior, 28,* 971–978.
Bovbjerg, D., Ader, R., & Cohen, N. (1982). Behaviorally conditioned suppression of a graft-vs-host response. *Proceedings of the National Academy of Sciences of the USA, 79,* 583–585.
Bovbjerg, N., Ader, R., & Cohen, N. (1984). Acquisition and extinction of conditioned suppression of a graft-vs-host response in the rat. *Journal of Immunology, 132,* 111–113.
Bovbjerg, D., Cohen, N., & Ader, R. (1987). Behaviorally conditioned enhancement of delayed-type hypersensitivity in the mouse. *Brain Behavioral Immunity, 1,* 64–71.
Brookshire, K. H. (1974). Changes in rats' preference for saccharin and sodium chloride solutions following injection of alloxan monohydrate. *Journal of Comparative and Physiological Psychology, 87,* 1061–1068.
Castonguay, T. W., Smith, L., & Stern, J. S. (1985). Corticosterone self-administration by adrenalectomized rats. *Federation Proceedings* (Abstract No. 6718).
Davis, H., & Levine, M. W. (1977). A model for the control of ingestion. *Psychological Review, 84,* 379–412.
Dolinsky, Z. S., Hardy, C. A., Burright, R. G., & Donovick, P. J. (1985). The progression of behavioral and pathological effects of the parasite *Toxocara canis* in the mouse. *Physiology and Behavior, 35,* 33–42.
Eikelboom, R., & Stewart, J. (1982). Conditioning of drug-induced physiological responses. *Psychological Review, 89,* 507–528.
Felten, D. L., Felten, S. Y., Bellinger, D. L., Carlson, S. L., Ackerman, K. D., Madden, K. S., Olschowka, J. A., & Livnat, S. (1987). Noradrenergic sympathetic neural interactions with the immune system: Structure and function. *Immunological Review, 100,* 225–260.
Forster, M. J., Popper, M. D., Retz, K. C., & Lal, H. (1987). Age differences in acquisition and retention of one-way avoidance learning in C547BL/6Nnia and autoimmune mice. *Behavioral and Neural Biology, 49,* 139–151.

Garcia, J., Hankins, W. G., & Rusiniak, K. W. (1974). Behavioral regulation of the milieu interne in man and rat. *Science, 185,* 824–831.
Gorczynski, R. M., Macrae, S., & Kennedy, M. (1982). Conditioned immune response associated with allogenic skin grafts in mice. *Journal of Immunology, 129,* 701–709.
Gorczynski, R. M., Macrae, S., & Kennedy, M. (1984). Factors involved in the classical conditioning of antibody responses in mice. In R. Ballieux, J. Fielding, & A. L'Abbatte (Eds.), *Breakdown in human adaptation to stress: Towards a multidisciplinary approach.* Boston: Martinus Nijhof.
Grota, L. J., Ader, R., & Cohen, N. (1987). Taste aversion learning in autoimmune Mrl-lpr/lpr and Mrl +/+ mice. *Brain Behavior and Immunity, 1,* 238–250.
Hoffman, S. A., Shucard, D. M., Harbeck, R. J., & Hoffman, A. A. (1978). Chronic immune complex disease: Behavioral and immunological correlates. *Neuropathology and Experimental Neurology, 37,* 426–436.
Hotchin, J., & Seegal, R. (1977). Virus-induced behavioral alteration of mice. *Science, 196,* 671–674.
Hotchin, J., Benson, L., & Gardner, J. (1970). Mother-infant interaction in lymphocytic choriomeningitis virus infection of the newborn mouse: The effect of maternal health on mortality of offspring. *Pediatric Research, 4,* 194–200.
Hughes, G. R. V. (1982). Systemic lupus erythematosus. In P. Lockman & D. Peters (Eds.), *Aspects of immunology,* (Vol. 2). London: Blackwell.
Klosterhalfen, W., & Klosterhalfen, S. (1983). Pavlovian conditioning of immunosuppression modifies adjuvant arthritis in rats. *Behavioral Neuroscience, 97,* 663–666.
Kusnecov, A. W., Sivyer, M., King, M. G., Husband, A. J., Cripps, A. W., & Clancy, R. L. (1983). *Journal of Immunology, 130,* 2117–2120.
Livnat, S., Felten, S. Y., Carlson, S. L., Bellinger, D. L., & Felten, D. L. (1985). Involvement of peripheral and central catecholamine systems in neural-immune interactions. *Journal of Neuroimmunology, 10,* 5–30.
Lysle, D. T., Cunnick, J. E., Fowler, H., & Rabin, B. S. (1988). Pavlovian conditioning of shock-induced suppression of lymphocyte reactivity: Acquisition, extinction, and preexposure effects. *Life Sciences, 42,* 2185–2194.
McCoy, D. F., Roszman, T. L., Miller, J. S., Kelly, K. S., & Titus, M. J. (1986). Some parameters of conditioned immunosuppression: Species differences and CS-US delay. *Physiology and Behavior, 36,* 731–736.
McFarland, D. J., & Hotchin, J. (1983). Host genetics and the behavioral sequelae to herpes encephalitis in mice. *Physiology and Behavior, 30,* 881–884.
McFarland, D. J., & Hotchin, J. (1984). Behavioral sequelae to early postnatal cytomegalovirus infection in mice. *Physiology and Behavior, 12,* 45–47.
McFarland, D. J., Sikora, E., & Hotchin, J. (1981). Age at infection as a determinant of the behavioral effects of herpes encephalitis in mice. *Physiology and Behavior, 9,* 87–89.
Miller, N. E. (1969). Learning of visceral and glandular responses. *Science, 163,* 434–445.
Miller, N. E., DiCara, L. V., & Wolf, G. (1968). Homeostasis and reward: T-maze learning induced by manipulating antidiuretic hormone. *American Journal of Physiology, 215,* 684–686.
Murphy, E. D., & Roths, J. B. (1978). Autoimmunity and lymphoproliferation. Induction by mutant gene lpr, and accelerated by a male-associated factor in strain BXSB mice. In N. R. Rose, P. E. Bigazzi, & N. L. Warner (Eds.), *Genetic control of autoimmune disease.* New York: Elsevier/North Holland.
Nandy, K., Lal, H., Bennett, M., & Bennett, D. (1983). Correlation between a learning disorder and elevated brain-reactive antibodies in aged C57BL/6 and young NZB mice. *Life Sciences, 33,* 1499–1503.

O'Reilly, C. A., & Exon, J. H. (1986). Conditioned suppression of the natural killer cell response in rats. *Physiology and Behavior, 37,* 759–764.

Peck, J. W. (1978). Rats defend different body weights depending on palatability and accessibility of their food. *Journal of Comparative Physiology and Psychology, 92,* 555–570.

Peeke, H. V. S., Ellman, G., Dark, K., Salfi, M., & Reus, V. I. (1987). Cortisol and behaviorally conditioned histamine release. *Annals of the New York Academy of Sciences, 496,* 583–587.

Plaut, S. M., & Friedman, S. B. (1981). Psychosocial factors in infectious disease. In R. Ader (Ed.), *Psychoneuroimmunology.* New York: Academic Press.

Rogers, M. P., Reich, P., Strom, T. B., & Carpenter, C. B. (1976). Behaviorally conditioned immunosuppression: Replication of a recent study. *Psychosomatic Medicine, 38,* 447–451.

Roszman, T. L., Jackson, J. C., Cross, J., Titus, M. J., Markesbery, W. R., & Brooks, W. H. (1985). Neuroanatomic and neurotransmitter influences on immune function. *Journal of Immunology, 135,* 769s–772s.

Rozin, P., & Kalat, J. W. (1971). Specific hungers and poison avoidance as adaptive specializations of learning. *Psychological Review, 78,* 459–486.

Russell, M., Dark, K. A., Cummins, R. W., Ellman, G., Callaway, E., & Peeke, H. V. S. (1984). Learned histamine release. *Science, 225,* 733–734.

Satinoff, E., & Henderson, R. (1977). Thermoregulatory behavior. In W. K. Konig, & E. R. Staddon (Eds.), *Handbook of operant behavior.* Englewood, NJ: Prentice-Hall.

Sato, K., Flood, J. F., & Makinodan, T. (1984). Influence of conditioned psychological stress on immunological recovery in mice exposed to low-dose x-irradiation. *Radiation Research, 98,* 381–388.

Shek, P. N., & Sabiston, B. H. (1983). Neuroendocrine regulation of immune processes: Change in circulating corticosterone levels induced by the primary antibody response in mice. *International Journal of Immunopharmacology, 5,* 23–33.

Shiraki, M., Fujiwara, M., & Tomura, S. (1984). Long term administration of cyclophosphamide in MRL/l mice: I. The effects on the development of immunological abnormalities and lupus nephritis. *Clinical and Experimental Immunology, 55,* 333–339.

Smith, H. R., & Steinberg, A. D. (1983). Autoimmunity—A perspective. *Annual Review of Immunology, 1,* 175—210.

Smith, H. R., Chused, T. M., & Steinberg, A. D. (1984). Cyclophosphamide-induced changes in the MRL-lpr/lpr mouse: Effects upon cellular composition, immune function, and disease. *Clinical Immunology and Immunopathology, 30,* 51–61.

Solvason, H. B., Ghanta, V. K., & Hiramoto, R. N. (1988). Conditioned augmentation of natural killer cell activity: Independence from nociceptive effects and dependence on Interferon-β. *Journal of Immunology, 140,* 661–665.

Stein, M., Schleifer, S. J., & Keller, R. E. (1981). Hypothalamic influences on immune responses. In R. Ader (Ed.), *Psychoneuroimmunology.* New York: Academic Press.

Tan, E., & Rothfield, N. F. (1978). Systemic lupus erythematosus. In M. Samter (Ed.), *Immunologic diseases* (Vol. 2, pp. 1038–1060). Boston: Little, Brown.

Wayner, E. A., Flannery, G. R., & Singer, G. (1978). Effect of taste aversion conditioning on the primary antibody response to sheep red blood cells and *Brucella abortus* in the albino rat. *Physiology and Behavior, 21,* 995–1000.

Zahorik, D. M., Maier, S. F., & Pies, R. W. (1974). Preference for tastes paired with recovery from thiamine deficiency in rats: Appetitive conditioning or learned safety? *Journal Comparative Physiology Psychology, 87,* 1083–1091.

CHAPTER 10

Behavioral Intervention and Disease
Possible Mechanisms

Nicholas R. S. Hall and Robert Kvarnes

Introduction

Over 30 years ago a patient with severe cancer insisted that he be treated with an experimental drug called Krebiozen. At that time it was regarded by its proponents to be a miracle cure for the type of cancer that the patient had. After a single treatment the patient's cancer "melted like snowballs on a hot stove," and within a short period of time he was able to resume his normal activities. However, upon the patient's reading articles that revealed Krebiozen to be ineffective, his condition once again worsened and his cancer began to metastasize. His physician encouraged his patient not to believe the studies that he had read about and introduced a new and improved version of the same drug. Following the administration of this new and improved form of Krebiozen the patient's condition improved significantly. The new and improved drug was merely water, and his doctor was Bruno Klopfer (1957), who reported this case history in the *Journal of Projective Techniques*.

This case represents one of countless examples of the dramatic impact that placebo treatments can have. On a larger scale, a classic example of a surgically induced placebo effect was the internal ligation of the

---

Nicholas R. S. Hall • Department of Psychiatry and Behavioral Medicine, University of South Florida, Tampa, Florida 33613, USA.   Robert Kvarnes • Washington School of Psychiatry, Washington, D.C., USA.

mammary artery to relieve the pain of angina pectoris. Although surgeons who were skeptical of the operation's effectiveness reported only moderate success with the procedure, others found that it could significantly relieve the pain in up to 75% of the patients so treated. In a subsequent double-blind study it was determined that internal ligation was no more beneficial than sham surgery in which skin incisions alone were made (Beecher, 1961). Both objective and subjective measures revealed that the placebo surgery was just as effective as the real surgery, with a larger number of patients who received sham operations reporting subjective improvement. In addition, placebo surgery was found to be correlated with a reduced utilization of nitroglycerin to relieve pain, an increased ability to exercise, and increased work tolerance (Cobb, Thomas, Dillard, Merendino, & Bruce, 1959). Numerous other conditions have proven responsive to placebo treatment and range from organic brain disorders, such as Parkinson's disease, to allergies and rheumatoid arthritis. Psychiatric disorders including depression, anxiety, and, in some instances, schizophrenia can also be alleviated through the use of placebos. These have been reviewed in a recent volume by White, Tursky, and Schwartz (1985).

Today a growing number of physicians and researchers acknowledge that placebos are not simply manifestations of noise in the system that serve only to confound clinical trials of drug efficacy. While they differ as to how various placebos should be categorized, most physicians agree that factors pertaining to the individual as well as to the physician are critical in order for the patient to maximally benefit from the prescribed treatment. It is also known that environmental as well as cultural factors are important and have to be considered when evaluating the effects of a treatment. Even the large pharmaceutical companies acknowledge the beneficial effect of placebos and for that reason usually package medical stimulants in red or pink capsules because they work better than blue ones (Evans, 1984). Unfortunately, placebos can also mimic active drugs in adverse ways. They have been found to produce toxic reactions as well as other undesirable side effects (Lasagna, Laties, & Dohan, 1958). It is in this framework that behavior-based strategies as intervention for chronic disease should be evaluated.

Emotions and Health

As early as the 2nd century A.D. Galen noted that one's emotional state could be correlated with disease susceptibility. He observed in his writings that melancholy individuals are more susceptible to cancer than are sanguine individuals. The correlation of specific emotional states with disease susceptibility was a refinement of an earlier view that had been put forth by Hippocrates in the 4th century B.C. It was Hippocrates' view that virtually all bodily functions could be influenced by emotions. It was not until 1637 that this view was challenged. During a period in our history when the Inquisition was taking place it was prudent to propose a model that allowed for the preservation of the soul after the demise of the body. Thus emerged the dualistic view of Descartes, which made a distinction between the mind in which resided the soul and the body. The body came to be viewed as a machine that could be repaired, thus paving the way for the technically oriented practice of medicine that exists today in Western society. In many medical circles a role for emotional state in modifying the course of somatic illness is at best tolerated and at worst rejected outright.

In the reductionist atmosphere that prevails today it is difficult to endorse phenomena such as placebo effects as well as those associated with improved health correlated with behavioral interventions. Mechanisms related to cause and effect are simply not known. However, not understanding the mechanism by which a phenomenon occurs should not be taken to mean that the phenomenon itself does not exist. Nor should it prevent the protocol from being utilized if beneficial effects may be forthcoming. A classic example occurred during the previous century when Jenner embarked upon his studies of vaccination protocols. By injecting material derived from the scabs of cowpox victims into healthy individuals, he discovered a potential cure for smallpox. To this day, we do not understand all of the complex interrelationships that enable subsets of lymphocytes to interact and ultimately rid the body of harmful pathogens. But through our proceeding with a protocol that today would probably be rejected on the basis of bioethical considerations, a lethal disease has been all but eliminated from the face of the planet.

The use of behavioral-based interventions as adjunct therapies in treating chronic disease is met with considerable resistance, in part because of the lack of understanding of the precise mechanism that transduces an emotional state into an immunomodulatory signal. In addition, many behavioral-based interventions are difficult to replicate. Nonetheless, through the use of varied model systems there does appear to be a firm association between emotional states and disease susceptibility and outcome. The placebo effect, which is well documented, although poorly characterized, is one such example. Others include miraculous healing and guided imagery.

Miraculous Healing, Guided Imagery, and Health

It has been suggested that the placebo response may, in part, work as a result of positive emotions (White, Tursky, and Schwartz, 1984). Miraculous healing also appears to be related to emotional state. Motivated by the expectation that something positive will occur, over 4 million pilgrims journey to the shrine of Bernadette in Lourdes each year. Of the cures claimed by 6000 individuals, 64 have been judged to be miraculous by the Vatican (Dowling, 1984). These include not only hyperplastic disorders but also infectious diseases and autoimmune disease. It is noteworthy that some of the chronic diseases that are remedied as a consequence of religious belief also have a high rate of spontaneous remission based upon those criteria (O'Regan, personal communication).

A different type of behavioral intervention was popularized in 1978. It involved relaxation and positive mental imagery by cancer patients (Simonton, Matthews-Simonton, & Creighton, 1978). Imagery has been successfully used in the field of advertising as well as in athletics for several decades (Schorr, Sobel-Whittington, Robin, & Connella, 1983). Cancer patients apply it by visualizing the destruction of their cancer. In some instances in our own studies, patients have visualized images based upon immune system involvement. Thus, natural killer cells are pictured along with appropriate lymphocytes as they destroy the cancer. Other individuals adopt a metaphoric approach, viewing their cancer as a weed that has to be removed from a garden, or as some other object that the patient can readily visualize. The use of the immune system as a component of the image may not be entirely valid. While animal models as well as *in vitro* protocols clearly indicate a role for the immune system in combating certain types of tumors, the evidence that the immune system plays a major role in eliminating cancer that occurs spontaneously in humans is not substantiated. Despite the reported observation that cancer patients using guided imagery can have a mean survival that is almost double that of control subjects (Simonton, Matthews-Simonton, & Sparks, 1980), the technique has been widely criticized.

Criticism is based, in part, upon the lack of evidence to substantiate the speculation of the Simontons and their colleagues that guided imagery was working by augmenting the ability of the immune system to combat the cancer. In order to address this specific criticism, a study was initiated in 1980 in collaboration with the late Dr. Robert Kvarnes. Initially, a group of six patients was recruited for the purpose of correlating changes in the immune system with the practice of relaxation and guided imagery. Because it was a double-blind study, no information was provided to the patients as to how they were progressing in response to the guided imagery, and consequently, we were unable to offer any incentive to remain in the study. After a period of 4 weeks only one patient remained; however, that individual was evaluated for a period in excess of 1 year during which blood samples were collected at either biweekly or monthly intervals for the purpose of evaluating the numbers of lymphocytes as well as circulating levels of the thymic peptide, thymosin alpha 1. The latter peptide is thought to have hormone-like properties and has been reported to augment the activity of T helper lymphocytes (Goldstein et al., 1981). Although the results were based upon a sample of one and therefore are far from being definitive, the pilot data that were collected were consistent with the conclusions that had been reported by the Simontons.

The single patient who remained in the study was a 66-year-old male who had metastatic cancer of the prostate. On December 5, 1980, a bone scan revealed spread of the tumor to the spinal column, skull, multiple ribs in both projections, both shoulders, intratrochanteric regions of both femurs, the upper shaft of the left femur, and the medial part of both iliac bones. An independent interpretation of the scan by the patient's oncologist was as follows: "So-called superscan suggestive of extensive metastases from carcinoma of the prostate. Compared to the last scan on 12/3/79, there is remarkable deterioration in scintographic picture." A few months later, on February 20, 1981, another scan revealed continued spread in the spine, skull, multiple ribs, femurs, and pelvis, as observed previously. New lesions were observed in the skull and the left humerus. The independent interpretation was as follows: "Scan continues to suggest extensive bone metastases. New lesions indicate internal deterioration compared to 12/5/80." It was at this point that the patient began to practice guided imagery and relaxation. The protocol involved relaxation while listening to music, followed by the conjuring up of mental images depicting the cancer being destroyed by various physiological processes. On November 27, 1981, 9 months after the previous bone scan, another was made and revealed decreased tracer uptake in several of the previously abnormal areas. The interpretation, which was independent of any knowledge that the patient had been engaged in guided imagery, was as follows: "Metastatic bone disease demonstrating overall improvement since 2/20/81." During the course of the imagery the subject had blood withdrawn on regular intervals, either every other week or once a month. White blood count and differentials were determined for the purpose of assessing the percentage of circulating lymphocytes, and circulating levels of thymosin alpha 1 were determined by radioimmunoassay. While not conclusive, it was observed that during periods when the subject reported in his diary that he was doing the imagery and doing it well, it corresponded with elevated levels of thymosin alpha 1. This also corresponded with elevated numbers of lymphocytes. During periods when the subject reported that the imagery was either discontinued or that he was not doing it well, the levels of thymosin alpha 1 dropped to below detectable limits and the number of lymphocytes was also found to be decreased.

Interpretation of these data was severely limited by the fact that there was only a single subject, as well as by the lack of a control group in order to compare seasonal changes as well as possible interassay variability. By themselves the results would be meaningless. However, the data did support the conclusions of the Simontons. In a subsequent study that has recently been reported (Gruber, Hall, Hersh, & Dubois, 1988), these observations have been extended. Although the initial observation with respect to thymosin alpha 1 was not observed in the latter study, we did find that several measures of lymphocyte function were elevated compared with baseline samples.

Adverse Effects of Imagery

As important as the data that were collected during the course of the original pilot study were the insights that resulted from working closely with patients in an investigation of this nature. It is commonly accepted that behavioral intervention strategies can pose no threat to the patient provided that the protocol adopted is not used as a substitute for other proven modes of treatment. This is simply not true. During the course of this early pilot study, and evaluating very closely the reasons why many individuals dropped out before the completion of the project, several potential side effects have been identified.

The first one has also been reported by others working in this field. It is associated with the feeling of guilt that some individuals experience as they become aware of such studies. An extension of the premise that by changing one's mental outlook and behavior one can alter the progression of a chronic disease such as cancer is the assumption that the disease was brought on as a consequence of a maladaptive thought process or behavior. Thus, the patient begins to experience a feeling of guilt that he or she did something to precipitate the onset of the disease. Sometimes, the resentment becomes directed toward a close friend or family member who might be perceived to have done something that triggered the emotional upheaval that the patient experienced. One of the patients in our initial pilot study became convinced that her spouse was the cause of her cancer as a consequence of her preoccupation with his smoking, subsequent emphysema, and demise. Also related to this outcome is the guilt that is sometimes experienced by friends or family members feeling that they were the cause of the patient's disease. Consequently, for certain individuals the mere act of engaging in a behavioral intervention study with a strong belief that by changing one's behavior in a positive manner one can effectively reduce the spread of disease can result in the opposite outcome.

A second side effect that has been identified is related to the specific nature of the image. One subject in the original pilot study was a Roman Catholic priest who was diagnosed as having a mesothelioma. Because of his religious training he had a very difficult time imagining that he was destroying a living cell that his God had created. Each time he attempted to relax and engage in an imaging protocol that required the destruction of his cancer, he experienced a feeling of uneasiness that he was engaging in a behavior that was counter to what his religious training had instilled in him. When we realized what was happening we met with the patient and learned that he enjoyed gardening as a hobby. In light of this knowledge, we instructed the subject to conjure an image in which his body was viewed as a garden. The healthy cells were viewed as flowers while the cancerous cells were the weeds. Instead of destroying the weeds, the patient imagined that nutrients were simply being given to the healthy cells and that the weeds were being ignored. Whether this process was responsible or not will never be known; however, the subject lived several years longer than the original prognosis had predicted.

A third potential side effect is preoccupation with the imaging process. Some goal-oriented individuals can become so obsessed with the protocol that they ignore all other activities in their lives. As a consequence of the preoccupation, the patient is constantly reminded that he or she has cancer. We have learned that some individuals appear to be better off simply using denial rather than engaging in activities that serve as a constant reminder that they suffer from a chronic illness.

Despite these potential side effects, one has to weigh the beneficial effects against the potential negative or adverse effects. Regardless of the medication, all forms of treatment have potential side effects. The fact that behavioral-based intervention strategies may have some should not be a reason to discourage certain patients from engaging in them. Instead, every attempt should be made to identify in advance those individuals who would best benefit from this type of procedure. During the course of the pilot study described above, it became apparent that only those patients who believed that the intervention was going to be beneficial volunteered for the study. Not only that, but individuals who have experienced guilt about the protocol have never appeared in our investigations. Concerns about guilt have arisen only when the results of such studies were presented at conferences. This particular side effect is more often the consequence of having read about the potential beneficial effects of such interventions rather than actually having engaged in them. Also identified have been cancer patients who have expressed the feeling that they did not want to have control over their disease. For certain individuals—but certainly not all—this was a major responsibility that they simply did not want to be burdened with. Again, this type of individual would rarely volunteer for a research protocol and so would not likely be identified during the course of a study. Thus, it is important to identify such individuals before encouraging them to engage in activity that may actually have more adverse effects than beneficial ones.

Physiological Processes That May Link Emotions with Health

There is now abundant evidence that the central nervous system is able to communicate with the immune system (Ader, 1981). Virtually all of the major lymphoid organs are innervated by projections from the central nervous system that include catecholaminergic as well as possibly cholinergic pathways (Bullock, 1985; Felten, Felten, Carlson, Olschovka, & Livnat, 1985). In addition to direct neuronal pathways, virtually all of the major hormonal circuits ultimately controlled by the brain are able to influence, either directly or indirectly, the various cells of the immune system. These include the hormones produced as part of the pituitary-adrenal axis (i.e., ACTH, beta-endorphin and glucocorticoids) as well as those hormones that are secreted as part of the pituitary-gonadal axis (i.e., LH, FSH, and gonadal steroids) (see Kiess & Hall, 1988, for a review).

Certain of these hormones, especially those associated with the pituitary-adrenal axis, are elevated when a stress-inducing situation exists. Since some stress-inducing protocols can be correlated with increased susceptibility to disease as well as to a diminished responsiveness involving some immune system measures, it is tempting to speculate that such hormones provide the link between emotions and the immune system. However, there is no evidence that such a role is played by these hormones. Nonetheless, there is very clear evidence that connections exist between the brain and the immune system. Most of these studies are based upon in vitro or animal models. In addition, there is evidence that, using certain experimental models, an association exists between the onset of some chronic diseases and negative emotional states. Some of these models have utilized bereaved individuals who have been found to have a depressed state of immunity (Stein, 1985) or medical students who have been found to have increased susceptibility to viral infections correlated with the stress of major examination periods (Kiecolt-Glaser, Garner, Speicher, Penn, & Glaser, 1984). Because anxiety and negative emotional states are often linked with increased secretion of ACTH and subsequently cortisol, the pituitary-adrenal axis is thought by many to serve as one of the conduits via which the brain is able to modulate the activity of the immune system. In addition, the autonomic nervous system is also activated during periods of distress (see Hall & Goldstein, 1984). Virtually all of the major immune system organs are extensively innervated by projections from the sympathetic branch of the autonomic nervous system, a topic that is reviewed elsewhere (Felten et al., 1985). Furthermore, all of the cells that constitute the immune system can be influenced either directly or indirectly by hormones produced by the pituitary gland (see Kiess & Hall, 1988). Because of the direct neuronal as well as endocrine links between the nervous system and the immune system, it is widely accepted, although far from proven, that these are the circuits via which emotional state is transduced into an immunomodulatory signal.

If the central nervous system is capable of modulating the course of an immune response via either neuroendocrine circuits and/or the autonomic nervous system, then one would postulate the existence of a feedback mechanism whereby activity within the immune system could be monitored by the brain. A number of chemical signals originating from within the immune system compartment have been identified with biological activity at the level of the brain (see Hall, McGillis, Spangelo, & Goldstein, 1985). For example, interleukin 1, a product of macrophages, has been found to be capable of stimulating slow wave sleep as well as a fever response (Krueger, Dinarello, Wolff, Chedid, & Walter, 1984). It is during the slow wave phase of sleep that growth hormone is released. It has tropic as well as growth-promoting effects that would be most beneficial for the host during a period when tissue repair would be required subsequent to infection. In addition, hyperthermia constitutes a microenvironment in which many microorganisms are unable to survive. C3a of the complement cascade has been found to mimic the effects of dopamine in the brain (Schupf, Williams, Hugh, & Cox, 1983). Other lymphokines such as interferons have also been found to have neuropsychiatric side effects that have complicated some ongoing clinical trials (Smedley, Katrak, Sikora, & Wheeler, 1983). Our own work as well as that of others has revealed that thymosin peptides, originally isolated from extracted thymus gland, are capable of activating a number of neuroendocrine pathways at the level of the brain and/or the pituitary gland. These include corticosterone and luteinizing hormone (Hall et al., 1982), luteinizing hormone releasing factor (Rebar, Miyake, Low, & Goldstein, 1981), as well as ACTH from cultured pituitary cells (McGillis, Hall, & Goldstein, 1988). In addition, beta-endorphin (Farah, Hall, Bishop, Goldstein, & O'Donohue, 1987), prolactin (Spangelo, Hall, Dunn, & Goldstein, 1987), and growth hormone (Spangelo, Judd, et al., 1987) are also stimulated. The release of certain of these immune system products may be responsible for the rise in corticosterone that has been observed to occur following the injection of Newcastle disease virus into mice (Dunn, Powell, Moreshead, Gaskin, & Hall, 1987) as well as during an immune response to foreign erythrocytes (Besedovsky, Sorkin, Keller, & Muller, 1975). Some of these changes in peptides are most likely the consequence of activation of neurotransmitters since both Newcastle disease virus and interleukin 1 have been found to alter the turnover rate of biogenic amines in discrete regions of the brain (Dunn, 1988; Dunn et al., 1987).

It is noteworthy that some of the neurotransmitters as well as neuropeptides that are stimulated by immune system products have been implicated in mediating certain behaviors as well as emotional states. These include the release of ACTH and glucocorticoids, which have been associated with arousal, as well as dopamine and other catecholamines, which have been implicated in the etiology of a number of psychiatric disorders. Thus, in addition to considering the role that emotional state might play upon the immune system, one must also consider the impact that the immune system may play in the etiology of certain psychiatric disorders. For example, rather than being due solely to a deficiency within the central nervous system, certain behavioral abnormalities may actually be due, in part, to abnormal production of lymphokines. The latter hypothesis is largely speculation since direct studies are only now being initiated in this laboratory. However, recent work using animal models suggests that this may, indeed, be the case. For example, it has been found that exposure of neonatal rodents to herpes virus is correlated with hyperactivity in adulthood (Crnic & Pizer, 1988). It has long been observed that individuals with a more aggressive outlook have a better prognosis than individuals who do not. It is quite possible that in some cases it is not the behavior that is improving the prognosis but a more efficient defense against a particular infection that happens to induce a particular type of behavioral pattern that may in turn be conducive to combating the infection.

Conclusion

It is quite clear that there are complex and numerous pathways that link the brain with the immune system. These are bidirectional circuits that enable the central nervous system and the immune system to communicate information to each other. In the past, emphasis has been placed upon the role that the nervous system plays in modulating the course of disease. It is noteworthy that all of the terms that have been coined to describe this general area of research begin with a designation referring to behavior or the brain—e.g., psychoneuroimmunology, neuroendocrinimmunology, psychosomatic medicine. In view of the evidence, however, it may be equally valid to propose that a healthy behavioral outlook may actually be part of our disease-fighting milieu and that this is all coordinated by the immune system. In simplistic terms, one might view the immune system as constituting a form of aggression, but directed against elements within the microbial environment as opposed to the macroenvironment. Thus, it would not be farfetched to propose that the hormonal systems that have evolved to increase the aggressiveness of the immune system may be the same ones that promote aggressive behaviors that increase survival of the individual within a social context. The evidence reviewed in this chapter indicates that this may indeed be the case and that they may be coordinated by some of the same events.

ACKNOWLEDGMENTS. Some of the studies described in this chapter were supported by a grant from the National Institutes of Health (NS21210). The first author is supported by an NIMH Research Scientist Development Award (MH00648). The excellent editorial assistance provided by Mrs. Cecilia Figueredo during the preparation of this manuscript is deeply appreciated.

References

Ader, R. (1981). *Psychoneuroimmunology* (p. 661). New York: Academic Press.
Beecher, H. (1961). Surgery as a placebo. *Journal of the American Medical Association, 176*, 1102–1107.
Besedovsky, H. O., Sorkin, E., Keller, M., & Muller, J. (1975). Changes in blood hormone levels during the immune response. *Proceedings of the Society for Experimental Biology and Medicine, 150*, 466–470.
Bulloch, K. (1985). Neuroanatomy of lymphoid tissue: A review. In R. Guillemin, M. Cohn, & T. Melnechuk (Eds.), *Neural modulation of immunity* (pp. 111–141). New York: Raven Press.

Cobb, L. A, Thomas, G. I., Dillard, D. H., Merendino, K. A., & Bruce, R. A. (1959). Evaluation of internal mammary artery ligation by double blind technique. *New England Journal of Medicine, 260,* 1115–1118.
Crnic, L. S., & Pizer, L. I. (1988). Behavioral effects of neonatal herpes simplex type 1 infection in mice. *Neurotoxicology and Teratology, 10,* 381–386.
Dowling, S. J. (1984). Lourdes cures and their medical assessment. *Journal of the Royal Society of Medicine, 77,* 634–638.
Dunn, A. J. (1988). Systemic interleukin-1 administration stimulates hypothalamic norepinephrine metabolism paralleling the increased plasma corticosterone. *Life Sciences, 43,* 429–435.
Dunn, A. J., Powell, M. L., Moreshead, W. V., Gaskin, J. M., & Hall, N. R. (1987). Effects of Newcastle disease virus administration to mice on the metabolism of cerebral biogenic amines, plasma corticosterone, and lymphocyte proliferation. *Brain Behavior and Immunity, 1,* 216–230.
Evans, F. (1984). Unravelling placebo effects: Expectations and the placebo response. *Advances, 1*(3), 11–20.
Farah, J. M., Jr., Hall, N. R., Bishop, J. F., Goldstein, A. L., & O'Donohue, T. L. (1987). Thymosin fraction-5 stimulates secretion of immunoreactive beta-endorphin in mouse corticotrophic tumor cells. *Journal of Neuroscience Research, 18,* 140–146.
Felten, D. L., Felten, S. Y., Carlson, S. L., Olschovka, J. A., & Livnat, S. (1985). Noradrenergic and peptidergic innervation of lymphoid tissue. *Journal of Immunology, 135,* 755s–765s.
Goldstein, A. L., Low, T. L. K., Thurman, G. B., Zatz, M. M., Hall, N. R., Chen, C-P, Hu, S-K, Naylor, P. H., & McClure, J. E. (1981). Current status of thymosin and other hormones of the thymus gland. *Recent Progress in Hormone Research, 37,* 369–415.
Gruber, B. L., Hall, N. R., Hersh, S. P., & Dubois, P. (1988). Immune system and psychologic changes in metastatic cancer patients while using ritualized relaxation and guided imagery: A pilot study. *Scandinavian Journal of Behavioural Therapy, 17,* 25–46.
Hall, N. R., & Goldstein, A. L. (1984). Endocrine regulation of host immunity. In R. L. Fenichel & M. A. Chirigos (Eds.), *Immune modulation agents and their mechanisms* (pp. 533–563). New York: Marcel Dekker.
Hall, N. R., McGillis, J. P., Spangelo, B. L., Palaszynski, E., Moody, T. W., & Goldstein, A. L. (1982). Evidence for a neuroendocrine-thymus axis mediated by thymosin polypeptides. *Developmental Immunology, 17,* 653–660.
Hall, N. R., McGillis, J. P., Spangelo, B. L., & Goldstein, A. L. (1985). Evidence that thymosins and other biological response modifiers can function as immunotransmitters. *Journal of Immunology, 135,* 806–811.
Kiecolt-Glaser, J. K., Garner, W., Speicher, C. E., Penn, G., & Glaser, R. (1984). Psychosocial modifiers of immunocompetence in medical students. *Psychosomatic Medicine, 46,* 7–14.
Kiess, W., & Hall, N. R. (1988). Psychoneuroimmunology and endocrine-mediated evolution of the immune system. In D. Hesch (Ed.), *Handbook of endocrinology* (Klinik der Gegenwart Series) (pp. 346–360). Baltimore: Urban & Schwarzenberg.
Klopfer, B. (1957). Psychological variables in human cancer. *Journal of Projective Techniques, 21,* 337–339.
Krueger, J., Dinarello, C., Wolff, M., Chedid, L., & Walter, J. (1984). Sleep-promoting effects of endogenous pyrogen (interleukin 1). *American Journal of Physiology, 246,* R994.
Lasagna, L., Laties, V., & Dohan, J. (1958). Further studies on the pharmacology of placebo administration. *Journal of Clinical Investigation, 37*(1), 533–537.

McGillis, J. P., Hall, N. R., & Goldstein, A. L. (1988). Thymosin fraction 5 (TF5) stimulates secretion of adrenocorticotropic hormone (ACTH) from cultured rat pituitaries. *Life Sciences, 42*, 2259–2268.
Rebar, R. W., Miyake, A., Low, T. L. K., & Goldstein, A. L. (1981). Thymosin stimulates secretion of luteinizing hormone-releasing factor. *Science, 214*, 669–671.
Schorr, J. E., Sobel-Whittington, T., Robin, P., & Connella, J. A. (1983). *Imagery: Theoretical and clinical implications* (p. 435). New York: Plenum Press.
Schupf, N., Williams, C. A., Hugh, T. E., & Cox, J. (1983). Psychopharmacological activity of anaphylatoxin C3a in rat hypothalamus. *Journal of Neuroimmunology, 5*, 305.
Simonton, C., Matthews-Simonton, S., & Creighton, J. (1978). *Getting well again*. Los Angeles: Tarcher.
Simonton, C., Matthews-Simonton, S., & Sparks, T. (1980). Psychological intervention in the treatment of cancer. *Psychosomatics, 21*, 226–233.
Smedley, H., Katrak, M., Sikora, K., & Wheeler, T. (1983). Neurological effects of recombinant human interferon. *British Medical Journal, 286*, 262–264.
Spangelo, B. L., Hall, N. R., Dunn, A. J., & Goldstein, A. L. (1987). Thymosin fraction 5 stimulates the release of prolactin from cultured GH3 cells. *Life Sciences, 40*, 283–288.
Spangelo, B. L., Judd, A. M., Ross, P. C., Login, I. S., Jarvis, W. D., Badamchian, M., Goldstein, A. L., & MacLeod, R. M. (1987). Thymosin fraction 5 stimulates prolactin and growth hormones release from anterior pituitary cells in vitro. *Endocrinology, 121*, 2035–2043.
Stein, M. (1985). Bereavement, depression, stress and immunity. In R. Guillemin, M. Cohen, & T. Melnechuk (Eds.), *Neural modulation of immunity* (pp. 29–44). New York: Raven Press.
White, L., Tursky, B., & Schwartz, G. E. (1984). Possible determinants of placebo response: A list. *Advances, 1*(3), 25.
White, L., Tursky, B., & Schwartz, G. (Eds.). (1985). *Placebos: Theory, research and mechanisms*. New York: Guilford Press.

CHAPTER 11

Altered Immunity through Behavioral Conditioning

Maurice G. King and Alan J. Husband

Table 1, compiled from our review of the immunoconditioning literature (Kusnecov, King, & Husband, 1989b), summarizes studies reported subsequent to Ader and Cohen's (1975) important observation of behaviorally conditioned immunosuppression using a taste aversion procedure. The summary is further confined to studies that have used drugs or biological substances as the UCS. Even within this homogeneous operational set there is evident a variety of relationships between the behavioral conditioning paradigm, predominantly taste aversion conditioning (CTA), and the concomitant immunoconditioning.

Conditioning of immunostimulation and of immunosuppression have been reported using the CTA procedure, but other conditioning procedures have also produced positive results. It is clear from Table 1 and consonant with the earlier Russian literature (see Ader, 1981, for a review) that taste aversion is neither a necessary nor a sufficient condition for immune conditioning. Evidence is starting to emerge suggesting that many UCSs, such as cyclophosphamide, antilymphocyte serum and levamisole, for instance, are more effective within a CTA procedure while others, such as BCG, sheep red blood cells, and Poly I:c, condition readily with strictly Pavlovian procedures. Alternatively, some components of the immune UCR—for example, serum antibody production—may be more readily conditionable by CTA than, say, the febrile component that in our hands seems to condition more readily using strict

---

Maurice G. King and Alan J. Husband • Department of Psychology, University of Newcastle, Newcastle, NSW 2308, Australia.

Table 1. *Effective Unconditioned Stimuli: Relationships between Conditioned Taste Aversion and Immunoconditioning*

Conditioned taste aversion	Strength of immunoconditioning		
	Strong	Medium	Nil
Strong	Lipopolysaccharide ∧	Cyclophosphamide ∨	Lithium chloride (?)
Mild	Antilymphocyte serum ∨ Levamisole ∧	?	?
Nil	Bacille Calmette-Guerin ∧	SRBC ∧	Water Lab chow

Note: ∧ = immunostimulation and ∨ = immunosuppression.

Pavlovian procedures. Attention has been drawn to a genetic dimension by Ader and Cohen (1982), who have reported important strain differences in CTA-induced immunoconditioning. These are all important observations that we, for our part, addressed by trying to determine what makes an effective UCS and which components of the UCR show an affinity for different conditioning procedures. It is clear, however, that a more extensive catalog of UCS outcomes than we have in Table 1 must be available before definitive statements can be made.

Effective UCSs in Immunoconditioning

Our recent review of immunoconditioning (Kusnecov, King, & Husband, 1989b) highlighted redirections that have occurred since Ader and Cohen's (1975) benchmark study. In the intervening years the majority of experimental reports on immunoconditioning have used a taste aversion procedure and within that procedure the SAC.CY (saccharin as a CS and cyclophosphamide as UCS) procedure has predominated. The main advantages of CY as a UCS are the robustness of conditioning and the reliability of the paradigm. Its main drawback is the toxicity of CY, which in an inverted way may be responsible in part for its success. If anything, then our only cavil with the SAC.CY procedure is that to date it may have been too successful, and that is really no criticism but rather an incitement to test alternative UCSs and procedures.

Alternative UCSs in Immunosuppression

As mentioned above, CY is highly toxic, and its potential for application is limited to a few diseases, such as leukemia, in which CY forms part of the regimen of chemotherapy. With wider clinical applications in mind, we sought to obtain taste aversion and immunoconditioning in a rodent model using an immunosuppressive UCS that would be generally acceptable in man. Gamzu (1977) had reviewed an increasing number of studies indicating that "neither emesis, nausea, gastrointestinal disturbance, nor 'sickness' in general are necessary consequences of treatments that are effective in producing taste aversions." In view of this, we tested the relatively "benign" biological immunosuppressant antilymphocyte serum (ALS). This serum was raised by immunizing New Zealand white rabbits with cells from rodent mesenteric lymph nodes, thus producing an ALS with antibodies to the full spectrum of cellular components of the rat immune system. Ip injection of 0.2 mls of the ALS (cytotoxicity 1/60) produced in rats a transient depletion of circulating lymph cells (lymphocytopenia) and a functional diminution of humoral and cellular immunoresponsivity.

Our next step was to show that ALS could produce taste aversion in the rat (Sivyer, King, Husband, Cripps, & Clancy, 1982). For this we used three groups: (1) the SAC.ALS group, an experimental group that drank a 0.3% sodium saccharin solution in tap water for 10 min/day (CS), which was followed by a 0.2-ml ip injection of the ALS (UCS); (2) the SAC.NRS group, a control group that also drank weak saccharin in water but received a 0.2-ml ip injection of noncytotoxic normal rabbit serum (NRS); and (3) the WAT.ALS group, a further control, which drank tap water and received a 0.2-ml injection of ALS. Following conditioning, rats were not treated again with ALS. For 2 weeks they were maintained on regularized drinking and ad lib access to feed. On the 14th day the groups were tested—groups (1) and (2) drank saccharin-flavored water, and group (3) was given their regular tap water. Only the experimental animals—group (1)—showed significant taste aversion, which is consistent with the observation of Gamzu (1977) that conditioning can occur in the absence of gastrointestinal upset.

Our next study (Kusnecov, Sivyer, King, Husband, Cripps, & Clancy, 1983) (1) attempted to replicate the SAC.ALS taste aversion and (2) tested for a concomitant conditioned immunosuppression. The conditioning and test procedures followed those described above (Sivyer et al., 1982) up to day 14, after which all rats were returned to ad lib feed and water for 7 days. On day 21 all groups were sacrificed, their mesenteric lymph nodes were harvested, and the cells were assayed for proliferative reactivity to antigen in a mixed lymphocyte culture.

As predicted from our previous study (Sivyer et al., 1982), ALS reliably conditioned taste aversion. More important, the SAC.ALS group exhibited a significant suppression *in vitro*, that is, in the mixed lymphocyte culture, of antigen-induced lymphocyte proliferation compared with the two control groups. We concluded that during the SAC.ALS pairing, in addition to taste aversion, there also occurred a concomitant conditioned immunosuppression to the taste of saccharin. This implies that on subsequent exposure of the rat to the CS alone, reenlistment of at least some ALS effects occurs without ALS. This demonstration of conditioned immunosuppression using ALS, a naturally occurring immunosuppressant with selective cytotoxicity for lymphocytes and with minimal acceptable side effects, opened the way for a broader clinical application of immunoconditioning.

If ALS were to be useful in an applied context, the immunoconditioning should not be ephemeral. Thus, we undertook a long-term study of ALS conditioning outcomes in our animal model. King, Husband, and Kusnecov (1987b) conditioned rats using the SAC.ALS procedure described above and tested for conditioned immunosuppression 14, 21, and 42 days later using the mixed lymphocyte culture test described above. *In vitro* suppression attributable to *in vivo* conditioning was present on days 14 and 21 postconditioning but had faded by day 42. Thus, ALS conditioning appears to have produced a learning effect on lymphocytes remarkable for its durability given that it is established with only one nontraumatic conditioning trial.

In the same study other rats were killed and exsanguinated following day 0 (Conditioning), or saccharin testing (CS alone) on day 14, day 21, or day 42. Their plasma was assayed for levels of corticosterone as an index of "stress." Their levels for the time of day were at the upper limit for resting controls and in other cases slightly elevated, which is consistent for a rat anticipating water and drinking (Yahaya bin Mahamood & King, 1985). The pattern however, is not consistent with a causal role for corticosterone, although it may indicate a permissive role.

We began this section by claiming that ALS was as effective as more noxious UCSs without producing marked gastrointestinal upset. Let me conclude the section by asking if there is any advantage to making ALS noxious. More specifically, is the taste aversion produced by ALS more pronounced if the ALS is endowed with unpleasant sensory qualities?

Using an extension of the SAC.ALS procedure described above, King, Husband, and Kusnecov (1987b) compared the relative extent of taste aversions produced by ALS alone, by a "cocktail" of 50 mg/kg lithium chloride (LiCl) and ALS together (ALS+LiCl), and by LiCl mixed with the control/vehicle solution, noncytotoxic normal rabbit serum

(NRS+LiCl). Groups were tested 14 days after conditioning for saccharin (CS) drinking: Each of the above groups drank significantly less than controls on the test day, indicating marked taste aversion for saccharin-flavored water. Within this main effect the extent of aversion was significantly different between each set of the three treatment groups. The ALS group drank 60% of their baseline intake, and the LiCl+NRS group drank 45% of their baseline. Since the SAC.NRS control did not differ significantly from other controls, it seems that, at the doses involved, LiCl is more effective than ALS as a UCS for taste aversion. However, the difference, while significant, was less (only about 15% of intake) than was anticipated. In another context, we (King, Husband, & Kusnecov, 1987a) have referred to ALS-induced CTA as conditioned taste "wariness" rather than aversion, and the present results are supportive of such a distinction.

Compared with ALS or (LiCl+NRS), the "cocktail" (ALS+LiCl) was significantly more suppressive as a UCS; the group drank only 33% of their baseline intake during testing with the CS. While both mean intake differences (ALS)−(LiCl+NRS) and (LiCl+NRS)−(ALS+LiCl), were significantly different in arithmetic terms, the sum of the ALS reduction and the LiCl+NRS reductions (95%) exceeded the ALS+LiCl "cocktail" reduction (66%). Arithmetically there was not even an additive effect on inhibition of intake. Having made this point arithmetically, it may not be physiologically meaningful since a 95% reduction would mean, in terms of expectation, virtually forgoing water for a further 24 hours.

We can conclude by answering the question posed: If ALS is made aversive, is the taste aversion stronger? The ALS+LiCl "cocktail" produced stronger conditioned inhibition than either ALS or LiCl alone. However, the relative difference between ALS and LiCl was only 15% of daily intake, which, though significant, is smaller than expected. Several important questions emerged from the data, and further behavioral studies are indicated. We are now in a position to address the important immunological hypothesis: Is the additional conditioned taste aversion produced by adding LiCl reflected in the accompanying conditioned immunosuppression?

Alternative UCSs in Immunostimulation

The drug levamisole has received considerable attention as a potential immunoenhancing agent (Fudenberg & Wybran, 1982), and we were successful in using a SAC.LEV procedure to induce conditioned taste aversion. Husband, King, and Brown (1986/1987) extended the study, showing that 3 mg/rat ip to rats produced 24 hours later a significant elevation in the T helper: T suppressor (Th:Ts) subset ratio. This occurred through a selective depression in the cytotoxic/suppressor subset.

Using a SAC.LEV conditioning regimen similar to the SAC.ALS procedure described above, taste aversion with LEV was confirmed to the CS alone 14 days after conditioning. In addition, the Th:Ts ratios were significantly elevated in the plasma of the experimental/conditioned animals. This study demonstrates behavioral conditioning of immunostimulation using an immunoenhancing drug in the CTA paradigm. For the most part, other reports of conditioned immunoenhancement have used strictly Pavlovian procedures. Olfactory CSs have been successfully applied to the classical conditioning of an enhanced histamine response to BSA in guinea pigs (Russell, Dark, Cummins, Ellman, Callaway and Peeke, 1984) and increased NK cell activity in mice when camphor odor was repeatedly paired with poly I:C injections (Ghanta, Hiramoto, Solvason, & Spector, 1985).

Biological Mediators of Immunoconditioning

Table 2 summarizes a set of experiments carried out in our laboratory using the SAC.CY taste aversion procedure in rats described by Ader and Cohen (1975, see also Chapter 9, this volume). Experimental groups were pretreated with dexamethazone (DEX 100 µg/kg ip; 4-hour delay) either before conditioning, before testing, or both. This dose of DEX blocks 75% of adrenal corticosterone produced by a stressor (etherization).

The effects of DEX blockade on conditioned taste aversion and con-

Table 2. *Effects of Dexamethasone Blockade on Conditioned Taste Aversion and Conditioned Immunosuppression*

	Conditioned taste aversion DEX pretest		Conditioned immunosuppression DEX pretest	
DEX preconditioning	Yes	No	Yes	No
Yes	TAV	TAV	NIL	NIL
No	TAV	TAV	CIS	CIS

ditioned immunosuppression are shown in Table 2. First, DEX blocking at 100 μg/kg ip had no effect on taste aversion regardless of whether it was given before conditioning or testing or both. In contrast to this, DEX blockade abrogated the conditioned immunosuppression if given before conditioning (or before conditioning and testing), which narrows down the blockade's action to conditioning (no effect on CIS if given only before testing). A major endocrine effect of DEX-blockade is inhibition of the pituitary secretion of ACTH and beta-endorphin.

To date we have established (a) links between immunoconditioning and the neuropeptides (ACTH, beta-endorphin) (Kusnecov, Husband, & King, 1989a) and (b) links between these neuropeptides and immune function (Kusnecov, Husband, Pang, Smith, & King, 1987).

In summary, we have described two lines of investigation proceeding in our laboratory. First, we have demonstrated that even within the taste aversion conditioning paradigm, ALS is an effective alternative to CY as a UCS. Of equal importance is our demonstration of conditioned immunostimulation using levamisole as the UCS. In both cases, conditioned immunostimulation using levamisole and conditioned immunosuppression with ALS, the minimizing of aversion to "wariness" raises interesting questions about the role of the UCS in immunoconditioning. Second, the susceptibility of conditioned immunosuppression to DEX pretreatment has led us to investigate the role of the pituitary neuropeptides, ACTH, and beta-endorphin in immune conditioning.

References

Ader, R. (Ed.). (1981). *Psychoneuroimmunology*. New York: Academic Press.
Ader, R., & Cohen, N. (1975). Behaviorally conditioned immunosuppression. *Psychosomatic Medicine, 37*, 333–340.
Ader, R., & Cohen, N. (1982). Behaviorally conditioned immunosuppression and murine systemic lupus erythematosous. *Science, 215*, 1534–1536.
Fudenberg, H. H., & Wybran, J. (1982). Experimental immunotherapy. In D. P. Stites, J. D. Stobo, H. H. Fudenberg, & J. V. Wells (Eds.), *Basic and clinical immunology* (4th ed.). Los Altos, CA: Medical Publications.
Gamzu, E. (1977). The multifaceted nature of taste-aversion-inducing agents: Is there a single common factor? In L. M. Barker, M. R. Best, & M. Domjan (Eds.), *Learning mechanisms in food selection*. Waco, TX: Baylor University Press.
Ghanta, V. K., Hiramoto, R. N., Solvason, H. B., & Spector, N. H. (1985). Neural and environmental influences on neoplasia and conditioning of NK activity. *Journal of Immunology, 135* (Suppl.), 848–852.

Husband, A. J., King, M. G., & Brown, R. (1986/1987). Behaviorally conditioned modification of T cell subset ratios in rats. *Immunology Letters, 14,* 91–94.

King, M. G., Husband, A. J., & Kusnecov, A. W. (1987a). Behavioural conditioning of the immune system: From laboratory to clinical application. In J. L. Sheppard (Ed.), *Advances in behavioural medicine* (Vol. 4). Sydney, Australia: Cumberland College Press.

King, M. G., Husband, A. J., & Kusnecov, A. W. (1987b). Behaviorally conditioned immunosuppression using antilymphocyte serum: Duration of effect and role of corticosteroids. *Medical Science Research, 15,* 407–408.

Kusnecov, A. W., King, M. G., & Husband, A. J. (1989). Immunomodulation by behavioral conditioning. *Biological Psychology, 28,* 25–39.

Kusnecov, A. W., Sivyer, M., King, M. G., Husband, A. J., Cripps, A. W., & Clancy, R. L. (1983). Behaviorally conditioned suppression of the immune response by antilymphocyte serum. *Journal of Immunology, 130,* 2117–2120.

Kusnecov, A. W., Husband, A. J., Pang, G., Smith, R., & King, M. G. (1987). *In vivo* effects of beta-endorphin on lymphocyte proliferation and Il-2 production. *Brain Behavior and Immunity, 2,* 88–97.

Kusnecov, A. W., Husband, A. J., & King, M. G. (in press). The influence of dexamethazone on behaviorally conditioned immunomodulation and plasma corticosterone. *Brain Behavior and Immunity.*

Russell, M., Dark, K. A., Cummins, R. W., Ellman, G., Gallaway, G., & Peeke, H. V. S. (1984). Learned histamine release. *Science, 225,* 733–734.

Sivyer, M., King, M. G., Husband, A. J., Cripps, A. W., & Clancy, R. L. (1982). Antilymphocyte serum produces conditioned taste aversion in rats. *IRCS Medical Science, 10,* 553.

Yahaya, Mahamood, & King, M. G. (1985). Extinction of a partially reinforced free operant behaviour: A comparison of methods of food withdrawal and their biochemical consequences. *Sains Malaysiana, 14,* 385–397.

PART IV

Pain

In this final section, on pain, five chapters deal with some of the complexities and applications of recent work in this area. G. F. Gebhart provides an overview of opioid analgesia in descending systems of pain modulation. Wolfgang Larbig provides us with an update on Melzack and Wall's gate control theory of pain. J. Peter Rosenfeld and James G. Broton summarize some interesting studies on orofacial pain mechanisms in the rat. Masamichi Satoh goes into detail on the role of neuropeptides and nociception in the spinal cord. And last, Lang Yan Xia and his colleagues, J. Peter Rosenfeld and Kun Hou Huang, review a set of fascinating findings pointing to the role of the neocortex in pain control through acupuncture.

In Chapter 12, Gebhart summarizes some of the key recent studies in the control of pain from a physiological perspective. He points out that the discovery of opiate receptors, stimulation-produced analgesia, and endogenous opioid peptides, in particular, contributed to recent progress in this area. Gebhart also discusses applications of recent animal studies in the control of pain at the human level. The use of electrical stimulation and spinal injections of opioids, as well as the use of external stimuli to achieve neurotransmitter effects are some of the possibilities. This overview of the field provides an excellent and up-to-date introduction to the subsequent papers in this section on pain control.

In Chapter 13, Larbig reviews recent evidence relative to Melzack and Wall's gate control theory of pain perception. This widely known theory maintains that the effects of peripheral neural impulses upon the central nervous system are facilitated by small fiber inputs (that open the gate) and inhibited by larger fiber inputs (that close the gate). In general, predictions from the theory concerning the "opening" system have not been substantiated, whereas the descending gate control system has received voluminous support through studies discussed here (and in Chapter 12 by Gebhart). Larbig's clear and interesting review puts gate control theory into proper perspective, in terms of the limitations of the model as well as its import for the self-regulation of pain.

Rosenfeld and Broton describe several studies in Chapter 14 that challenge widely held views concerning the perception of pain stimulation in the brainstem, in particular within the area termed the trigeminal nuclear complex. The significance of Rosenfeld and Broton's observation is, in part, in demonstrating the role of controlled animal models in helping to modify an old theory of pain processing that was based largely on clinical observations. With the identification of actual—rather than conjectural—neural pathways for pain reception and perception, future attempts at pain intervention with methods of self-regulation can be more accurately understood.

In Chapter 15, Satoh explores some of the functions of neuropeptides in the spinal cord (specifically, the spinal dorsal horn), thus filling in detail for the earlier overviews of the role of neuropeptides in pain perception in other chapters in this section. The effects he observes using a variety of methods implicate the role of substance P during mechanical noxious stimulation and somatostatin during thermal noxious stimulation. While the relationship between the results obtained with Satoh's animal model and the self-regulation of pain perception at the human level is not yet known, such fine studies as these on the role of neurotransmitters in the spinal cord advance our fundamental knowledge of pain perception and control.

In Chapter 16, Xia, Rosenfeld, and Huang provide a review of their own evidence and that of others to demonstrate the relationship between events in the cortex and electrical stimulation of a variety of acupuncture points, termed "acupuncture analgesia." The authors summarize an assortment of observations that provide indirect support for the involvement of the cortex in acupuncture analgesia in pain sensation and inhibition, inhibition of responses to noxious stimuli, and effects due to conditioned somatosensory cortical evoked potentials. These and other results consistently support the Xia et al. notion that the cortex is involved in acupuncture analgesia, and help to bridge the gulf between ancient monistic views of mind and body and current neural and biochemical mechanisms of pain management. This work highlights the importance of attempts such as this to internationalize meetings of researchers in the field of self-regulation.

CHAPTER 12

Opioid Analgesia and Descending Systems of Pain Control

G. F. Gebhart

Introduction

The control of pain has long been a primary concern of man. Our current knowledge about pain and its control derives from studies of the anatomy and physiology of pain and its pharmacological control. The recent intensified research into and significant progress in the control of pain arose from several nearly simultaneous key discoveries: opiate receptors, stimulation-produced analgesia, and endogenous opioid peptides.

Present understanding of the sites and mechanisms of opioid-produced analgesia was stimulated by the discovery in the early 1970s of receptors specific for opioids. Interest in an endogenous, descending system for pain control can be traced to the first demonstration by Reynolds (1969) of stimulation-produced analgesia. Coupled with these two seminal developments, endogenous opioid peptides were soon discovered, and it was demonstrated that opioids given directly into the central nervous system produced analgesia. We know today that opioids such as morphine produce analgesia in part by engaging descending systems of pain control and that endogenous opioid peptides likely mediate some aspects of these descending systems. Developments in this field have been rapid and have led directly to new and better methods for pain relief.

G. F. Gebhart • Department of Pharmacology, College of Medicine, University of Iowa, Iowa City, Iowa 52242, USA.

Opioids and Analgesia

Receptors and Mechanisms of Action

Opioids are the most efficacious drugs known for relief from pain. Although their use has a long history, both our understanding of their sites and mechanisms of action and new drug developments in this field were limited until receptors for opioid action were demonstrated (Pert & Snyder, 1973; Simon, Hiller, & Adelman, 1973; Terenius, 1973). The binding of opioids to their receptors was established as stereospecific, saturable, and reversible. That is, only the pharmacologically active isomers of opioids bound to the receptors, the receptors were limited in number, and binding was competitive between agonists and antagonists. These receptors were found to be distributed nonhomogeneously throughout the brain and spinal cord as well as in other tissues where opioids have important pharmacological actions (e.g., smooth muscle of the gastrointestinal tract). It has since been demonstrated that there are several opioid receptor subtypes, the principal subtypes being *mu*, *kappa*, and *delta* opioid receptors. Each of these different receptor subtypes has a unique distribution in the central nervous system, and all are believed to mediate different effects of opioids. The *mu* receptor is believed to mediate the analgesia and respiratory depression produced by opioids. Action at *kappa* and *delta* opioid receptors is also believed to contribute to the analgesia produced by opioids, but probably at sites anatomically different from opioid actions at *mu* receptors (e.g., spinal cord). In addition to analgesia and respiratory depression, opioids produce a number of other effects (e.g., sedation, euphoria, suppression/stimulation of a variety of hormones) mediated by opioid receptors both within and outside of the central nervous system. For example, opioids increase the tone of the smooth muscle of the gastrointestinal tract and decrease its motility, producing a constipating effect mediated by opioid receptors.

In addition to *mu*, *delta*, and *kappa* opioid receptors, opioid receptors named *epsilon* and *sigma* have also been described. A role for an *epsilon* receptor has not been established, and it is believed that the endogenous opioid peptide β-endorphin may produce its central actions at an *epsilon* receptor. The *sigma* receptor, originally considered an opioid receptor, has subsequently been determined to bind a group of hallucinogenic chemicals typified by phencyclidine ("angel dust"). Opioids often produce dysphoric effects, and these effects are believed to be mediated by the *sigma* receptor, although the *sigma* receptor is not considered to be an opioid receptor per se.

The molecular mechanisms by which opioids produce their effects have also been clarified. Using *in vitro* preparations, a number of investigators have demonstrated that opioids affect both Ca^{++} and K^+ ionic conductances in neurons. The effects of opioids in the central nervous system are generally considered to be inhibitory. Thus, opioids would be expected to depress neuronal activity. By increasing a K^+ conductance in neurons, opioids lead to a hyperpolarization of the neuronal membrane, thus making it more difficult for neurons to be excited. Similarly, by decreasing a Ca^{++} conductance, neuronal activity is suppressed. Ca^{++} must be conducted into nerve terminals for neurotransmitters to be released. When the Ca^{++} conductance is decreased by drugs such as opioids, less neurotransmitter is released by the neuron and its activity is thus suppressed.

The receptors themselves are also the focus of concentrated investigation, and molecular biological methods will soon reveal their structure, the genomic regulation of their expression, their number (more than seven have been proposed), and whether they are derived from several genes or are the product of differential, tissue-specific processing of a single gene.

Endogenous Opioid Peptides

After their discovery (Hughes, 1975), opioid peptides were intensively studied, and they are probably now among the best understood peptides in the central nervous system. Initial interest focused on their role in the modulation of pain. Indeed, when analogues of these peptides are administered systemically, an analgesia is produced. However, how opioid peptides endogenously participate in the modulation of pain is not understood. For instance, stimulation-produced analgesia (see below) was initially associated with release of a humoral factor, possibly β-endorphin (e.g., see Meyerson, 1983), but the involvement of endogenous opioids in stimulation-produced analgesia is controversial.

There are three different families of endogenous peptides, each derived from different, larger parent peptides. The best characterized parent peptide is proopiomelanocortin (POMC), which gives rise to the 31 amino acid peptide β-endorphin. In addition, POMC gives rise to adrenocorticotropin hormone (ACTH) and melanocyte-stimulating hormone, as well as other, less well characterized opioid peptides. The pentapeptide opioid peptides, lucine and methionine enkephalin, are derived from proenkephalin, while the dynorphins are derived from prodynorphin. Like the opioid receptors, opioid peptides are distributed nonhomogeneously in the brain. It has been generally believed that the different opioid peptides selectively interact with different opioid receptors. However, the correspondence between the distribution of *mu, delta,* and *kappa* opioid receptors and the opioid peptides does not support that assumption (e.g., see Mansour, Khachaturian, Lewis, Akill, & Watson, 1988). While it is known that some opioid peptides exhibit relative selectivity for certain of the opioid receptors (e.g., lucine enkephalin for delta receptors), opioid peptides derived from proenkephalin and prodynorphin can bind to all three opioid receptors: *mu, delta,* and *kappa.*

Thus, it does not appear that the action of an opioid peptide can be correlated with only one opioid receptor, and it is likely that differential, local processing of peptide precursors is important to opioid peptide–receptor interactions.

Sites of Action

Before opioid receptors were discovered, it had been demonstrated that opioids produced analgesia when administered directly into the ventricular spaces of the brain and also when injected directly into the brain parenchyma. The sites in the brain most sensitive to opioids were found to be the midbrain periaqueductal gray matter (PAG), particularly its ventrolateral aspect, and the rostral, ventral medulla (RVM), including the nucleus raphe magnus and adjacent nucleus paragigantocellularis (for review, see Yaksh & Rudy, 1978). The PAG has since become identified as a nodal point in descending systems of pain control (see below). When microinjected in the PAG, opioids produce an analgesia in a variety of test procedures across species (see Yaksh & Rudy, 1978) and inhibit spinal neuron responses to noxious stimuli—that is, produce a descending inhibition (for review, see Gebhart & Jones, 1988). These effects were established to arise from the PAG and not from redistribution of drug to the systemic circulation, for example. Thus, how opioids given in the PAG or RVM produce analgesia and descending inhibition has been an important focus of investigation.

Yaksh demonstrated that morphine microinjected into the PAG released the spinal neurotransmitter serotonin (5-hydroxytryptamine, 5-HT) and that the analgesia produced by morphine given in the PAG could be antagonized by the injection of a serotonin receptor antagonist, methysergide, into the spinal subarachnoid space (i.e., intrathecally) (Yaksh & Tyce, 1979; Yaksh & Wilson, 1979). The intrathecal injection of a selective opioid receptor antagonist, naloxone, had no effect on the analgesia produced by morphine microinjected into the PAG. Subsequent work established that the effects of morphine given in the PAG were mediated by both spinal serotonergic and adrenergic receptors (e.g., Jensen & Yaksh, 1986). Similarly, when microinjected into the RVM, opioids produce an analgesia mediated by spinal serotonergic and adrenergic receptors (e.g., Jensen & Yaksh, 1986).

These results and those from converging investigation of stimulation-produced analgesia (see below) strongly supported the existence of an endogenous system of pain control upon which opioids acted, contributing to their significant analgesic effect. Thus, in addition to direct actions at opioid receptors in the brain and spinal cord—actions that are competitively antagonized by the opioid receptor antagonist naloxone—opioids also engage an endogenous system of pain control mediated by spinal 5-HT and norepinephrine (NE) acting at their respective receptors. Clinically, manipulations that increase 5-HT and/or NE in the central nervous system, by blocking their reuptake with antidepressant drugs, for example, enhance the analgesia produced by opioids. Similarly, the coadministration of morphine with amphetamine or like drugs that enhance noradrenergic neurotransmission also enhances the analgesic effect of morphine (Forrest et al., 1979).

As indicated above, there are opioid receptors in the spinal cord. Their presence there has been exploited by administering opioids intrathecally or epidurally to produce analgesia in man (e.g., Cousins, 1988). When given systemically, opioids produce respiratory depression and sedation in addition to the desired analgesia. When opioid action is limited to the spinal cord, the analgesic effect can be retained while the sedation and respiratory depression can be reduced, if not eliminated. Studies related to these developments and the involvement of spinal adrenergic receptors in pain control discussed above establish that the intrathecal administration of drugs acting at α-adrenergic receptors also produce analgesia. In a variety of animal tests, α_2-adrenoceptor agonists such as clonidine and ST-91 produce a potent analgesia (e.g., Yaksh & Stevens, 1988). In complementary electrophysiological studies, clonidine and morphine both have been demonstrated to significantly attenuate the responses of spinal cord dorsal horn neurons to noxious cutaneous and visceral stimuli (Ness & Gebhart, 1988). Recent investigations suggest that *mu* opioid and α_2-adrenergic receptors in the spinal cord interact in their ability to mediate the analgesia produced by these drugs (Solomon & Gebhart, 1988; Stevens, Monasky, & Yaksh, 1988). As with opioids, clonidine has been given into the cerebrospinal fluid in man for pain relief (Coombs, Saunders, Gaylor, LaChance, & Jensen, 1984; Tamsen & Gordh, 1985). Thus, the combination of opioids with drugs like clonidine raises the possibility of reducing the rate of development of tolerance to opioids while maintaining analgesic efficacy.

Stimulation-Produced Analgesia

Reynolds (1969) was the first to report that focal electrical stimulation in the PAG produced an analgesia sufficient to permit surgery in rats. The demonstration of stimulation-produced analgesia (SPA) suggested that there existed an endogenous system for control of pain. It was subsequently demonstrated that stimulation in the ventral, lateral PAG produced an analgesia in a variety of animal species and was free of other sensory or motoric effects (for review, see Mayer, 1979). This basic work in nonhuman animals quickly led to demonstrations in man that stimulation in the brain was efficacious and useful for relief from otherwise intractable pain (for review, see Meyerson, 1983). Stimulation in the PAG was also shown to produce a powerful descending inhibition of spinal cord dorsal horn neurons responsive to noxious stimulation (for review, see Gebhart, 1986). In both electrophysiological and behavioral experiments, the data were interpreted initially to provide evidence of selectivity of stimulation-produced effects for nociception (pain) and nociceptive neurons. It has been subsequently established, however, that SPA does not selectively inhibit only noxious inputs to the central nervous system, but rather is only relatively selective. The effects of SPA on nonnoxious inputs are evident, but are less in magnitude than effects on noxious inputs (for review, see Gebhart, 1986).

Because both stimulation and morphine produced potent analgesia and descending inhibition when given in the ventral, lateral PAG, they were initially considered to influence the same endogenous systems of pain control. There is supportive evidence for a common mechanism in the PAG: Repeated administration of morphine or of stimulation in the PAG leads to analgesic tolerance, SPA can be partially antagonized by the opioid receptor antagonist naloxone, and some cross-tolerance develops between stimulation and morphine given in the PAG (for reviews, see Gebhart, 1983, Mayer, 1979). In addition, SPA from the PAG is antagonized by the intrathecal administration of serotonergic and adrenergic receptor antagonists, but not by naloxone. Given these similarities and anatomical evidence that spinopetal efferents from the PAG directly to the spinal cord are few in number (see below), the endogenous descending system proposed and upon which investigation focused required a bulbar relay in the RVM between the PAG and the spinal cord (Basbaum & Fields, 1984).

Stimulation in the proposed relay site (the nucleus raphe magnus, NRM) produces an analgesia and attenuates responses of spinal neurons to cutaneous and visceral noxious stimulation (Ness & Gebhart,

1987; for review, see Gebhart, 1986). The analgesia produced by stimulation, morphine, or glutamate given in the NRM, like that produced by stimulation, morphine, or glutamate given in the PAG, is antagonized by the intrathecal administration of serotonergic and/or adrenergic receptor antagonists (e.g., Aimone, Jones, & Gebhart, 1987; Jensen & Yaksh, 1984, 1986). These and other converging results clearly establish that the PAG → NRM → spinal cord pathway is at least one component of an endogenous pain control system (for review, see Basbaum & Fields, 1984).

That there are likely multiple components of descending systems important in pain modulation is supported by a large and growing body of evidence. It was found soon after the initial demonstration of SPA that descending inhibition of spinal neurons could be produced from areas in the midbrain that did not produce analgesia (Liebeskind, Guilbaud, Besson, & Oliveras, 1973). It has since been documented that stimulation in widespread areas in the brain produces powerful descending inhibition of spinal neurons as well as nociceptive reflexes (for review, see Gebhart, 1986, 1988). Stimulation in some of these sites has been established to produce inhibition parametrically different from that produced by stimulation in the PAG. Indeed, stimulation in the NRM produces effects on the same spinal neurons that are both quantitatively and qualitatively different from the effects produced by stimulation in the PAG (Gebhart, Sandkühler, Thalhammer, & Zimmermann, 1983a). Results such as these led to an examination of how descending systems are organized (see below), and it was demonstrated that either permanent or reversible inactivation of the NRM did not affect the descending inhibition from the PAG (e.g., Gebhart, Sandkühler, Thalhammer, & Zimmerman, 1983b; Morton, Duggan, & Zhao, 1984; for review, see Gebhart, 1988), providing strong evidence for the existence of multiple descending systems of inhibition. Similarly, stimulation in the lateral hypothalamus, the midbrain reticular formation, including the nucleus cuneiformis and parabrachial area, the locus coeruleus, and the lateral reticular area in the caudal medulla, has been shown to powerfully inhibit spinal neurons and nociceptive reflexes. Where examined, spinal serotonergic and/or adrenergic receptors have been found to mediate the descending effects of stimulation (for review, see Gebhart, 1988). The results of these and other studies not reviewed here establish that multiple descending systems are present in the central nervous system and that descending serotonergic and adrenergic systems are coactivated and mediate the inhibition produced. Some of these descending systems are illustrated schematically in Figure 1. Opioids clearly can activate

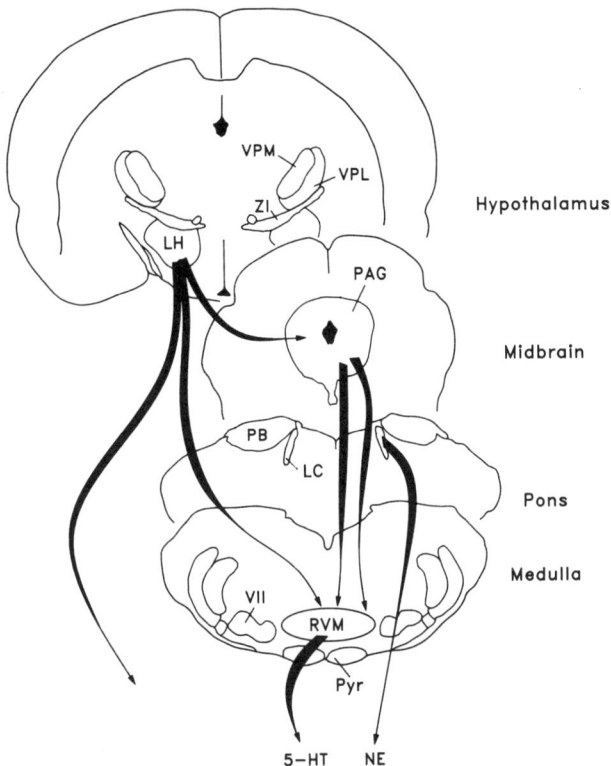

Figure 1. Illustration of the organization in the brainstem of descending systems of inhibition. The projections schematically illustrated are based on those established experimentally to be functionally important to descending modulation of pain. For example, descending projections from the lateral hypothalamus (LH) are directly to the spinal cord or indirectly to the periaqueductal gray (PAG) or nucleus raphe magnus in the medial rostroventral medulla (RVM). Projections from the RVM to the spinal cord are shown to be serotonergic (5-HT), while the locus coeruleus (LC) is shown to be the main source of norepinephrine (NE) to the spinal cord. Not shown in this illustration are projections from the RVM to the NE-containing A5 cell group, which also likely contributes descending NE-containing fibers to the spinal cord. See text for additional details. Other abbreviations: PB = parabrachial nuclei; Pry = pyramidal tract; VPL and VPM = nuclei ventralis posterior lateralis and medialis, respectively, of the thalamus; and ZI = zona incerta.

some of these descending systems and also have a direct analgesic effect mediated by opioid receptors. Despite the fact that enkephalin-containing interneurons are present in the spinal cord, convincing evidence for their involvement in the known descending systems of inhibition does not currently exist.

Organization of Descending Systems

The existence of multiple descending modulatory systems raises the issue of their independence. That is, are they parallel, independent systems or are they interdependent? That all systems studied to date are mediated by the same monoamine neurotransmitters in the spinal cord clearly points to their dependence on final common descending pathways.

As indicated above, there are only sparse direct spinopetal efferents from the PAG to the spinal cord (Mantyh & Peschanski, 1982; for reviews, see Basbaum & Fields, 1984; Gebhart, 1982). There is, however, both anatomical and electrophysiological evidence supporting functionally important projections from the PAG to the RVM (e.g., Abols & Basbaum, 1981; Behbehani & Fields, 1979; Beitz, Mullet, & Weiner, 1983). The projection from the PAG to the medial RVM, specifically the NRM, is not, however, essential to descending inhibition produced in the PAG since, as indicated above, conduction through the NRM can be interrupted without affecting SPA from the PAG. Thus, projections lateral to the NRM also are clearly important. Anatomical evidence that different neurons in the PAG project to the medial or to the lateral RVM has been provided by Beitz *et al.* (1983). Thus, as illustrated in Figure 1, descending inhibition from the PAG can relay in the medial *or* lateral RVM (as well as perhaps other nuclei in the brainstem).

It also has been demonstrated that descending inhibition from the locus coeruleus, a norepinephrine-containing group of cells in the dorsolateral pons, is independent of a relay in the NRM (Jones & Gebhart, 1987). Consistent with this finding, descending influences from the locus coeruleus are mediated by α_2-adrenoceptors in the spinal cord; serotonin receptor antagonists given intrathecally were without influence on SPA from the locus coeruleus (Jones & Gebhart, 1986). Descending inhibition from the caudal medullary lateral reticular nucleus is also predominantly α_2 noradrenergic in character, but includes a serotonergic component based on the partial effect of methysergide given intrathecally on SPA from the lateral reticular nucleus (Gebhart & Ossipov, 1986; Janss & Gebhart, 1987). In support, descending influences from the lateral reticular nucleus, like those from the NRM, were demonstrated to descend the spinal cord in the dorsolateral funiculi, whereas descending influences from the locus coeruleus, which are independent of serotonergic influences, descend the spinal cord in the ventrolateral funiculi (e.g., Jones & Gebhart, 1987).

Rostral to the PAG, the lateral hypothalamus also has been implicated in descending modulatory systems (e.g., Carstens, Frauenhoffer,

& Suberg, 1983), and descending influences from the LH are also mediated by spinal serotonin and adrenergic receptors (Aimone & Gebhart, 1987). In studies examining the relation of the lateral hypothalamus to descending influences produced in the PAG, locus coeruleus, and NRM, it was found that in addition to possible direct projections from the lateral hypothalamus to the spinal cord, relays in the PAG and the NRM, but not the LC, were functionally important (Aimone, Bauer, & Gebhart, 1988; see Figure 1).

The sources of spinal 5-HT and NE that mediate descending inhibition from the brainstem are limited to the 5-HT-containing B cell groups in the medullary raphe nuclei (NRM, n. raphe obscuris and n. raphe pallidus) and the NE-containing A cell groups in the medulla and pons (e.g., A5, A6 = locus coeruleus and A7). There are few or no endogenous sources of either 5-HT or NE in the spinal cord. When the spinal cord is transected, virtually all 5-HT and NE caudal to the transection disappears, demonstrating that 5-HT and NE in the spinal cord arises from long descending fibers whose cell bodies are located in the medulla and pons. Thus, stimulation or morphine given in the NRM increases the synthesis of 5-HT in the spinal cord (Bourgoin, Oliveras, Bruxelle, Hamon, & Besson, 1980; Vasko, Pang, & Vogt, 1984), while stimulation in the locus coeruleus increases the metabolism of NE in the spinal cord (Crawley, Roth, & Mass, 1979). Stimulation in and adjacent to the NRM also has been reported to increase the spinal content of NE as well as 5-HT (Hammond & Yaksh, 1985) and morphine given in the lateral RVM increases the metabolism of NE in the spinal cord (e.g., Kuraishi, Fukui, Shiomi, Akaike, & Takagi, 1978). Stimulation laterally in the RVM likely increases the content of NE in the spinal cord by activation of NE-containing fibers descending from the locus coeruleus. Stimulation in the medial RVM (i.e., the NRM), however, is believed to increase the content of NE in the spinal cord by activation of NE-containing neurons in the A5 cell group (for review, see Proudfit, 1988). This result is consistent with the ability of noradrenergic receptor antagonists administered intrathecally to partially attenuate the descending inhibitory effects of activation of 5-HT-containing neurons in the NRM (for review, see Proudfit, 1988). Thus, the likely sources of spinal 5-HT and NE influenced by SPA in the brainstem are known. The neurotransmitters mediating interactions between cell groups in the brainstem are less well understood.

The primary focus of investigations to date has been on the relay in the NRM. Two independent investigations have concluded that the neurotransmitter in the NRM mediating descending inhibition from the PAG is an excitatory amino acid, likely glutamate (Aimone & Gebhart,

1986; Wiklund et al., 1988). Using different experimental approaches, these investigators demonstrated that the descending inhibitory influences of stimulation in the PAG were blocked by selective glutamate receptor antagonists administered directly into the NRM. Other work suggests that a GABAergic inhibitory interneuron modulates the output neuron in the PAG (Moreau & Fields, 1986); a similar GABA-mediated inhibition is likely operative in the NRM (Drower & Hammond, 1988).

Summary

The preceding is but a brief review of important developments that have led to our present understanding of opioid analgesia and descending systems of pain control. Stimulation-produced analgesia can be demonstrated from widespread areas in the brain. These divergent areas share in common the fact that their descending influences, whether produced by stimulation or by morphine given into those sites, are mediated by spinal serotonergic and/or noradrenergic receptors. Opioid receptors and opioid peptides are located in all of these areas from which SPA can be produced as well as in the spinal cord. If endogenous opioid peptides are involved in these endogenous systems of control, and they likely are, it appears that such modulation occurs in the brain rather than in the spinal cord. The systems of pain control considered here are in a sense parallel but are not independent of each other. Rather, considerable evidence suggests that these systems are interdependent, and activation of the lateral hypothalamus or PAG, for example, also engages many of the other descending components discussed here.

The practical application of results in this field of research have led directly to improved pain control in man. For example, SPA is now used for relief of some otherwise intractable pains. The administration of opioids spinally reduces dosage, sedation, and respiratory depression in man without compromising the desired analgesic efficacy. The contributions of α-adrenoceptors to pain modulation are better understood and have led to the spinal use of clonidine and have clarified how adjuncts such as antidepressants can enhance pain relief. The discovery of opioid receptor subtypes has stimulated development of opioid receptor-selective drugs. It is hoped that such new drugs will retain analgesic efficacy but will possess reduced respiratory depressant effects or be free of the development of analgesic tolerance. Indeed, experimental data suggest that analgesic tolerance to one receptor-selective opioid does not necessarily develop to an opioid having a selective action at a different opioid receptor. Since the development of analgesic tolerance often limits pain relief in cases of chronic pain where long-term therapy is required, the ability to alternate successfully between different receptor-selective drugs will represent a very significant therapeutic advance.

It should also be emphasized that while only experimental activation of endogenous systems of pain control was discussed, environmental stimuli likely engage these same systems. For example, pain itself and stress have been demonstrated in experimental situations to produce analgesia, likely mediated by the systems reviewed here. An interaction between endogenous systems of pain control with those cardiopulmonary systems responsible for the modulation of blood pressure also has been established (e.g., see Randich & Maixner, 1984). Continued investigation into these and other areas will further enhance our understanding and improve our ability to control pain.

ACKNOWLEDGMENTS. The work of the author reported here has been supported by USPHS awards DA 02879, NS 19912, and NS 24598. The secretarial assistance of M. Kirkpatrick is gratefully acknowledged.

References

Abols, I. A., & Basbaum, A. I. (1981). Afferent connections of the rostral medulla of the cat: A neural substrate for midbrain-medullary interactions in the modulation of pain. *Journal of Comparative Neurology, 201*, 285–297.

Aimone, L. D., Jones, S. L., & Gebhart, G. F. (1987). Stimulation-produced descending inhibition from the periaqueductal gray and nucleus raphe magnus in the rat: Mediation by spinal monoamines but not opioids. *Pain, 31*, 123–136.

Aimone, L. D., & Gebhart, G. F. (1987). Spinal monoamine mediation of stimulation-produced antinociception from the lateral hypothalamus. *Brain Research, 403*, 290–300.

Aimone, L. D., Jones, S. L., & Gebhart, G. F. (1987). Stimulation-produced descending inhibition from the periaqueductal gray and nucleus raphe magnus in the rat: Mediation by spinal monoamines but not opioids. *Pain, 31*, 123–136.

Aimone, L. D., Bauer, C., & Gebhart, G. F. (1988). Brainstem relays mediating stimulation-produced antinociception from the lateral hypothalamus in the rat. *Journal of Neuroscience, 8*, 2652–2663.

Basbaum, A. I., & Fields, H. L. (1984). Endogenous pain control systems: Brainstem spinal pathways and endorphin circuitry. *Annual Review of Neuroscience, 7*, 319–338.

Behbehani, M. M., & Fields, H. L. (1979). Evidence that an excitatory connection between the periaqueductal gray and the nucleus raphe magnus mediates stimulation-produced analgesia. *Brain Research, 170*, 85–93.

Beitz, A. J., Mullet, M. A., & Weiner, L. L. (1983). The periaqueductal projections to the rat spinal trigeminal, raphe magnus, gigantocellular pars alpha and paragigantocellular nuclei arise from separate neurons. *Brain Research, 288*, 307–314.

Bourgoin, S., Oliveras, J. L., Bruxelle, J., Hamon, N., & Besson, J. M. (1980). Electrical stimulation of the nucleus raphe magnus in the rat: Effects on 5-HT metabolism in the spinal cord. *Brain Research, 194,* 377–389.

Carstens, E., Frauenhoffer, M., & Suberg, S. (1983). Inhibition of spinal dorsal horn neuronal responses to noxious skin heating by lateral hypothalamic simulation in the cat. *Journal of Neurophysiology, 50,* 192–204.

Coombs, D. W., Saunders, R., Gaylor, M., LaChance, D., & Jensen, L. (1984). Clinical trial of intrathecal clonidine for cancer pain. *Journal of Regional Anesthesiology, 9,* 34–35.

Cousins, M. J. (1988). The spinal route of analgesia for acute and chronic pain. In R. Dubner, G. F. Gebhart, & M. R. Bond (Eds.), *Proceedings of the Vth world congress on pain, Pain research in clinical management* (Vol. 3, pp. 454–471). Amsterdam: Elsevier.

Crawley, J. N., Roth, R. H., & Mass, J. W. (1979). Locus coeruleus stimulation increases noradrenergic metabolite levels in rat spinal cord. *Brain Research, 166,* 180–184.

Drower, E. J., & Hammond, D. L. (1988). GABAergic modulation of nociceptive threshold: Effects of THIP and bicuculline microinjected into the ventral medulla of the rat. *Brain Research, 450,* 316–324.

Forrest, W. H., Brown, B. W., Brown, C. K., Defalque, R., Gold, M., Gordon, H. E., James, K. E., Katz, J., Mahler, D. L., Schroff, P., & Teutsch, G. (1979). Dextroamphetamine with morphine for the treatment of postoperative pain. *New England Journal of Medicine, 296,* 712–715.

Gebhart, G. F. (1982). Opiate and opioid peptide effects on brainstem neurons: Relevance to nociception and antinociceptive mechanisms. *Pain, 12,* 93–140.

Gebhart, G. F. (1983). Recent developments in the neurochemical bases of pain and analgesia. In R. M. Brown, T. M. Pinkert, & J. Ludford (Eds.), *Contemporary research in pain and analgesia* (pp. 19–35). National Institute on Drug Abuse, Research Monograph 45. Washington, DC: U.S. Government Printing Office.

Gebhart, G. F. (1986). Modulatory effects of descending systems on spinal dorsal horn neurons. In T. L. Yaksh (Ed.), *Spinal afferent processing* (pp. 391–416). New York: Plenum.

Gebhart, G. F. (1988). Descending inhibition of nociceptive transmission. In J. Olesen & L. Edvinsson (Eds.), *Basic mechanisms of headache* (pp. 201–212). Amsterdam: Elsevier.

Gebhart, G. F., & Jones, S. L. (1988). Effects on morphine given in the brainstem on the activity of dorsal horn nociceptive neurons. In H. L. Fields & J. M. Besson (Eds.), *Pain modulation* (Progress in Brain Research, Vol. 77, pp. 229–243). Amsterdam: Elsevier.

Gebhart, G. F., & Ossipov, M. H. (1986). Characterization of inhibition of the nociceptive tail flick reflex in the rat from the medullary lateral reticular nucleus. *Journal of Neuroscience, 6,* 701–713.

Gebhart, G. F., Sandkühler, J., Thalhammer, J. G., & Zimmerman, M. (1983a). Quantitative comparison of inhibition in the spinal cord of nociceptive information by electrical stimulation in the periaqueductal gray and the nucleus raphe magnus of the cat. *Journal of Neurophysiology, 50,* 1433–1445.

Gebhart, G. F., Sandkühler, J., Thalhammer, J. G., & Zimmerman, M. (1983b). Inhibition of spinal nociceptive information by stimulation in the midbrain of the cat is blocked by lidocaine microinjected in nucleus raphe magnus and the medullary reticular formation. *Journal of Neurophysiology, 50,* 1446–1457.

Hammond, D. L., & Yaksh, T. L. (1985). Efflux of 5-hydroxytryptamine and noradrenaline into spinal cord superfusates during stimulation of the rat medulla. *Journal of Physiology (London), 359,* 151–162.

Hughes, J. (1975). Isolation of an endogenous compound from the brain with pharmacological properties similar to morphine. *Brain Research, 88,* 295–308.

Janss, A. J., & Gebhart, G. F. (1987). Spinal monoaminergic receptors mediate the anti-

nociceptive effects of glutamate in the lateral reticular nucleus. *Journal of Neuroscience, 7*, 2862–2873.
Jensen, T. S., & Yaksh, T. L. (1984). Spinal monoamine and opioid systems partially mediate analgesia induced by glutamate at brainstem sites. *Brain Research, 321*, 285–293.
Jensen, T. S., & Yaksh, T. L. (1986). II. Examination of spinal monoamine receptors through which brainstem opiate-sensitive systems act in the rat. *Brain Research, 363*, 114–127.
Jones, S. L., & Gebhart, G. F. (1986). Characterization of coeruleospinal inhibition of the nociceptive tail flick reflex in the rat: Mediation by spinal α-adrenoceptors. *Brain Research, 364*, 315–330.
Jones, S. L., & Gebhart, G. F. (1987). Spinal pathways mediating tonic, coeruleospinal and raphespinal descending inhibition in the rat. *Journal of Neurophysiology, 58*, 138–159.
Kuraishi, Y. Fukui, K., Shiomi, H., Akaike, A., & Takagi, H. (1978). Microinjection of opioids into the nucleus reticuluris gigantocellurlaris in the rat: Analgesia and increase in the normetanephrine level in the spinal cord. *Biochemical Pharmacology, 27*, 2756–2758.
Liebeskind, J. C., Guilbaud, G., Besson, J. M., & Oliveras, J. L. (1973). Analgesia from electrical stimulation of the periaqueductal gray matter in the cat: Behavioral observations and inhibitory effects on spinal cord interneurons. *Brain Research, 50*, 441–446.
Mansour, A., Khachaturian, H., Lewis, M. E., Akill, H., & Watson, S. J. (1988). Anatomy of CNS opioid receptors. *Trends in Neuroscience, 11*, 308–314.
Mantyh, P. W., & Peschanski, M. (1982). Spinal projection from the periaqueductal gray and dorsal raphe, cat and monkey. *Neuroscience, 7*, 2769–2776.
Mayer, D. J. (1979). Endogenous analgesia systems: Neural and behavioral mechanisms. In J. J. Bonica, J. Liebeskind, & D. Albe-Fessard (Eds.), *Advances in pain research and therapy* (Vol. 3, pp. 385–410). New York: Raven Press.
Meyerson, B. A. (1983). Electrostimulation procedures: Effects, presumed rationale and possible mechanisms. In J. J. Bonica, U. Lindblom, & A. Iggo (Eds.), *Advances in pain research and therapy* (Vol. 5, pp. 495–534). New York: Raven Press.
Moreau, J. L., & Fields, H. L. (1986). Evidence for GABA involvement in midbrain control of medullary neurons that modulate nociceptive transmission. *Brain Research, 397*, 37–46.
Morton, C. R., Duggan, A. W., & Zhao, Z. Q. (1984). The effects of lesions of medullary midline and lateral reticular areas on inhibition in the dorsal horn produced by periaqueductal gray stimulation in the cat. *Brain Research, 301*, 121–130.
Ness, T. J., & Gebhart, G. F. (1987). Quantitative comparison of inhibition of visceral and cutaneous spinal nociceptive transmissions from the midbrain and medulla in the rat. *Journal of Neurophysiology, 58*, 850–865.
Ness, T. J., & Gebhart, G. F. (1988). Inhibition of visceral and cutaneous spinal nociceptive transmission by morphine and clonidine: Differential effects on intensity coding. In R. Dubner, G. F. Gebhart, & M. R. Bond (Eds.), *Proceedings of the Vth world congress on pain, Pain research in clinical management* (Vol. 3, pp. 442–448). Amsterdam: Elsevier.
Pert, C. B., & Snyder, S. H. (1973). Properties of opiate receptor binding in rat brain. *Proceedings of the National Academy of Sciences (Washington), 70*, 2243–2247.
Proudfit, H. K. (1988). Pharmacologic evidence for the modulation of nociception by noradrenergic neurons. In H. L. Fields & J. M. Besson (Eds.), *Pain modulation* (Progress in Brain Research, Vol. 77, pp. 357–370). Amsterdam: Elsevier.
Randich, A., & Maixner, W. (1984). Interactions between cardiovascular and pain regulatory systems. *Neuroscience and Biohavioral Reviews, 8*, 343–367.
Reynolds, D. V. (1969). Surgery in the rat during electrical analgesia induced by focal brain stimulation. *Science, 164*, 444–445.

Simon, E. J., Hiller, J. M., & Adelman, I. (1973). Stereospecific binding of the potent analgesic [³H]etorphine to rat brain homogenate. *Proceedings of the National Academy of Sciences (Washington), 70,* 1947–1949.

Solomon, R. E., & Gebhart, G. F. (1988). Intrathecal morphine and clonidine: Antinociceptive tolerance and cross-tolerance and effects on blood pressure. *Journal of Pharmacology and Experimental Therapeutics, 245,* 444–454.

Stevens, C. W., Monasky, M. S., & Yaksh, T. L. (1988). Spinal infusion of opiate and α_2-agonists in rats: Tolerance and cross-tolerance studies. *Journal of Pharmacology and Experimental Therapeutics, 244,* 63–70.

Tamsen, A., & Gordh, T. (1984). Epidural clonidine produces analgesia. *Lancet, ii,* 231–232.

Terenius, L. (1973). Characteristics of the "receptor" for narcotic analgesics in synaptic plasma membrane fraction from rat brain. *Acta Pharmacologica, 33,* 337–384.

Vasko, M. R., Pang, I. H., & Vogt, M. (1984). Involvement of 5-hydroxytryptamine-containing neurons in the antinociception produced by injection of morphine into nucleus raphe magnus or onto spinal cord. *Brain Research, 306,* 341–348.

Wiklund, L., Behzadi, G., Kalan, P., Headley, P. M., Nicolopoulos, L. S., Parsons, C. G., & West, D. C. (1988). Autoradiographic and electrophysiological evidence for excitatory amino acid transmission in the periaqueductal gray projection to nucleus raphe magnus in the rat. *Neuroscience Letters, 93,* 158–163.

Yaksh, T. L., & Rudy, T. A. (1978). Narcotic analgesics: CNS sites and mechanisms of action as revealed by intracerebral injection techniques. *Pain, 4,* 299–359.

Yaksh, T. L., & Stevens, C. W. (1988). Properties of the modulation of spinal nociceptive transmission by receptor-selective agents. In R. Dubner, G. F. Gebhart, & M. R. Bond (Eds.), *Proceedings of the Vth world congress on pain, Pain research and clinical management* (Vol. 3, pp. 417–435). Amsterdam: Elsevier.

Yaksh, T. L., & Tyce, G. M. (1979). Microinjection of morphine into the periaqueductal gray evokes the release of serotonin from spinal cord. *Brain Research, 171,* 176–181.

Yaksh, T. L., & Wilson, P. R. (1979). Spinal serotonin terminal mediates antinociception. *Journal of Pharmacology and Experimental Therapeutics, 208,* 446–453.

CHAPTER 13

Gate Control Theory of Pain Perception
Current Status

Wolfgang Larbig

Introduction

While we are awake our brain is constantly processing a continuous stream of sensory stimuli, including even more or less small injuries within the body and aversive social events, of which we are not aware and do not take the slightest notice. Yet we feel no pain. For example, the mechanism of suppressing sensory input can be clearly observed during strenuous sports or during wartime.

Melzack and co-workers (Melzack, Wall, & Ty, 1982) demonstrated that out of 138 patients with serious civilian injuries, 37% did not feel pain at the time of injury. The delays of pain perception varied from 1 to 9 hours after the injury. Similar results were demonstrated by Beecher (1959) in his famous study showing that 66% of wounded soldiers did not experience any pain sensation.

What are the mechanisms by which nerve activity is suppressed in normal and in special pain-evoking circumstances (i.e., after heavy injuries or during stress)? Melzack and Wall were the first to give a plausible answer to questions about the nature and underlying mechanisms of the suppression of pain across a variety of circumstances.

Wolfgang Larbig • Psychological Institute, University of Tübingen, D 7400 Tübingen 1, Federal Republic of Germany.

The Gate Control Theory of Pain

In 1965 the stage was set for Melzack and Wall's introduction of a psychophysiological pain-suppression concept known as the "gate control theory." This hypothesis revived the old duality theory of Head (Head & Sherren, 1905), who maintained that the epicritic afferent system inhibits the protopathic afferent system of nerves. More specifically, fast conducting fibers (epicritic) inhibit slow fibers (protopathic).

Melzack and Wall's theory very clearly illustrates pain-modulating principles and also makes the idea of pain-inhibitory mechanisms understandable. Therefore, this concept has gained wide acceptance but has also been subject to much criticism. The theory proposes that a neural mechanism in the spinal cord acts like a "gate" that can facilitate or inhibit the flow of nerve impulses from peripheral fibers to the central nervous system. Somatic input is therefore subjected to the modulating influences of the gate before it evokes pain perception—that is, before the afferent flow of nerve impulses exceeds a critical level.

In neurophysiological terms, the gate control model views pain perception and response as complex phenomena, resulting from the interaction of large-fiber activities that could modulate small-fiber transmission by activating inhibitory cells in the substantia gelatinosa (SG) of the spinal cord. The theory suggests that large-fiber inputs tend to close the gate while smaller-fiber inputs generally open it, and that the gate is profoundly influenced by descending influences from the brain.

Pain is generated by small high-threshold A-delta and C fibers when tissue damage occurs. The inputs presynaptically potentiate synaptic transmission by hyperpolarizing the central terminals of primary afferent neurons—this is the "gate opening" part of the mechanism. The sensory input depolarizes the central terminals of dorsal root fibers via low-threshold large-diameter A fibers, thus producing presynaptic inhibition of pain—this is the "gate closing" part of the gate theory (see Figure 1).

On the basis of experimental evidence, this difference in the action of large myelinated and small nonmyelinated fibers at the spinal level led Melzack and Wall (1965) to postulate that a gate control mechanism resides in the spinal gray matter. According to the theory, afferent impulses mediated by large fibers have activating effects on inhibitory "T-cells" in the SG of the spinal cord, including presynaptic inhibition of posterior root fibers by closing the gate. The onward transmission from all sensory neurons, including those with both large- and small-diameter fibers is reduced or inhibited.

Small fibers, however, open the gate by inhibiting the T-cells, thus

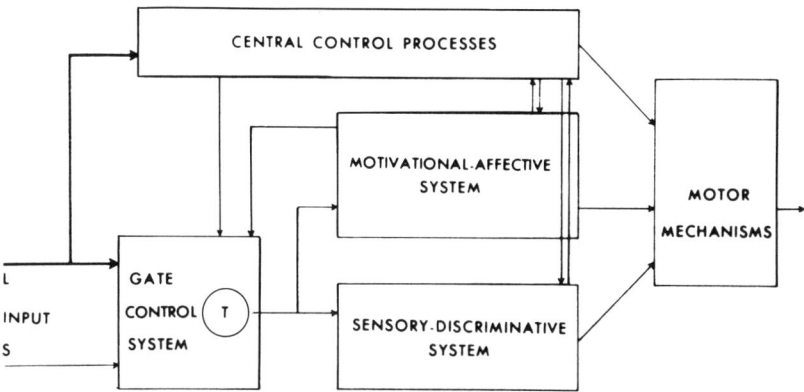

Figure 1. Schematic diagram of the gate control model. Pain is generated by small (s) fibers. Adjacent large (l) fibers could modulate pain transmission by activating inhibitory cells (T) in the substantia gelatinosa of the spinal cord as well as the sensory-discriminative and motivational-emotional system. Central control processes in the brain further modulate pain by means of corticofugal fibers carrying signals to the gate to inhibit the transmission of nociception. All systems interact with one another, and project to the motor system. (Adapted from Melzack & Dennis, 1978.)

facilitating onward transmission of painful stimuli to the brain coming from the periphery. Presynaptic control could control the depth and distribution of arriving impulses over dendrites and cell bodies of the receiving cells in the spinal cord. In other words, the output of dorsal horn cells at successive synapses throughout the projection from the spinal cord to the brain is determined by the balance of large and small fiber activity on account of their presynaptic effects (Figure 1), thereby affecting pain experience and response. The theory further postulates that large fibers of the fast-conducting systems of the posterior columns activate central control processes, and that these events occur before the input to the brain from more slowly conducting pathways arrives. Melzack and Wall also proposed that the entire gating system is modulated by means of corticofugal fibers that carry transmission of nociception.

Spinal Pain Modulation: Further Research and Criticism

In his evaluation of the gate control theory, Noordenbos (1974) stated:

the name gate admirably expressed the mode of action and was acceptable in our modern computer society. But although it was supported by clinical and experimental evidence, it was still a theory. The diagram was simple: it had to be in order to make it understandable. This is always the trouble when discussing the nervous system: you have to simplify in order to be able to talk about it at all. Criticism was bound to come; details were lacking and modification would no doubt have to be made. More important was the fact that it led directly to therapeutic methods. (p. 334)

Similarly, in 1979, Noordenbos commented: "Many critics seem to spend more time on the model, which is a gross simplification of which the authors were well aware, than on the conception that gave rise to it" (p. 322).

Some critics focused their attention solely on controversial aspects of neural transmission processes in the dorsal horn of the spinal cord, and failed to consider that Melzack and Wall also claimed the importance of experimentally well confirmed corticofugal pain-modulatory components. Pre- or postsynaptic inhibition occurs at every segment at the endings of large afferent fibers at the posterior column nucleus, thus blocking pain transmission from entering fibers into the terminal arborization. This is one component on which the gate theory is built that is generally accepted by all research groups in the field (Nathan, 1976). On the other hand, the mechanisms by which these inhibitory depolarizing processes occur remain in doubt.

The other part of the spinal balance system between large and small fibers became the most controversial aspect of the theory—that activation or "opening" of small fibers causes hyperpolarization, thus producing presynaptic facilitation and counteracting any effects of presynaptic inhibition.

Hyperpolarization is indicated by two positive waves, called dorsal root potential (DRP), of which the first wave is due to the *delta* fiber's input and the second wave to the C fiber's input (Mendell, 1970; Mendell & Wall, 1964). In numerous electrophysiological studies, clear cut positive DRPs could be seen after stimulation of small fibers (Hodge, 1972; Mendell, 1970). Other physiological experiments, however, have presented evidence for depolarization (negative DRPs) of a fiber's terminal ending (Franz & Iggo, 1968; Janig & Zimmermann, 1971; Schmidt, 1972), results that are not consistent with the gate-opening part of the theory. For example, Whitehorn and Burgess (1973) found that noxious stimuli tended to depolarize or hyperpolarize central endings of small fibers. This result contradicts an essential proposed feature of the gate control theory—namely, that small fiber activation inhibits interneurons mediating primary afferent depolarization in nociceptor terminals.

Whitehorn and Burgess investigated changes in terminal polarization of nociceptor fibers produced by noxious skin stimulation using a single-unit-recording method with microelectrodes. Various types of natural stimuli were applied to the skin outside of each fiber's receptive field. Depolarization or hyperpolarization of a fiber's terminal ending was tested by determining the current required to discharge it antidromically by microstimulation within the dorsal horn. According to the gate theory, noxious or high-intensity natural stimuli should produce either hyperpolarization (i.e., increased neurotransmitter release) or a reduced depolarization (i.e., reduced neurotransmitter release). It was found, however, that noxious stimuli tended to depolarize and, presumably, presynaptically inhibit the central endings of the A-*delta* mechanical nociceptors. That is, the hyperpolarization postulated by the gate theory was not demonstrated. Primary afferent hyperpolarization (PAH) occurred only *after* the termination of the stimulation, thus challenging the "gate opening" mechanism of the gate-control hypothesis.

Several studies by other physiologists (Franz & Iggo, 1968; Janig & Zimmermann, 1971; Schmidt, 1972) also are not consistent with the opening part of the theory. These investigators observed only negative DRPs following C-fiber stimulation.

Several recent studies (Dubner & Sessle, 1971; Hodge, 1972; Mendell, 1972; Young & King, 1972) have presented additional evidence for a PAH-action of small fibers. Also Mendell (1970) has shown clear-cut positive DRPs (i.e., hyperpolarization) after stimulation of smaller *delta* and C fibers. Mendell's later work (1972, 1973) shows that both depolarization (PAD) and PAH in small and large fibers can occur depending on stimulus strength (increased PAH) and frequency (reduced PAH).

Hodge (1972) obtained similar results using intracellular recordings instead of much less certain measures of DRPs—the latter represent a mass effect in many fibers owing to the averaging effect. Hodge stated that the DRP is thus a less reliable source of information about processes occurring inside single afferent fiber terminals compared with intracellular recordings. DRPs as mass effects can represent prominent PAD that masks PAH, and vice versa. Hodge's results show directly that small-diameter cutaneous and muscle nerves cause hyperpolarization and further that this hyperpolarization causes facilitation. This indicates a presynaptic gating mechanism of pain perception. The PAH, however, was not distributed equally to small-diameter afferents—only about one-third of the afferents studied were subject to small-fiber-induced PAH.

Hodge came to an interesting conclusion concerning a fine- and well-tuned specificity of presynaptic pain control at the spinal level. He speculates that there exists a complex selective distribution of PAH and PAD, indicating a functional presynaptic interaction depending either upon the type of peripheral information they transmit or upon the central pathways they activate. Such functional interaction would allow finer control of some selected peripheral events. (It is of interest that the trigeminal system also displays a somewhat selective distribution of both PAH and PAD; Dubner & Sessle, 1971.) Summarizing these results, a number of different studies support the "gate opening" mechanism of the theory, others do not.

Recently, Wall (1984) has described a neuroanatomical model that represents the anatomical and neurophysiological structure of the "gate," emphasizing that the dorsal horn is a significant synaptical relay station of the whole neural pain system. The structure of the dorsal column consists of six laminae, stratified in a dorsal-ventral direction, that run the entire length of the cord, each one having a particular histological structure. The sensory input arriving through dorsal roots shows a rigid scheme of laminar distribution. Wall (1984) proposed one possible overall plan for segmental circuitry, a "cascade model," with a general flow of excitation and inhibition from ventral to dorsal linking all laminae (see Figure 2). There is some disagreement as to which layers are driven primarily by C, A-*delta*, and A-*beta* fibers. The smallest C fibers end in lamina I and II (labeled as the substantia gelatinosa, SG), the largest terminate in Lamina VI. The SG represents a band of densely packed neurons, also containing the hypothetical T-cells, thought to have a major role in nociceptive transmission. These cells as well as other nociceptive cells do not function independently but rather are under the control of the concomitant peripheral barrage from larger fibers, firing patterns of local interneurons, and influences of descending pathways (Wall, 1984).

The nociceptive signals arriving at the dorsal horn must cross a synapse and ascend the spinal cord through one of several pathways to higher centers to evoke pain. The cells for such spinothalamic transmission can be separated into four types: low-threshold neurons, wide-dynamic-range neurons, high-threshold neurons, and deep neurons responding to deep-tissue receptors (Willis, 1984).

Nociception depends primarily on high-threshold and wide-dynamic-range neurons. Stimulation of wide-dynamic-range neurons can elicit qualitative and affective dimensions of pain. The class of spinothalamic tract (STT) neurons can be inhibited by peripheral stimulation, consistent with the gate-closing mechanism of the gate-control hypothesis (Willis, Trevino, Coulter, & Manuz, 1974). The monosynaptic termination of nociceptive afferents on cells is concentrated in laminae,

GATE CONTROL THEORY

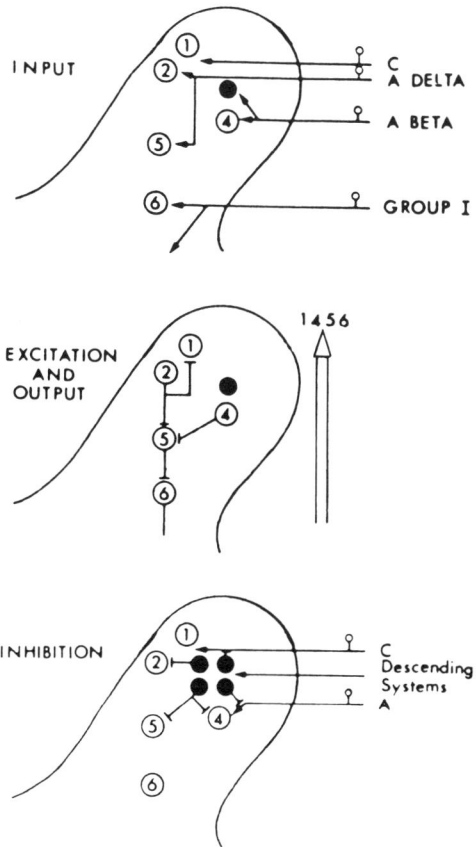

Figure 2. Diagrams of the dorsal horn. The circles represent groups of neurons in the six laminae of the dorsal horn. Dark circles represent inhibitory interneurons. Input shows the scheme of the laminar distribution of primary afferents with small fibers (C) ending in lamina I and II, and the largest, the group 1 afferents from muscle, ending in lamina VI. Excitation and output show the cascade model of excitatory activity. Lamina I, IV, V and VI project to the brain. In inhibition, interneurons (dark circles) receive input from descending systems and from local interneurons. They project presynaptically onto the terminals of A and C fibres and postsynaptically on to dorsal horn cells. (Adapted from Fields & Basbaum, 1984.)

I, II, and V, representing nociceptive neurons. These contain, for example, the wide-dynamic-range neurons with low threshold fast-conducting axons (Willis *et al.*, 1974) or the nociceptive high-threshold STT neurons (Foreman, Beall, Applebaum, Coulter, & Willis, 1976). Groups of local inhibitory interneurons (see Figure 2) receive inputs from afferent fibers, from descending systems, and from local interneurons projecting presynaptically onto the terminals of A and C fibers, and postsynaptically onto dorsal horn cells. Compared with the observed complex multiplicity of interconnections at the dorsal horn, the gate control theory seems to represent a very simple but clear model.

Descending Pain Control System

The existence of a specific supraspinal descending pain modulating system was first clearly proposed in the gate control theory, but evidence of centrifugal control was limited at that time. The early central control postulates have been amply confirmed by the discovery of the phenomenon called "stimulation-produced analgesia (SPA)" (Mayer & Liebeskind, 1974, Reynolds, 1969). SPA is a powerful and highly selective suppression of pain-related behavior produced by electrical stimulation of periaqueductal gray areas (PAG).

At each level of the neuraxis receiving ascending sensory input there are neurons with descending processes capable of influencing the input into that area. SPA appears to inhibit the nociceptive components of high-threshold STT and of wide-dynamic range neurons of laminae I and V of the spinal dorsal horn (Fields & Basbaum, 1984). Analgesia at the first synapse also depends upon corticofugal pathways extending from the frontal cortex and hypothalamus through PAG to the rostral ventromedial medulla (RVM), including the nucleus reticularis paragigantocellularis (RPG) and nucleus raphe magnus (NRM). The pathways then extend to the superficial layers of the dorsal horn via the dorsolateral funiculus (DLF), as shown in Figure 3 (Fields & Basbaum, 1984).

A parallel important breakthrough in pain research was the discovery of the endogenous opioid peptides, shown to be widely distributed along the entire neuraxis involved in the control of pain. This analgesia system functions as a negative feedback loop for nociception: It is activated by noxious stimuli and, in turn, it suppresses pain transmission.

Both enkephalins and dynorphin terminals and cells are present in the dorsal horn forming a dense network in Laminae I–II and V. Enkephalin-containing interneurons inhibit the release of substance P, a putative neurotransmitter of nociceptive sensory afferents (Jessell & Iversen, 1977; see Figure 4).

The neurotransmitter serotonin (5-HT) also plays a prominent role in analgesia, whereas norepinephrine has been shown to depress analgesic effects. To understand the neural mechanisms of corticofugal pain control at the spinal level, a detailed map of local circuits in the super-

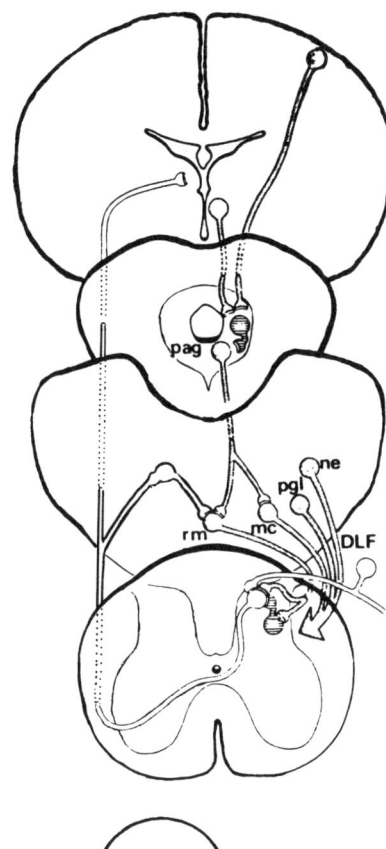

Figure 3. Diagram of pain modulating corticofugal structures extending from frontal cortex and hypothalamus to the midbrain periaqueductal grey (pag) to the medullary nucleus raphe magnus (rm)/reticularis magnocellularis (mc) and, via the dorsolateral funiculus (DLF), to the spinal cord dorsal horn. Additional pathways potentially relevant to analgesia arise from the nucleus paragigantocellularis (pgl) which also receives input from pag and noradrenergic medullary cell groups (ne). (Adapted from Fields & Basbaum, 1984.)

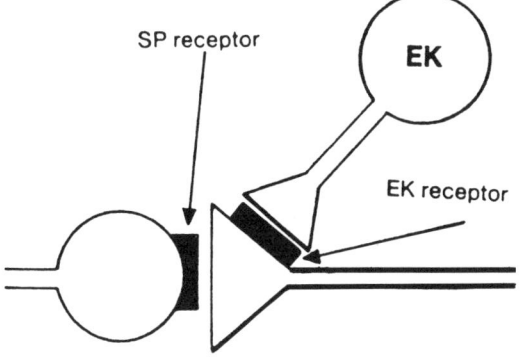

Figure 4. Enkephalin interneurons of the substantia gelatinosa exert a postsynaptic control of nociceptive transmission. Enkephalin-containing terminals synapsing on specific opiate receptors appear to inhibit the release of substance P, which is thought to transmit noxious impulses via unmyelinated fibers to the brain. Enkephalins function not only as neuro transmitters in the dorsal horn. They have also been found in higher areas of the brain, i.e., in the nucleus raphe magnus. (Adapted from Costa & Trabucchi, 1978.)

ficial dorsal horn is required. Two classes of neurons predominate in lamina I and SG, stalk and islet cells, receiving nociceptive input, some of them containing pain-modulating peptides (GABA, enkephalin, neurotensin). These cells are regarded to be the best candidates for the local inhibitory interneurons, the so called T-cells of the gate theory. These are believed to control the nociceptive projection neurons, both pre- and postsynaptically. The fact that spinal naloxone blocks the analgesic effects of descending pain-modulation circuits suggests a medullary connection to opioid-releasing interneurons in the cord (Fields & Basbaum, 1984; see Figures 5 and 6).

Clinical Implications: The Psychological Management of Pain

The gate theory has given us a new picture of the functional, neuroanatomical, neurophysiological, pharmacological, and behavioral bases of pain and has stimulated clinical research investigating and using the patient's own inborn neurophysiological pain control mechanisms. In addition to pharmacological and surgical treatment of clinical pain, the gate model has made it clear for the first time that pain-

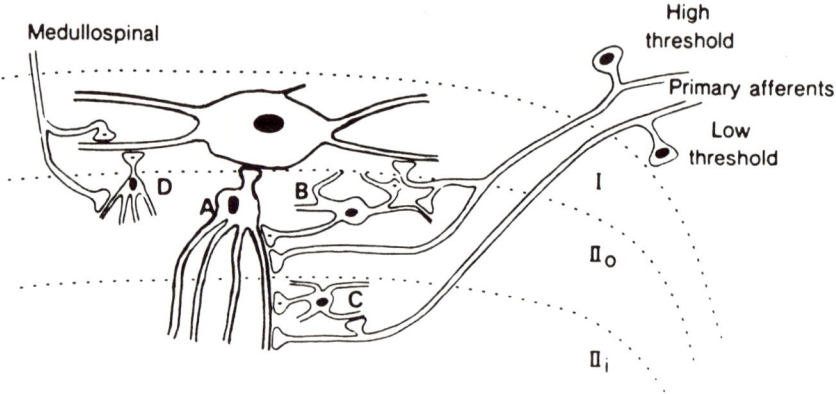

Figure 5. Diagram of afferent terminals and local circuitry in the dorsal horn illustrates that nociceptive input via high threshold primary afferent fibres excite neurons of lamina I, dendrites of stalk cell interneurons (A) and inhibitory islet interneurons (B) of lamina IIo. Low threshold fibres provide non-nociceptive input to stalk cells in lamina IIi. In contrast, non-nociceptive input to islet cell interneurons of lamina IIi (C) may contribute to the inhibitory control of nociceptive marginal neurons. Descending medullospinal axons may excite inhibitory interneurons (D), which postsynaptically control nociceptive projection neurons. (Adapted from Fields & Basbaum, 1984.)

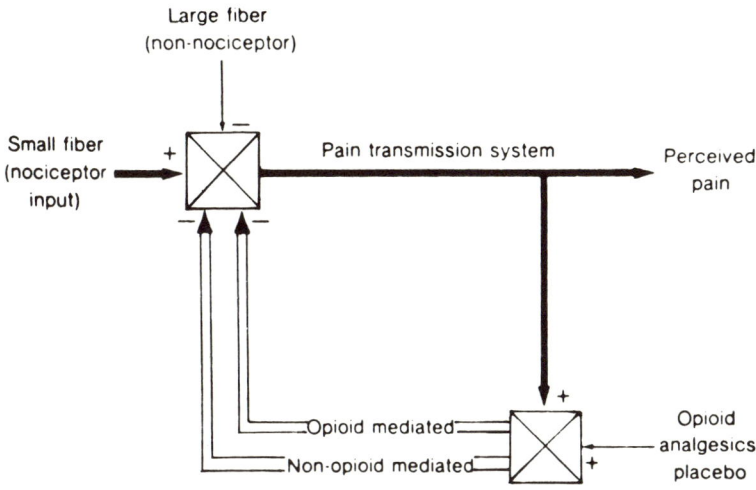

Figure 6. Diagram of pain modulating systems. The pain transmission system, activated by nociceptor input, creates a negative feedback loop and can be enhanced by narcotic (opioid and non-opioid) analgesics and modulated by non-nociceptive primary efferents. (Adapted from Fields & Basbaum, 1984.)

modulating systems possibly can be triggered by psychological and physical methods.

Stimulation Therapies

Transcutaneous electrical stimulation (TENS), electrical acupuncture, and other counterirritational treatments (such as direct peripheral nerve stimulation, dorsal column stimulation, and vibration) have been employed in chronic pain patients. TENS has successfully diminished acute postoperative pain (Tyler, Caldwell, & Ghia, 1982), pain during delivery (Augustinsson et al., 1977), and sports-related pain (Roeser, Meeks, Venis, & Strickland, 1976). It has been shown to have benefits in over 60% of all patients, and in cases of intractable severe pain, refractory to all conventional treatments, it may benefit up to 30% of patients (Woolf, 1984).

Recent neurophysiological experiments have clearly demonstrated the combination of central and peripheral inhibitory mechanisms that would be responsible for mediating the analgesia produced by TENS. Confirming the early major predictions of the gate theory, it was found that the activation of low-threshold primary A-*beta* afferents selectively inhibit C fibers and noxious evoked responses in dorsal horn neurons. This is accomplished by presynaptic and probably postsynaptic mechanisms (Fitzgerald & Woolf, 1981). Moreover, naloxone has been shown to reverse pain-relieving effects of TENS, indicating a clear role for endogenous opioid peptides in mediating the analgesia produced by TENS (Sjölund & Eriksson, 1979). (Other authors, using high-frequency TENS, have not found the same analgesia-antagonizing effects. These discrepancies may be explained by the involvement of several subclasses of opiate receptors, as described by Woolf, 1984, and by different descending inhibitory pathways.)

Psychological Interventions

The pain-relieving effects of psychological treatment also confirm essential features of the gate control theory, that somatic input is subjected to the modulating influences of cognitive, affective, attentional, and other behavioral processes before it evokes pain perception. Cognitive, behavioral, or social interventions, as well as suggestion in the form of either hypnosis or placebo therapy, can also be remarkably effective, even for severe clinical pain. These psychological approaches to the management of pain may be used alone or in combination with other therapies. Psychologically, pain patients are enabled to restructure perceptual and thought processes involved in suffering by altering appraisals of the threat, ability to control the quality of noxious sensations, and level of emotional arousal. Psychological procedures maximize beliefs regarding self-control, and minimize anxiety, helplessness, and depression. Psychological methods that modulate affective, cognitive, and operant factors may thus prevent the development of chronic pain, abolish it entirely, or at least reduce the intensity of noxious sensations.

The regulation of attention is also a major factor in psychological pain therapies. Recent experimental findings confirm early speculations that attention, arousal, learned helplessness, and environmental and conditioning factors activate different analgesia-producing systems (Mayer, 1982).

Pathological Conditions

An obvious testing ground for the gate control theory is pathology. There exists some clinical evidence elucidating the peripheral aspects of the gate control theory. In a detailed study on postherpetic neuralgia, it was shown that intercostal nerve biopsy specimens had a preferential loss of large unmyelinated fibers. This suggested that the heavy pain was a consequence of a selective loss of inhibition normally provided by the large fibers (Noordenbos, 1959). However, other clinical studies concerning pathological conditions of peripheral nerves do not fit the gate theory (Nathan, 1976).

Concluding Remarks

Summarizing our review, neurophysiological, pharmacological, and clinical work has tended to support the gate control theory of pain, although some aspects of the theory remain speculative and subject to criticism. In particular, the "gate opening" mechanism of the gate control hypothesis has not been supported in several neurophysiological studies. In Wall's terms, "That a gate control exists is no longer open to doubt but its functional role and its detailed mechanism remain open for speculation and for experiment" (1978, p. 14).

As our knowledge of sensory and physiological factors that activate pain-modulating neurons increases, the tools for pain management can be refined and extended. Thus, future research on pain-modulating systems holds promise not only for greater understanding of the variability of the pain experience but for significant advances in pain management as well.

References

Augustinsson, L. E., Bohlin, P., Bundsen, P., Carlsson, C. A., Forssmann, L., Sjöberg, P., & Tyreman, N. O. (1977). Pain relief during delivery by transcutaneous electrical nerve stimulation. *Pain, 4*, 59–65.
Beecher, H. K. (1959). *Measurement of subjective responses. Quantitative effects of drugs.* New York: Oxford University Press.
Costa, E., & Trabucchi, M. (1978). *The endorphins.* New York: Raven Press.
Dubner, R., & Sessle, B. J. (1971). Presynaptic excitability changes of primary afferent and corticofugal fibers projecting to trigeminal brain stem nuclei. *Experimental Neurology, 30*, 223–238.
Fields, H. L., & Basbaum, A. I. (1984). Endogenous pain control mechanisms. In P. D. Wall & R. Melzack (Eds.), *Textbook of pain* (pp. 142–152). Edinburgh: Churchill Livingstone.
Fitzgerald, M., & Woolf, C. J. (1981). Effects of cutaneous nerve and intraspinal conditioning on C fiber afferent terminals excitability in decerebrate spinal rats. *Journal of Physiology, 318*, 25–39.
Foreman, R. D., Beall, J. E., Applebaum, A. E., Coulter, J. D., & Willis, W. D. (1976). Effects of dorsal column stimulation on primate spinothalamic tract neurons. *Journal of Physiology, 39*, 534–546.
Franz, D. N., & Iggo, A. (1968). Dorsal root potentials and ventral reflexes evoked by non-myelinated fibers. *Science, 162*, 1140–1142.

Head, H., & Sherren, J. (1905). The consequence of injury to the peripheral nerves in man. *Brain, 28,* 116.
Hodge, C. J. (1972). Potential changes inside central afferent terminals secondary to stimulation of large- and small-diameter peripheral nerve fibers. *Journal of Neurophysiology, 35,* 30–43.
Janig, W., & Zimmermann, M. (1971). Presynaptic depolarization of myelinated afferent fibers evoked by stimulation of cutaneous C fibers. *Journal of Physiology, London, 214,* 29–50.
Jessell, T. M., & Iversen, L. L. (1977). Opiate analgesia inhibit Substance P release from rat trigeminus nucleus. *Nature, 268,* 549–551.
Mayer, D. J., & Liebeskind, J. C. (1974). Pain reduction by focal electrical stimulation of the brain: An anatomical and behavioral analysis. *Brain Research, 68,* 73–93.
Mayer, M. I. (1982). Periaqueductal gray neuronal activity: Correlation with EEG arousal evoked by noxious stimuli in the rat. *Neuroscience Letters, 28,* 297–301.
Melzak, R., & Dennis, S. G. (1978). Neurophysiological foundations of pain. In R. A. Sternback (Ed.), *The psychology of pain* (pp. 1–26). New York: Raven Press.
Melzack, R., & Wall, P. D. (1965). Pain mechanisms: A new theory. *Science 197,* 1351–1354.
Melzack, R., Wall, P. D., & Ty, T. C. (1982). Acute pain in an emergency clinic: Latency of onset and descriptor patterns related to different injuries. *Pain, 14,* 33–43.
Mendell, L. (1970). Positive dorsal root potentials produced by stimulation of small diameter muscle afferents. *Brain Research, 18,* 375–379.
Mendell, L. (1972). Properties and distribution of peripherally evoked presynaptic hyperpolarization in cat lumbar spinal cord. *Journal of Physiology, London, 226,* 769–792.
Mendell, L. (1973). Two negative dorsal root potentials evoke a positive dorsal root potential. *Brain Research, 55,* 198–202.
Mendell, L., & Wall, P. D. (1964). Presynaptic hyperpolarization: A role for fine afferent fibers. *Journal of Physiology, London, 172,* 274–294.
Nathan, P. (1976). The gate-control theory of pain. A critical Review. *Brain, 99,* 123–158.
Noordenbos, W. (1959). *Pain.* Amsterdam. Elsevier.
Noordenbos, W. (1974). Pathologic aspects of central pain states. In J. J. Bonica (Ed.), *Advances in neurology. Pain* (Vol. 4, pp. 333–337). New York: Raven Press.
Noordenbos, W. (1979). Mechanisms of pain. In J. W. F. Beks (Ed.), *The management of pain* (pp. 317–327). Amsterdam: Excerpta Medica.
Reynolds, D. V. (1969). Surgery in the rat during electrical analgesia induced by focal brain stimulation. *Science, 164,* 444–445.
Roeser, W. M., Meeks, L. W., Venis, R. G., & Strickland, A. T. C. (1976). The use of transcutaneous nerve stimulation for pain control in athletic medicine: A preliminary report. *American Journal of Sports Medicine, 4,* 210–213.
Schmidt, R. F. (1972). The gate control theory of pain. An unlikely hypothesis. In R. Janzen, W. D. Keidel, A. Herz, & C. Steichele (Eds.), *Pain* (pp. 124–127). London: Churchill Livingstone.
Sjölund, F., & Eriksson, M. (1979). The influence of naloxone on analgesia produced by peripheral conditioning stimulation. *Brain Research, 173,* 295–301.
Tyler, E., Caldwell, C., & Ghia, J. N. (1982). Transcutaneous electrical stimulation: An alternative approach to the management of postoperative pain. *Anesthetic Analgesia, 61,* 449–456.
Wall, P. D. (1979). The role of substantia gelatinosa as a gate control. In J. J. Bonica (Ed.), *Pain* (pp. 205–231). New York: Raven Press.
Wall, P. D. (1984). The dorsal horn. In P. D. Wall & R. Melzack (Eds.), *Textbook of pain* (pp. 80–87). Edinburgh: Churchill Livingstone.

Whitehorn, D., & Burgess, P. R. (1973). Changes in polarization of central branches of myelinated mechanoreceptor and nociceptor fibers during noxious and innocuous stimulation of the skin. *Journal of Neurophysiology, 36,* 226–237.

Willis, W. D. (1984). The origin and destination of pathways involved in pain transmission. In P. D. Wall & R. Melzack (Eds.), *Textbook of pain* (pp. 88–99). Edinburgh: Churchill Livingstone.

Willis, W. D., Trevino, D. L., Coulter, J. D., & Manuz, R. A. (1974). Responses of primate spinothalamic tract neurons to natural stimulation of hindlimb. *Journal of Neurophysiology, 37,* 358–372.

Woolf, C. J. (1984). Transcutaneous and implanted nerve stimulation. In P. D. Wall & R. Melzack (Eds.), *Textbook of pain* (pp. 679–690). Edinburgh: Churchill Livingstone.

Young, R. F., & King, R. B. (1972). Excitability changes in trigeminal primary afferent fibers in response to noxious and non-noxious stimuli. *Journal of Neurophysiology, 35,* 87–95.

CHAPTER 14

Behavioral–Anatomical Studies of the Central Pathways Subserving Orofacial Pain

J. Peter Rosenfeld and James G. Broton

Somatosensory information (concerning, e.g., touch, pressure, pain) from the head, face, and oral cavity are received by the endings of primary afferent neurons with processes in the fifth cranial (trigeminal) nerve, and with cell bodies in the trigeminal (or Gasserian) ganglion. The central axon terminals of these ganglion neurons synapse within the trigeminal nuclear complex (TN) in the brainstem (see Figure 1). This complex is a long, sausage-shaped set of subnuclei extending from the caudal pons to the caudal medulla. Its two major histologically defined subdivisions include the most rostral nucleus principalis or main sensory trigeminal nucleus (MTN) and the immediately caudal spinal nucleus of the fifth cranial nerve (SPV). SPV itself has been subdivided into three subnuclei, which from rostral to caudal levels, respectively, include subnucleus oralis (SO), subnucleus interpolaris (SI), and subnucleus caudalis (SC). The primary afferent fibers entering the brainstem from the trigeminal ganglion descend laterally along side of the entire long nuclear complex in the primary descending trigeminal tract (TT), projecting terminating fibers into the nuclear complex from MTN to the most caudal SC region of SPV. Axons of secondary afferent neurons in TN relay the information and sweep medially through the brainstem mostly to the contralateral side as they ascend to the ventrobasal complex of thalamus for final relay to somatosensory cortex.

J. Peter Rosenfeld and James G. Broton • Cresap Neuroscience Laboratory, Northwestern University, Evanston, Illinois 60208, USA.

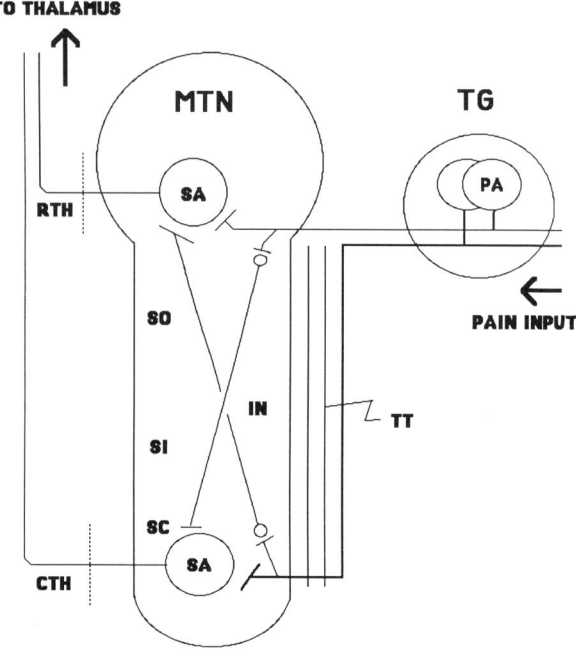

Figure 1. A diagram of the major connections of the trigeminal nuclear complex (TN), the central oblong shape consisting of MTN + SO + SI + SC (see text for further definitions). The perspective of the figure is rostral to caudal from top to bottom; i.e., the MTN part of the TN is closer to the top of the head than to the tail; the reverse is true for SC. Also, lateral is to the right, medial to the left. Two primary afferent (PA) neurons are shown with cell bodies in the trigeminal ganglion (TG). The terminals of one are at the level of the primary descending subnucleus oralis (SO). The axonal process of the other descends the length of trigeminal tract (TT), which runs down the lateral aspect of TN. (Other axonal fibers are suggested running alongside those whose cell bodies are shown. In Figure 2, the close proximity of TT and TN can be seen in regular coronal section.) SA labels cell bodies of secondary afferent neurons whose efferents run medially and rostrally in the secondary ascending trigeminal tract to connect with thalamus. Rostral (RTH) and caudal (CTH) efferents constituting the secondary tract are shown; the dashed vertical lines indicate the intended locations of the saggital knife cuts in Broton and Rosenfeld (1982, 1986). PA cells synapse on SA cells, but also may have collateral branches synapsing on interneurons (IN) that interconnect rostral and caudal levels.

It is worth additionally emphasizing that within TN, interneurons interconnect the rostral and caudal sections (Carpenter & Hannah, 1961; Falls, 1984; Gobel & Purvis, 1972; Hockfield & Gobel, 1982; Ikeda, Matsushita, & Tanami, 1982; Kruger, Saporta, & Feldman, 1977; Panneton & Burton, 1982; Stewart & King, 1963). There is considerable evidence of functional significance of the SC connections to MTN and NO (Greenwood & Sessle, 1976; Khayyat, Yu, & King, 1975; Scibetta & King, 1969; Sessle & Hu, 1981). We shall be drawing attention to these intranuclear connections below.

From the early 1900s to about the 1970s it was widely believed that there existed in TN a *submodality segregation* or *labeled line* coding scheme such that the most rostral portions (MTN and SO) processed innocuous (nonpainful) orofacial information, whereas the more caudally situated neurons in SC processed orofacial pain signals. This chapter discusses recent evidence from the authors' and other labs that is not consistent with this simple view.

The submodality segregation model arose partly from our tendency to (often correctly) reason that principles of somatosensory organization that explain somatic sensation and perception from structures in the lower body (below the neck) may be appropriately generalized to the trigeminally mediated orofacial sensations. Since there is some degree of submodality segregation in the spinal cord—with conscious proprioception and other spinal sensations handled mostly by the dorsal column system and nociception (pain) handled largely by the lateral spinothalamic tract (Mountcastle, 1980)—the desire among neuroscientists for simple order tended to encourage models of orofacial nociception along the lines of lower body sensory representation. Also, there were relevant clinical data (Kunc, 1970; Walker, 1939; Weinberger & Grant, 1943): In the treatment of trigeminal neuralgia, an excruciatingly painful condition of man known also as *tic douloureux*, section of the TT (tractotomy) was at one time not uncommonly used to alleviate the neuralgia. It was sometimes observed that when the section was made at lower levels of the tract (so as to avoid cerebellar inputs that are just lateral to TT at higher levels and whose section would produce undesirable motoric side effects), the pain sensation would be reduced while nonpainful sensation was preserved. Since lower tractotomies tended to denervate SC but not MTN and SO, it was thought that the surgical results were consistent with a functional role for MTN and SO in orofacial innocuous sensation and for SC in orofacial nociception. The inconsistencies of the clinical results, however, were often de-emphasized. Moreover, control histology was frequently unavailable with these clinical cases. Finally, the nature of the surgical procedure—a knife cut in a sagittal plane through the lateral aspect of the medulla, assuring a concomitant section of the medially underlying trigeminal nuclear tissue, thus interrupting caudal–rostral interconnections—made it impossible to rigorously conclude from the clinical data which TN structures were really necessary for orofacial nociception (see Figure 2). Nevertheless the clinical studies inspired an extensive electrophysiologically oriented program of research in which workers searched for

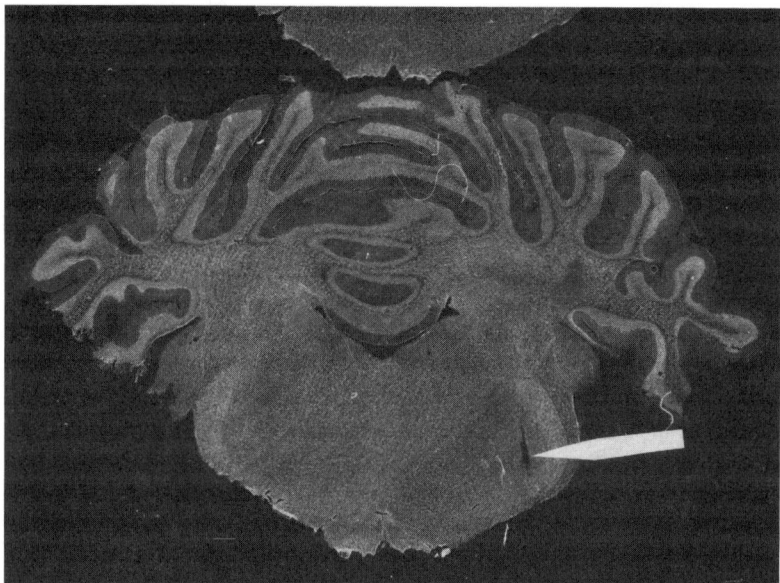

Figure 2. An unstained coronal cross section through the cerebellum (top) and brainstem at the level of lower MTN and upper SO. On the lower right side of the figure from right to left (outside/lateral to inside/medial) are shown, respectively, the spinocerebellar tract, the inwardly concave TT, which is wrapped closely about the rostral TN areas. An electrode track is seen at right in the center of TN. It is indicated with a marker.

exclusive nociceptors in SC with projections to thalamus. While this search was nonproductive at first, the searched-for units were eventually found in SC (Bushnell, Duncan, Dubner, & He, 1984; Hoffman, Dubner, Hayes, & Medlin, 1981; Hu, Dostrovsky, & Sessle, 1981; Price, Dubner, & Hu, 1976). These neurons' existence was consistent with a role for SC in orofacial nociception, but such data are never conclusive. Actually, SC could play a role in orofacial nociception even if *non*exclusively nociceptive neurons connecting to the thalamus via *non*direct projections (i.e., via a synaptic interruption) had been the only nociception-relevant SC neurons seen. However, the presence of either exclusively or nonexclusively nociceptive neurons in SC with either direct or indirect connections to thalamus does not prove the necessity of SC for orofacial pain any more than the documented existence of such neurons in MTN and SO (Eisenman, Landgren, & Novin, 1963, Eisenman, Fromm, Landgren, & Novin, 1964; Sessle & Greenwood, 1976; Sessle & Hu, 1981; Woda, Azerald, & Albe-Fessard, 1977) proves the necessity of these rostral regions. Because of the interconnections of rostral and caudal areas, either area could be necessary with the response of the other being epiphenomenal; this limitation inheres in all electrophysiological data, despite the fact that neurons in SC with the necessary response properties for representation of the sensory-discriminative aspect of pain have been demonstrated and, indeed, ought to be present in structures purported to encode this specialized orofacial nociception (Dubner, 1985). Nevertheless, to prove that a structure is necessary for a given function, one must show that its exclusive removal removes the normal progress of the function. As of the 1970s, there were no such data in any species regarding orofacial nociception.

Our laboratory became interested in TN function by chance: To test certain hypotheses about opiate analgesia mechanisms, we needed to be able to electrically stimulate primary-to-secondary synaptic regions subserving somatic sensation in awake, freely moving, chronically implanted rats (Rosenfeld & Vickery, 1976). There are of course only two such areas. The one in the dorsal horn nucleus of the spinal cord, we felt, presented an unnecessarily daunting technical challenge for chronic implantation in a small animal, leaving the homologous area, TN (whose caudalmost part, SC, is indeed increasingly referred to as the "dorsal horn of the medulla"), as our ultimate choice. Had we in 1976 known well the literature summarized above concerning putative submodality segregation in TN, we probably would have been careful to use SC as our primary target. Instead we aimed for MTN and SO since these are larger, easier-to-target areas. Our pilot work showed us that at very low levels of MTN and SO stimulation (10–50 uA, p-p), the rats would display signs of discomfort and facial distress, e.g., squealing, urinating, freezing, and, in particular, rubbing at the perioral facial region, so we proceeded to assess effects of opiates on the aversive reactions produced by stimulation of trigeminal and other brain loci (Rosenfeld & Holtzman, 1977; Rosenfeld & Stocco, 1980, Rosenfeld & Vickery, 1976). As these data became available, our colleagues asked us why we chose to stimulate MTN and SO rather than SC since it was the latter that most individuals tended to implicate in orofacial nociception. These repeated questions alongside our findings of low aversive stimulation thresholds in MTN and SO prompted us to look through the literature to see if anyone had ever shown rigorously (via experimental lesions) that MTN and SO were *not* necessary for orofacial nociception, as was commonly believed. Not finding answers in the literature, we decided to seek them ourselves.

The first challenge was to develop a reliable and valid index of orofacial pain. What we developed was a heater mounted on the rat's face (analogue cheek area) by attachment to a standard, chronically installed socket whose pins could be used for stimulation and/or recording (see Figure 3). The device (detailed in Rosenfeld, Broton, & Clavier, 1978a; Rosenfeld, Clavier, & Broton, 1978b) was a 10-ohm resistor, which, when overdriven with DC current, would become aversively hot, causing a vigorous, face-rub (FR) escape response. The latency of this response was our inverse pain index, inverse because the *greater* the time to FR response, the *lower* the pain sensitivity.

Once we had the FR device operational, we posed our first empirical question: Are MTN and/or SO involved in orofacial pain and are they necessary? Despite the amount of time that ablation methods have existed, and despite their sometimes alleged crudeness, the only way to show that MTN and SO are not necessary for orofacial pain is to ablate them and note no change in pain function. Thus, we electrolytically destroyed these regions in rats and observed the effect on FR latency ipsi- and contralateral to the lesion. Also, we observed tail-flick and paw-lick latencies to noxious heat. Only the ipsilateral FR should have

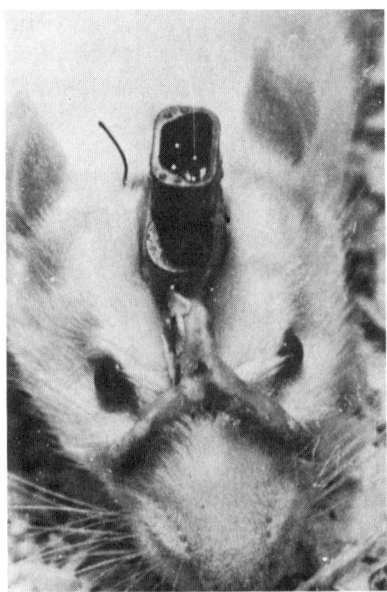 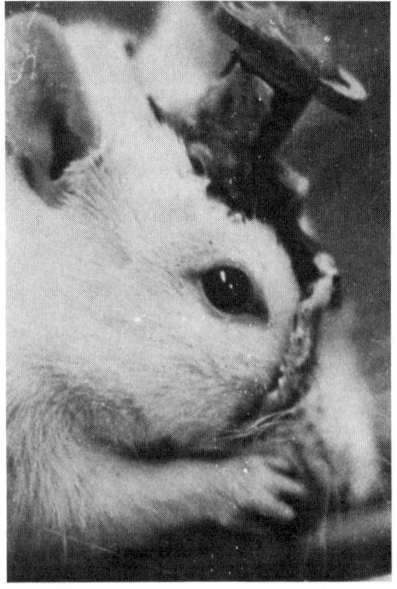

Figure 3. Left: The face-rub (FR) test device in place. Right: A rat executing an FR.

been affected if MTN and SO are involved in the nociceptive sensory aspects of the FR response, since a given side of a rat's face is ipsilaterally represented in MTN and SO. The other behavioral tests were used to control for motoric, arousal, or other nonspecific effects of the lesions.

In making these lesions, there was one other potentially serious methodological problem of which we had to be aware: Since the descending TT is just lateral to the TN (see Figures 1, 2, and 4), a large, laterally expansive TN lesion at the level of MTN or SO could spread into TT, thus denervating SC. Subsequent changes in facial pain could then not be unambiguously and exclusively attributed to MTN or SO damage, since the lateral lesion would have also deprived SC of normal input. We utilized a special histological control procedure to monitor this possible confound. We stained alternative sections of the brainstem caudal to the lesion with a compound that would reveal any degenerating fibers and terminals in TT below the level of the lesion (Fink & Heimer, 1967). Thus, even if routine inspection of Nissl-stained cross sections through TN and TT did not *clearly* show an exclusively nuclear (versus nuclear plus tract) lesion, the Fink-Heimer procedures would settle the matter (see Figure 4).

Not unexpectedly, some of our lesions were nicely localized to MTN and/or SO (sometimes including more *medial* areas) and some strayed out into the tract. The behavioral results are shown in Table 1 (Rosenfeld, 1978b).

It is seen that for the group with the well-placed rostral nuclear lesions, ipsilateral FR is more than double (i.e., 219.3%) the prelesion value, whereas the other means are unchanged. This ipsilateral FR is significantly different (at $p < .05$) from each of the other means in the group. For the rats with tract damage, there was also significant effect on FR ipsilaterally ($p < .05$). (There was also in rats with TT damage an additional incidental effect on contralateral FR, which we replicated in Pickoff-Matuk, Rosenfeld, & Broton, 1986.) *The main point of this first study, however, was that rostral areas of TN were shown to be clearly necessary for orofacial pain.*

Both rostral (SO and MTN) and caudal (SC) regions of TN send forth efferent fibers medially and rostrally which mostly cross midline to ascend in the contralateral secondary, ascending, trigeminal tract connecting to thalamus. Our next question concerning the central pathways subserving orofacial pain asked whether rostrally exiting and caudally exiting TN efferents continued the pain path from SO, MTN, and possibly SC. One might quickly jump to the conclusion that since we showed that SO and MTN are necessary for orofacial nociception, efferents from these loci must also be necessary. The trigeminothalamic efferents, how-

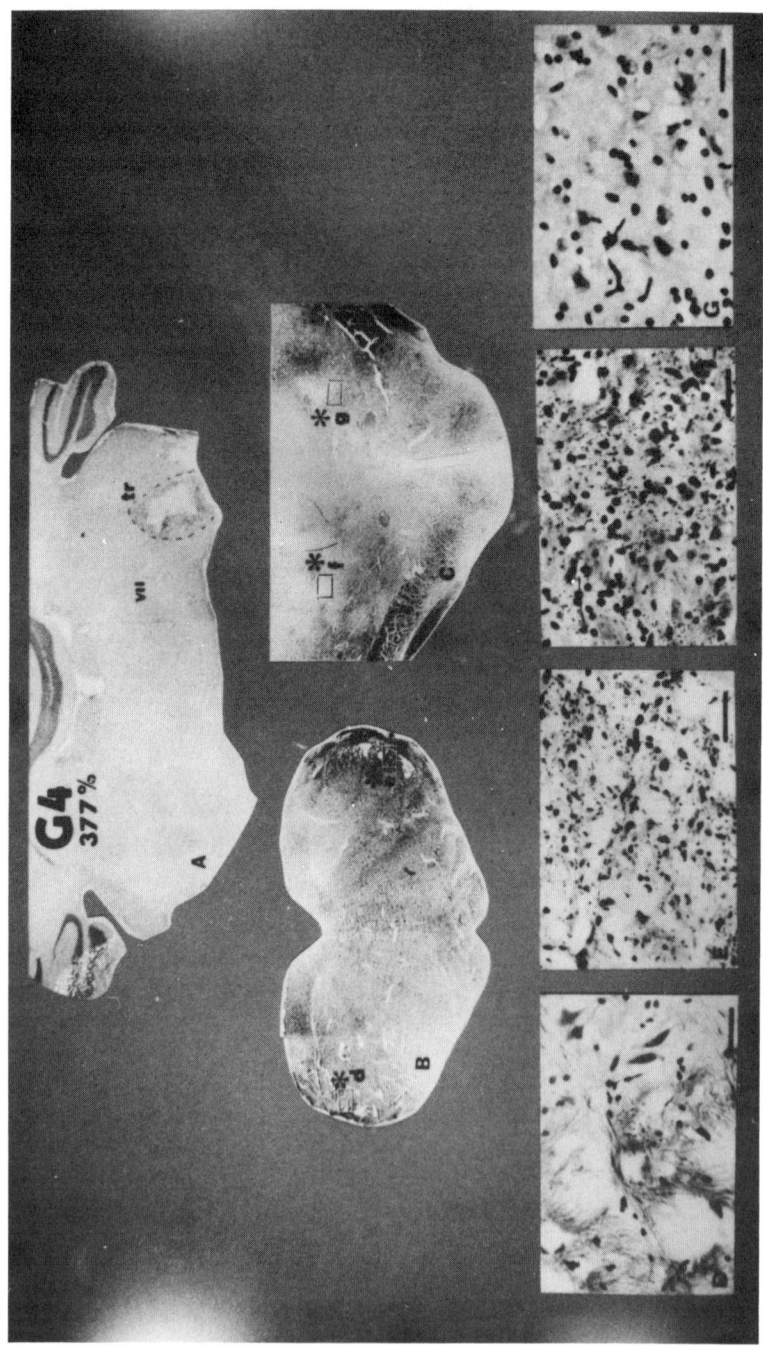

Table 1. *Effects of Rostral Trigeminal Nuclear and Tract Lesions on Mean % Change Scores after Lesions ± SE on Indicated Responses[a]*

	Ipsilateral face rub	Contralateral face rub	Tail flick	Paw lick
Nuclear damage only (n and prelesion mean latencies [sec] in parentheses)	219.3 ± 35.3 ($n = 7$; 4.8 ± 0.6)	109.2 ± 5.6 ($n = 6$; 4.3 ± 1.2)	114.4 ± 5.0 ($n = 7$; 16.9 ± 1.2)	100.8 ± 23.1 ($n = 5$; 9.9 ± 2.1)
Nucleus and tract damage, ($n = 5$ in all cases, prelesion mean latencies [sec] in parentheses)	244.8 ± 33.6 (7.8 ± 2.7)	184.8 ± 47.0 (6.4 ± 3.3)	132.0 ± 5.1 (13.6 ± 0.97)	118.4 ± 4.0 (5.0 ± 1.4)

[a] For each rat the 4-day postlesion mean was divided by the 4-day prelesion mean to yield a % of baseline change score (i.e., 100% = no change). Averages of these are shown at tops of cells with actual prelesion latencies (sec) shown directly underneath in parentheses.

ever, are not the only ones leaving rostral TN areas. It will be recalled (Figure 1) that rostral areas also send interneurons to connect with SC (Falls, 1984; Hockfield & Gobel, 1982). Our first study thus did not allow one to choose between the following two possible and non-mutually exclusive central routes for orofacial pain:

1. MTN/SO → rostral trigeminothalamic efferents → thalamus
2. MTN/SO → SC → caudal trigeminothalamic efferents → thalamus

Of course, SC could also be an orofacial pain processing area. Since it also connects via interneurons to rostral areas (many references cited

←

Figure 4. (a, top) Cross section through rostral trigeminal SO in rat G4 from Rosenfeld, Clavier, & Broton (1978b). A piece of ventral brainstem is missing, but one sees the lesion at right outlined in dotted line, just medial to TT (labeled tr here). In the middle row of two cross sections, the one at left (b) is taken from the level of SC to show where left and right Fink-Heimer-stained trigeminal tract sections were examined. The two left panels at bottom (d, e) show contralateral (leftmost) and ipsilateral (second to left) reconstructions. The contralateral tract is of course clear, but the tract ipsilateral to and below the level of the lesion shows fine black stipplings, which are degenerating axons and terminals, indicating that the TN lesion higher up impinged on the tract (TT), thus denervating SC along with SO. The cross section in the middle row at right is through thalamus; (f) and (g) indicate areas magnified at bottom extreme right (g) and second from right (f). As expected, thalamus contra- but not ipsilateral to the lesion shows degeneration. The number 377% refers to the percent elevation of FR latency over baseline seen in this rat.

above), there are at least two other possible central routes which are not only nonmutually exclusive but which also are not mutually exclusive with routes 1 and 2, just described:

3. SC → caudal trigeminothalamic efferents → thalamus
4. SC → MTN/SO → rostral trigeminothalamic efferents → thalamus

To get at these possibilities, we utilized a knife cut technique designed to cut in a sagittal plane the efferents leaving TN at rostral levels (including MTN and SO, from 3 to 6 mm rostral to obex) as well as at caudal levels (SC and SI from 2.5 mm behind obex to 1.5 mm above obex). Figure 1 shows with dashed vertical lines the regions of these cuts. We also generated a control group in which all surgical procedures were followed, but cuts weren't made. Using behavioral methods as before, we obtained the results shown in Table 2 (from Broton & Rosenfeld, 1982).

It is clear that the rostral efferent cuts are the only lesions having specific effects on orofacial nociception, which tends to eliminate pathways 2 and 3, above. On the one hand, these results are arresting when one bears in mind the great numbers of studies searching for SC units with direct trigeminothalamic projections. On the other hand, our caudal cuts could have been not caudal enough to sever the intended fibers, and had we been able to sever the lowest level of SC efferents, we might have seen effects. It should be noted, however, that our caudal cuts must have severed some population of SC-thalamic fibers, since our

Table 2. Changes in Response Latencies to Nociception Tests after Knife Cuts

	Rostral cuts ($n = 6$)	Caudal cuts ($n = 6$)	Control ($n = 6$)
Ipsilateral FRR	233.0 ± 88.8^{a,c,d}	103.3 ± 19.9^a	89.0 ± 20.8^a
	(5.5 ± 1.9)^b	(3.8 ± 0.8)^b	(4.8 ± 0.9)^b
Contralateral FRR	114.5 ± 34.8	104.3 ± 33.7	98.7 ± 21.7
	(4.9 ± 0.8)	(3.5 ± 0.7)	(5.0 ± 1.9)
Tail flick	112.2 ± 21.8	112.5 ± 22.2	114.8 ± 18.3
	(11.6 ± 2.7)	(11.8 ± 3.1)	(11.6 ± 1.4)
Hotplate paw lick	133.3 ± 51.2)	132.6 ± 26.9	126.2 ± 52.3
	(104.4 ± 4.8)	(8.5 ± 1.6)	(105 ± 4.5)

^{a}Mean percent + 1SD.
^{b}Baseline mean ± 1SD (sec).
^{c}Conservative estimate. Includes two rats that did not respond after cuts in time allotted.
$^d p < .05$.

Fink-Heimer stained sections of thalamus revealed degeneration patterns that would be expected with trigeminothalamic fiber section.

Our next study (Broton & Rosenfeld, 1985) strengthened the case for pathway 1, above (and further weakened the case for routes 2 and 3) We performed rat tractotomies (TT sections) that were somewhat analogous to the manipulations made in the old clinical studies. Our cuts were made at the level of SI; i.e., they were designed to denervate lower SI and SC. The results were complex, but basically we found that tractotomies extending medially into TN caused 7 of 20 (35%) possible significant elevations in FR latency, whereas the most lateral lesions (i.e., mostly involving TT and being purer tractotomies although none of our lesions destroyed all of TT while sparing all of TN) caused only 2 of 16 possible elevations (12.5%). The two salient features here were that (1) most tractotomies were without effect and (2) transecting nuclear areas and thus presumably disconnecting rostral and caudal areas of TN was more damaging than denervation of SC—which is largely without effect. Others have shown also that the lower TN and TT are not necessary for orofacial pain reactions in cats (Ikegami & Kawamura, 1979; Vyklicky, Keller, Jastrchoff, Vyklicky, & Butkhuzi, 1977), which is consistent with our 1985 study just described. Taken together, all these results strongly argue that MTN and SO in Pathway 1 are critical for orofacial pain perception in rats and cats. Pathway 4 may also be involved, thus implicating SC, if not its trigeminothalamic efferents, but the greater effects of Pathway 1 interruptions, relative to those of Pathway 4 interruptions, tend to support a case for the predominant role of Pathway 1. However besides the possible exceptions to this view already noted, there is another possible principle that could yet leave an important role for SC and its trigeminothalamic efferents, and this is the possibility that only certain parts of the face depend on Pathway 1, leaving Pathways 2 and 3 to possibly subserve nociception from other facial areas.

In fact, in our most recent study (Broton & Rosenfeld, 1986), we tested five sites on the rat's face (see Figure 5) for FR sensitivity before and after saggital knife cut lesions of rostral trigeminothalamic efferents, as in our earlier study (Broton & Rosenfeld, 1982). The results were that only Sites 1 and 2 were significantly affected (see Table 3). This nicely replicated Broton and Rosenfeld (1982), who utilized only Site 1 in the earlier paper, but it also implied that other areas of TN—perhaps SC and its efferents and/or other rostral regions and their efferents—are involved in signaling orofacial pain from more dorsal-caudal regions of face (i.e., Sites 3,4,5).

In this most recent report, we also looked in a preliminary way at the effects of rostral knife cut lesions on *innocuous* facial sensation. This

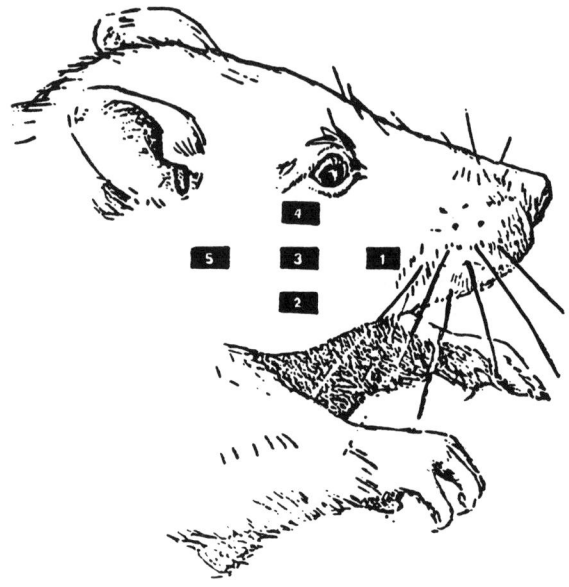

Figure 5. A drawing of a rat showing the tested sites in Broton and Rosenfeld (1986).

had never been done before, probably because it is difficult to study nonnoxious facial somatic sensation in a rat. Rats show innate escape responses to pain, but to very mild stimulation they are typically unreactive, which usually forces an interested experimenter to develop a complex discrimination paradigm. We took a different approach:

It is known that when higher mammals pass from drowsiness to

Table 3. Effects of Rostral Knife Cuts on Face-Rub Response Latencies

	FR latencies (sec)	
Facial site	Precut mean + SEM ($N = 11$)	Postcut mean + 1 SEM ($N = 11$)
1	7.8 + 2.6	13.6 + 8.2[a]
2	6.8 + 2.7	17.6 + 10.5[a]
3	5.8 + 3.0	9.4 + 6.9
4	6.9 + 3.3	7.6 + 7.8
5	5.9 + 1.8	11.4 + 8.4

[a]$p < .05$.

heightened alertness or arousal, while there may be minimal outward behavioral signs of the exact onset of the aroused state, the cortical electroencephalogram (EEG) will go from low-frequency, high-amplitude synchronized waves to assynchronous, high-frequency, low-amplitude waves during the transition. We thus installed a 5-nozzle air hose on the rat's skull installation, each nozzle aimed at a different facial position (see Figure 5). After waiting (sometimes up to 3 hours!) for the onset of the drowsy state EEG pattern, mild air puffs of 5 seconds' duration were presented to the rat's face at increasing air pressures until we saw the EEG arousal response. (The threshold air puffs in all rats were at clearly nonpainful levels as confirmed on our own lips.) We noted the response latencies from air puff onset before and after lesions. The results are shown for three rats (15 sites on face) in Table 4. (We had only three rats in the sample because of the extraordinary amounts of wait time involved in this study.) Only one of the 15 innocuous perception tests even approached ($p < .06$) significance following the same rostral knife cut lesions that produced profound effects on facial nociception.

Table 4. *Effects of Sagittal Knife Cuts on Response Latencies to Nonnoxious Facial Stimuli*

		Air puff response latencies	
Rat	Site	Precut mean (sec + 1 SD)	Postcut (sec)
A	1	0.43 + 0.23	0.62
	2	0.33 + 0.11	0.38
	3	0.63 + 0.06	0.62
	4	0.27 + 0.06	0.50
	5	0.37 + 0.12	0.58
B	1	0.47 + 0.15	0.60
	2	0.43 + 0.16	0.48
	3	0.49 + 0.24	0.52
	4	0.23 + 0.05	0.28
	5	0.25 + 0.09	0.40
C	1	0.43 + 0.11	0.52
	2	0.71 + 0.19	0.32
	3	0.39 + 0.10	1.80[a]
	4	0.35 + 0.13	0.32
	5	0.41 + 0.09	0.44

[a] $p < .06$.

The most parsimonious interpretation of these data is that there may indeed be a submodality segregation scheme operating in rat TN, but with rostral efferents being necessary for normal nociception and not for normal nonnoxious facial perception, it appears to be the reverse of the scheme so widely believed! Of course, as always, these early data need confirmation in future larger-scale studies. All our studies to date, however, along with other recent papers (cited here), and most recently in Dallel, Raboisson, Aurou, & Woda, 1988), raise serious doubts about the well-known putative submodality segregation scheme that grew out of some often cited and, of necessity, inadequately controlled clinical reports dating back to the turn of the century.

ACKNOWLEDGMENT. This work was supported by NIH grant DE07905.

References

Broton, J. G., & Rosenfeld, J. P. (1982). Rostral trigeminal projections signal perioral facial pain. *Brain Research, 243*, 395–400.

Broton, J. G., & Rosenfeld, J. P. (1985). Effects of trigeminal tractotomy on facial thermal nociception in the rat. *Brain Research, 333*, 63–72.

Broton, J., & Rosenfeld, J. P. (1986). Cutting rostral trigeminal nuclear comex projections preferentially affects perioral nociception in the rat. *Brain Research, 397*, 1–8.

Bushnell, M. C., Duncan, G. H., Dubner, R., & He, L. F. (1984). Activity of trigeminothalamic neurons in medullary dorsal horn of awake monkeys trained in a thermal discrimination task. *Journal of Neurophysiology, 52*, 170–187.

Carpenter, M. B., & Hanna, G. R. (1961). Fiber projections from the spinal trigeminal nucleus in the cat. *Journal of Comparative Neurology, 117*, 117–132.

Dallel, R., Raboisson, P., Aurou, P., & Woda, A. (1988). The rostral part of the trigeminal sensory nucleus is involved in orofacial nociception. *Brain Research, 448*, 7–19.

Dubner, R. (1985). Specialization in nociceptive pathways. In H. L. Fields *et al.* (Eds.), *Advances in pain research and therapy* (pp. 111–137). New York: Raven Press.

Eisenman, J., Landgren, S., & Novin, D. (1963). Functional organization in the main sensory trigeminal nucleus and in the rostral subdivision of the nucleus of the spinal trigeminal tract in the cat. *Acta Physiologica Scandinavica, 59* (Suppl. 214), 1–44.

Eisenman, J., Fromm, G., Landgren, S., & Novin, D. (1964). The ascending projections of trigeminal neurons in the cat investigated by antidromic stimulation. *Acta Physiologica Scandinavica, 60*, 337–350.

Falls, W. M. (1984). Termination in trigeminal nucleus oralis of ascending intratrigeminal axons originating from neurons in the medullary dorsal horn: An HRP study in the rat employing light and electron microscopy. *Brain Research, 290*, 136–140.

Fink, R. P. & Heimer, L. (1967). Two methods for selective silver impregnation of degenerating axons and their synaptic endings in the central nervous system. *Brain Research, 4*, 369–374.

Gerard, M. W. (1923). Afferent impulses of the trigeminal nerve. *Archives of Neurological Psychiatry, 9*, 306–338.

Gobel, S., & Purvis, M. B. (1972). Anatomical studies of the organization of the spinal V nucleus: The deep bundles and the spinal V tract. *Brain Research, 48*, 27–44.

Greenwood, F., & Sessle, B. J. (1976). Inputs to trigeminal brain stem neurones from facial, oral, tooth pulp and pharyngolaryngeal tissues. II. Role of trigeminal nucleus caudalis in modulating responses to innocuous and noxious stimuli. *Brain Research, 117*, 227–238.

Hockfield, S., & Gobel, S. (1982). An anatomical demonstration of projections to the medullary dorsal horn (trigeminal nucleus caudalis) from rostral trigeminal nuclei and the contralateral caudal medulla. *Brain Research, 252*, 203–211.

Hoffman, D. S., Dubner, R., Hayes, R. L., & Medlin, T. P. (1981). Neuronal activity in the medullary dorsal horn of awake monkeys trained in a thermal discrimination task. I. Responses to innocuous and noxious thermal stimuli. *Journal of Neurophysiology, 46*, 409–427.

Hu, J. W., Dostrovsky, J. O., & Sessle, B. J. (1981). Functional properties of neurons in cat trigeminal subnucleus caudalis (medullary dorsal horn). I. Responses to oral-facial noxious and nonnoxious stimuli and projections to thalamus and subnucleus oralis. *Journal of Neurophysiology, 45*, 173–192.

Ikeda, M., Matsushita, M., & Tanami, T. (1982). Termination and cells of origin of the ascending intranuclear fibers in the spinal trigeminal nucleus of the cat. A study with the horse-radish peroxidase technique. *Neuroscience Letters, 31*, 215–220.

Ikegami, S., & Kawamura, H. (1979). Avoidance conditioning to tooth pulp stimulation in the cat after bulbar transection. *Physiology and Behavior, 23*, 593–596.

Khayyat, G. F., Yu, Y. J., & King, R. B. (1975). Response patterns to noxious and nonnoxious stimuli in rostral trigeminal relay nuclei. *Brain Research, 97*, 47–60.

Kruger, L., Saporta, S., & Feldman, S. G. (1977). Axonal transport studies of the sensory trigeminal complex. In D. J. Anderson & B. Matthews (Eds.), *Pain in the trigeminal region* (pp. 191–201). Amsterdam: Elsevier.

Kunc, Z. (1970). Significant factors pertaining to the results of trigeminal tractotomy. In R. Hassler & A. E. Wakloer (Eds.), *Trigeminal neuralgia* (pp. 90–98). Philadelphia: W. B. Saunders.

Mountcastle, V. B. (1980). Neural mechanisms in somesthesia. In V. B. Mountcastle (Ed.), *Medical physiology*. St. Louis: C. V. Mosby.

Panneton, W. M., & Burton, H. (1982). Origin of ascending intratrigeminal pathways in the cat. *Brain Research, 236*, 463–470.

Pickoff-Matuk, J. F., Rosenfeld, J. P., & Broton, J. G. (1986). Lesions of the mid-spinal trigeminal complex are effective in producing perioral thermal hypoalgesia. *Brain Research, 382*, 291–298.

Price, D. D., Dubner, R., & Hu, J. W. (1976). Trigeminothalamic neurons in nucleus caudalis responsive to tactile, thermal and nociceptive stimulation of the monkey's face. *Journal of Neurophysiology, 39*, 936–953.

Rosenfeld, J. P., & Stocco, S. (1980). Differential effects of systemic versus intracranial injection of opiates on central, orofacial and lower body nociception: Somatotypy in bulbar analgesia systems. *Pain, 9*, 307–318.

Rosenfeld, J. P., & Vickery, J. L. (1976). Differential effects of morphine on trigeminal nucleus versus reticular aversive stimulation: Independence of negative effects from stimulation parameters. *Pain, 2*, 405–416.

Rosenfeld, J. P., & Holzman, B. S. (1977). Differential effect of morphine on stimulation of primary versus higher order trigeminal terminals. *Brain Research, 124*, 367–372.

Rosenfeld, J. P., Broton, J. G., & Clavier, R. M. (1978a). A reliable facial nociception device for unrestrained awake animals. *Physiology and Behavior, 21*, 287–290.

Rosenfeld, J. P., Clavier, R. M., & Broton, J. G. (1978b). Bilateral and unilateral antinociceptive effects of rostral trigeminal nuclear complex lesions in rats. *Brain Research, 157*, 147–152.

Scibetta, C. J., & King, R. B. (1969). Hyperpolarizing influence of trigeminal nucleus caudalis on primary afferent preterminals in trigeminal nucleus oralis. *Journal of Neurophysiology, 32*, 229–238.

Sessle, B. J., & Greenwood, L. F. (1976). Inputs to trigeminal brain stem neurones from facial, oral, tooth pulp and pharyngolaryngeal tissues. I. Responses to innocuous and noxious stimuli. *Brain Research, 117*, 211–226.

Sessle, B. J., & Hu, J. W. (1981). Raphe-induced suppression of the jaw-opening reflex and single neurons in trigeminal subnucleus oralis, and influence of naloxone and subnucleus caudalis. *Pain, 10*, 19–36.

Sjoquist, O. (1938). Studies on pain conduction in the trigeminal nerve. *Archives of Psychiatrica Scandinavica, 17* (Suppl.), 1–139.

Spiller, W. G. (1915). Remarks on the central representation of sensation. *Journal of Nervous Mental Diseases, 42*, 399–418.

Stewart, W. A., & King, R. B. (1963). Fiber projections from the nucleus caudalis of the spinal trigeminal nucleus. *Journal of Comparative Neurology, 121*, 271–286.

Vyklicky, L., Keller, O., Jastreboff, P., Vyklicky, L., Jr., & Butkhuzi, S. (1973). Spinal trigeminal tractotomy and nociceptive reactions evoked by tooth pulp stimulation in the cat. *Journal of Physiology (Paris), 73*, 379–386.

Walker, A. E. (1939). Anatomy, physiology and surgical considerations of the spinal tract of the trigeminal nerve. *Journal of Neurophysiology, 2*, 234–248.

Weinberger, L. M., & Grant, F. C. (1943). Experiences with intramedullary tractomy: III. Immediate and late neurological complications. *Archiches of Neurology and Psychiatry, 49*, 665–682.

Woda, A., Azerald, J., & Albe-Fessard, D. (1977). Mapping of the trigeminal sensory complex of the cat. Characterization of its neurons by stimulation of peripheral field, dental pulp afferents and thalamic projections. *Journal of Physiology (Paris), 73*, 367–378.

CHAPTER **15**

Neuropeptides and Nociception in the Spinal Cord

Masamichi Satoh

At the Beginning

Pain is the most common symptom that brings a patient to the physician. However, *pain* has no standard definition. It is helpful to consider that pain may have at least two components: physiologic and psychologic components. In fact, neurophysiologists and most neuropharmacologists use the word *pain* to mean the appropriate response of specific pathways within the nervous system to noxious stimuli, with the potential for producing tissue injury. On the other hand, clinical psychologists mean that an individual complains of pain, whether or not a physiological stimulus is identified.

As a neuropharmacologist, the author has been studying mechanisms of action of analgesic drugs and is particularly interested in physiological and neurochemical bases of pain perception of nociceptive transmission in the CNS. A focus of this chapter is on the involvement of neuropeptides in nociceptive transmission at the spinal dorsal horn.

Several neuropeptides are immunohistochemically revealed to be contained in the small-sized cells in the dorsal root ganglia and their axons, the small primary afferents that are known to convey nociceptive information. For example, substance P, which consists of 11 amino acid residues, is contained in 15 to 20% of the total small primary afferents. Somatostatin, consisting of 14 amino acids, is found in 5 to 10% of the

---

Masamichi Satoh • Department of Pharmacology, Faculty of Pharmaceutical Sciences, Kyoto University, Kyoto 606, Japan.

total (Dodd, Jahr, & Jessel, 1984). Substance P and somatostatin are reportedly contained in the separate populations of the primary afferents (Hökfelt, Elde, Johansson, Luft, Nilsson, & Arimura, 1976). More recently, calcitonin gene-related peptide (CGRP), consisting of 37 amino acids, was found to be formed by alternative splicing of mRNA of the calcitonin-coding gene (Amara, Jonas, Rosenfeld, Ong, & Evans, 1982). This peptide is contained in a large population of primary afferent neurons and in nerve terminals in the superficial layers of the dorsal horn, and at least in part coexists with substance P (Wiesenfeld-Hallin, Hökfelt, Lundberg, Frossmann, Reinecke, Tschopp, & Fischer, 1984). However, functional roles of these neuropeptides in the thin primary afferents have not been revealed. On the other hand, electrophysiological studies classified several peripheral nociceptors like high-threshold mechanoreceptors with Aδ and C fibers, thermonociceptors with Aδ and C fibers, and polymodal nociceptors with C fibers (Willis, 1985). However, neurotransmitters contained in the primary afferents with such nociceptors have not been elucidated.

Thus, we have been studying the neuropeptides involved in transmission of information from the various nociceptors to the spinal dorsal horn.

Experimental Methods

In Situ Perfusion of the Rabbit Spinal Dorsal Horn

Male rabbits (2.5–3.5 kg) under pentobarbital anesthesia were decerebrated at the rostral end of the diencephalon in light of ethical considerations. The spinal cord was fixed in a stereotaxic frame and exposed by laminectomy at the levels of L4–L7. A push-pull cannula (see Figure 1) devised by us (Kuraishi, Hirota, Sugimoto, Satoh, & Takagi, 1983) was unilaterally introduced into the dorsal horn (L5 level) with the tip in the dorsolateral area where neuropeptides like substance P, somatostatin, and CGRP are highly concentrated. The experiments were performed under conditions of gallamine immobilization and artificial ventilation. Two hours after these procedures, the spinal dorsal horn was perfused with 37°C perfusion medium (artificial cerebrospinal fluid) bubbled with O_2 95% + CO_2 5%, at a rate of 0.05 ml/min. Samples were collected at 20-minute intervals (1.0 ml/sample) for 3 to 5 hours, after preperfusion of 40 minutes. The amounts of substance P and/or somatostatin in each sample were determined by usual radioimmunoassay methods.

Natural stimuli, including noxious mechanical (pinch) and thermal

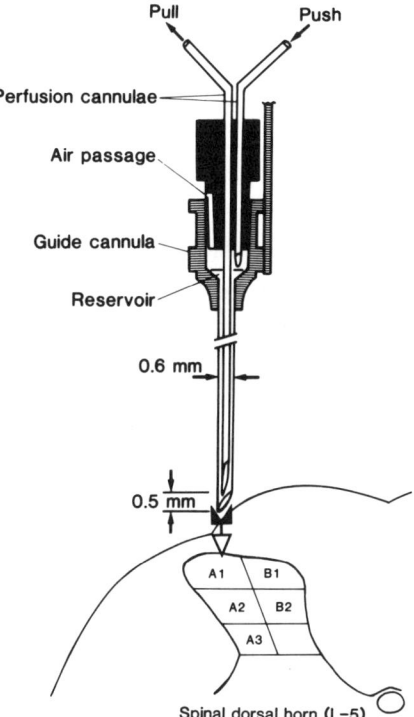

Figure 1. A method for the push-pull perfusion of the rabbit spinal dorsal horn *in situ*.

(radiant heat) stimulation given intermittently for 20 minutes, were applied to the clipped skin of the posterior region of the hind leg, ipsilateral to the perfusion site. Such noxious stimuli produced nociceptive behaviors like struggling and flexion reflex in freely moving rabbits.

In Vitro Superfusion of the Rat Spinal Dorsal Horn

The spinal cords of male Sprague-Dawley rats were removed immediately after decapitation and were place on ice. The dorsal halves of cervical and lumbar enlargements were dissected, minced into cubes of 1 mm^3 or less with a razor blade, and transferred to a superfusion chamber with a volume of 600 μl. The slices (Figure 2) were superfused with 37°C Krebs-bicarbonate medium (bubbled with O_2 95% + CO_2 5%) containing peptidase inhibitors (in μM: bestatin 10, captopril 5, leupeptin 1, and chymostatin 1) at a rate of 0.2 ml/min. Samples were collected every 6 minutes (1.2 ml/sample), after presuperfusion of 20 minutes.

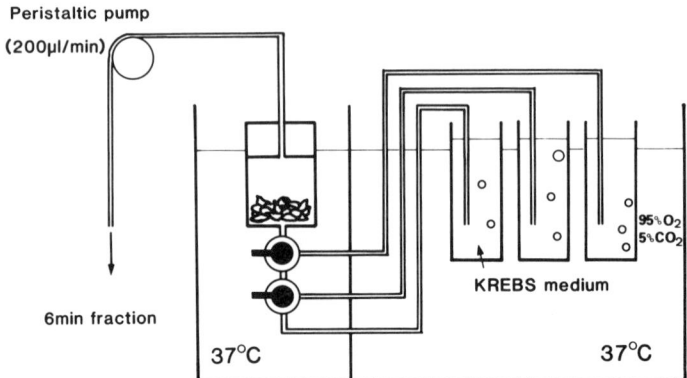

Figure 2. A method for superfusion of the spinal dorsal horn slices *in vitro*. Krebs medium contains bestatin (10 μM), captopril (5 μM), leupeptin (1 μM), and chymostatin (1 μM).

The amount of substance P in each sample was determined by the specific radioimmunoassay method.

Stimulations of the slices were performed by addition of 50 mM K^+ or 5×10^{-7}M capsaicin to the superfusion medium for the initial 3 minutes of a given 6-minute fraction. It is known that high K^+ stimulation nonselectively depolarizes every neuron, while capsaicin selectively acts on the unmyerinated primary afferents, and that both produce release of neurotransmitters from the nerve terminals in a Ca^{2+}-dependent manner.

Behavioral Measurements of Nociception in the Rat

Male Sprague-Dawley rats (200–250 g) were employed. Nociceptive responsiveness of the hind paws to thermal stimulation was measured using the hot-plate method, in which a copper plate was maintained at 52°C and licking of the hindpaw was used as nociceptive response. Nociceptive threshold of the hind paw for mechanical stimulation was measured by the paw-pressure method using an analgesimeter, in which struggling was used as nociceptive response.

Intrathecal injections of neuropeptides were given in a volume of 10 μl, according to the method described by Satoh, Yasui, Fujibayashi, and Takagi (1983). In brief, the rats were anesthetized with ether and the skin over the L2–L6 vertebrae was dissected. The next day, a stainless steel needle (25-gauge) connected to a microinjector was inserted into the subarachnoid space through the foramen intervertebrale, between L3 and L4.

Separate Roles of Substance P and Somatostatin

Thermal and mechanical noxious stimuli produced very contrastive influences on the release of immunoreactive substance P (iSP) and immunoreactive somatostatin (iSST) in the spinal dorsal horn. The amounts of iSP and iSST shown in Figure 3 were simultaneously determined following division of each sample into two parts. Therefore, the corresponding columns in the upper and lower graphs were obtained from the same samples. The ordinates indicate that magnitudes of release as percentages of spontaneous release, which were calculated by an average of the amounts in the first three samples. Heat (noxious thermal stimulation) did not increase the iSP release but did produce a marked and significant

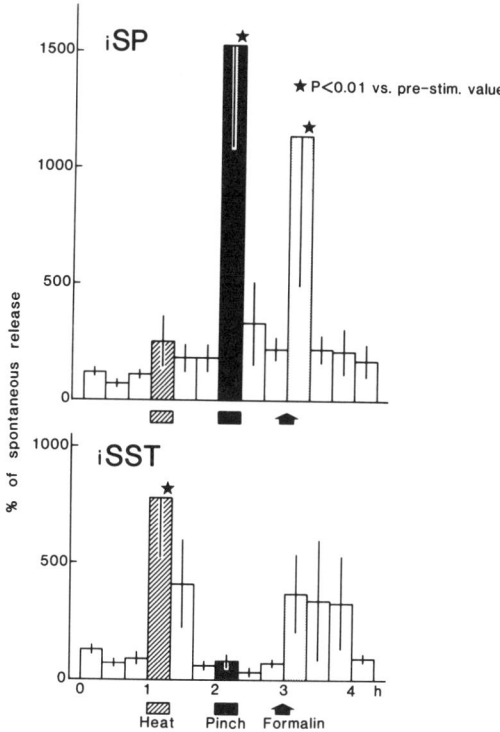

Figure 3. Selective effects of thermal (heat) and mechanical (pinch), and nonselective effect of chemical (subcutaneous injection of formalin), noxious stimuli on the release of immunoreactive substance P (iSP) and immunoreactive somatostatin (iSST) from the rabbit spinal dorsal horn *in situ*. A spontaneous release was calculated by an average of the amount of immunoreactive peptides released in the first three samples from each experiment and served as the control value (100%). Values represent in the mean and S.E.M.

increase in the iSST release. On the contrary, pinch (noxious mechanical stimulation) significantly increased the iSP release to about 10 times as large as the spontaneous release, while the same stimulation did not change the iSST release (Kuraishi, Hirota, Sato, Hino, Satoh, & Takagi, 1985). Subcutaneous injection of a diluted 5% formalin solution, which induces an inflammation, increased both iSP and iSST releases.

The noxious stimuli-induced increases in the releases of iSP and iSST were not observed when similar stimuli were given to the skin of the contralateral hind leg to the perfusion site (Figures 4 and 5), or when the perfusion was done with a Ca^{2+}-free and higher Mg^{2+}-containing medium. Such a result strongly suggests that the stimulus-induced release of iSP or iSST originates from the terminal of the primary afferents. Various innocuous stimuli given to the skin of the ipsilateral hind leg, such as blowing air, rubbing, and warming up to 40°C, did not cause any changes in the iSP and iSST releases. The ineffectiveness of the thermal or mechanical stimulation in increasing the release of iSP or iSST, respectively, is not due to an insufficient strength of the stimulation, since the same stimulation significantly increased the iSST or iSP release, respectively.

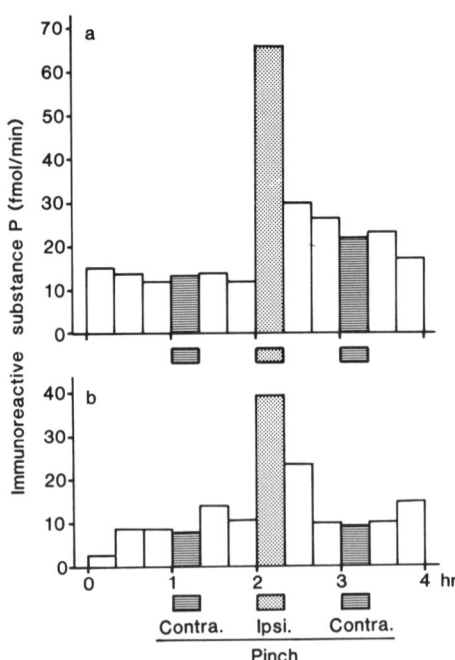

Figure 4. Ineffectiveness of noxious pinch stimulation of the hind leg contralateral to the perfusion site, on the release of immunoreactive substance P from the rabbit spinal dorsal horn *in situ*.

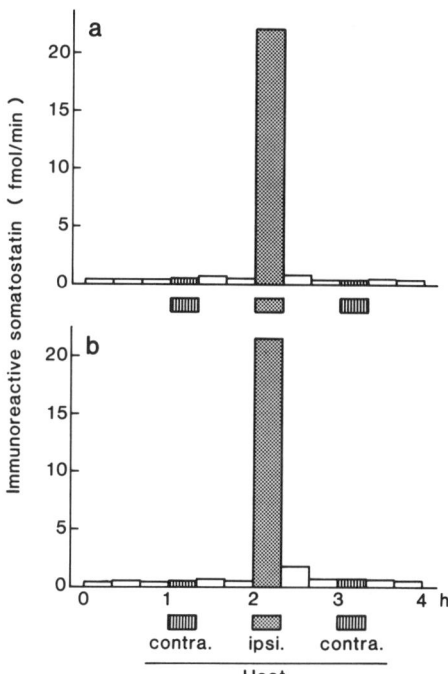

Figure 5. Ineffectiveness of noxious heat stimulation of the hind leg contralateral to the perfusion site, on the release of immunoreactive somatostatin from the rabbit spinal dorsal horn *in situ*.

The effects of substance P and somatostatin injected intrathecally on behavioral responsiveness to noxious stimuli were investigated using rats. Intrathecal injection of substance P in a dose of 0.1 nmol/rat produced a significant reduction of the threshold (hyperalgesia) in the paw-pressure test but rather hypoalgesia in the hot-plate test. The latter hypoalgesic effect of substance P became statistically significant when a dose of the peptide was increased to 1 nmol/rat. On the contrary, similar injection of somatostatin at a dose of 0.1 nmol/rat did not significantly change the nociceptive threshold in the paw-pressure test but did produce a significant shortening latency (hyperalgesia) in the hot-plate test.

Furthermore, in order to estimate physiological significance of endogenous substance P and somatostatin in nociceptive transmission, it is useful to examine the effects of intrathecal injections of antisera against substance P and somatostatin. Nance, Sawynok, and Nance (1987) reported that intrathecal injection of antisubstance P antiserum inhibited the mechanical, but not the thermal, nociceptive response of rats. We clearly demonstrated that intrathecal injection of antiserum against somatostatin significantly inhibited the nociceptive response to

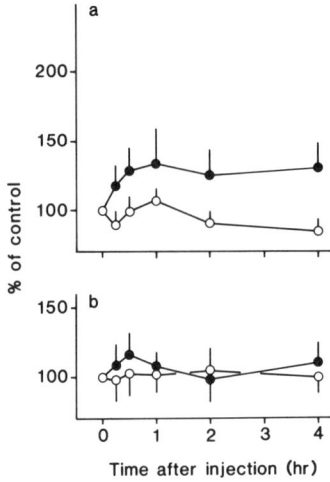

Figure 6. Differential effects of intrathecal injection of antisomatostatin antiserum on thermal(a) and mechanical(b) nociception in rats. The antiserum (filled circles) or the antiserum absorbed with synthetic somatostatin (open circles) was given in a volume of 10 μl at 0 time. The ordinates represent (a) change in latency of nociceptive responses in the hot-plate method, and (b) change in nociceptive threshold in the paw-pressure method. Latency (a) and threshold (b) of each animal before the injection served as control (100%). Values represent the mean and S.E.M. The effects of antisomatostatin antiserum ($n = 6$) were significantly ($F(1, 50) = 13.0647$, $p < .001$, ANOVA) different from those of the absorbed antiserum ($n = 6$) in (a) the hot-plate but not (b) the paw-pressure method.

thermal, but not mechanical, stimulation in rats (Figure 6; Ohno, Kuraishi, Minami, & Satoh, 1988).

From the above-described findings, the author hypothesizes as follows: (a) Noxious mechanical stimuli (pinch) given to the skin activate the substance P-containing, but not somatostatin-containing, primary afferents. Substance P is released from the nerve terminals and transmits the mechanonociceptive information to the secondary neurons in the spinal dorsal horn. On the other hand, (b) noxious thermal stimuli (radiant heat) excites the somatostatin-containing, but not substance P-containing, primary afferents. Somatostatin is released from the nerve terminals and transmits the thermonociceptive information to the secondary neurons in the spinal dorsal horn. Further, (c) chemical or inflammatory noxious stimuli like subcutaneous injection of formalin may activate both substance P-containing and somatostatin-containing primary afferents.

A Role of Calcitonin Gene-Related Peptide (CGRP)

Intrathecal injection of synthetic human CGRP (hCGRP) at a dose of 5 nmol/rat significantly lowered the nociceptive threshold for mechanical stimulation in the paw-pressure method (Figure 7) but produced few aversive responses such as caudally directed biting and scratching. On the other hand, similar injection of substance P produced the aversive responses and a decrease in the nociceptive threshold. When substance

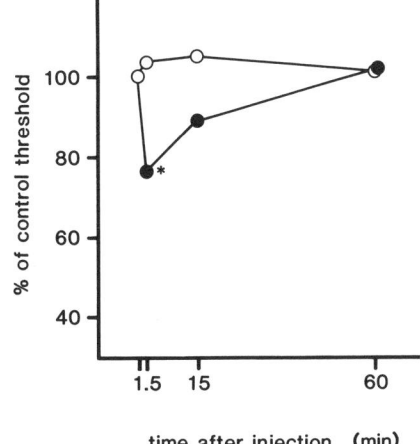

Figure 7. Hyperalgesia induced by intrathecal injection of CGRP (5 nmol/rat; filled circles). Vertical bars indicate S.E.M. The asterisk indicates a significant difference ($p < .05$, Student's t test) from vehicle group (open circles).

P and CGRP were simultaneously injected intrathecally, CGRP did not alter the number of aversive responses produced by substance P alone (Oku, Satoh, Fujii, Otaka, Yajima, & Takagi 1987).

Furthermore, intrathecal injection of anti-CGRP antiserum elevated the nociceptive threshold in the rat paw-pressure test, while 0.9% saline, preimmune serum, and anti-CGRP antiserum that was previously absorbed by synthetic CGRP were without effect (Figure 8; Kuraishi, Nanayama, Ohno, Minami, & Satoh, 1988).

In order to reveal a mechanism of hyperalgesia by CGRP in the paw-pressure test, we investigated the effect of CGRP on the release of substance P, which is suggested to transmit mechanonociceptive information in the spinal dorsal horn (Oku, Satoh, Fujii, Otaka, Yajima, & Takagi, 1987). For this purpose, a method of *in vitro* perfusion of the rat spinal dorsal horn was employed. The basal release of iSP—that is, the content of iSP in the superfusate in the absence of any particular stimuli—tended to decrease slowly (open column in Figure 9). When high K^+ (50 mM) or capsaicin (5×10^{-7}M) was added to the medium for 3 minutes, a significant increase in the amount of iSP was produced in the fraction including the stimulation period and the next fraction (Figure 9a, hatched columns). Therefore, the total amount of iSP in the two samples was regarded as the released iSP with each stimulus. The capsaicin-evoked release of iSP was markedly reduced in the lumbar dorsal horn slices prepared from rats in which the bilateral sciatic nerves had been cut 10 days before the experiment, thereby strongly suggesting that the capsaicin-evoked release of iSP was derived from the primary afferent terminals. An addition of CGRP (1 μM) to the medium did not

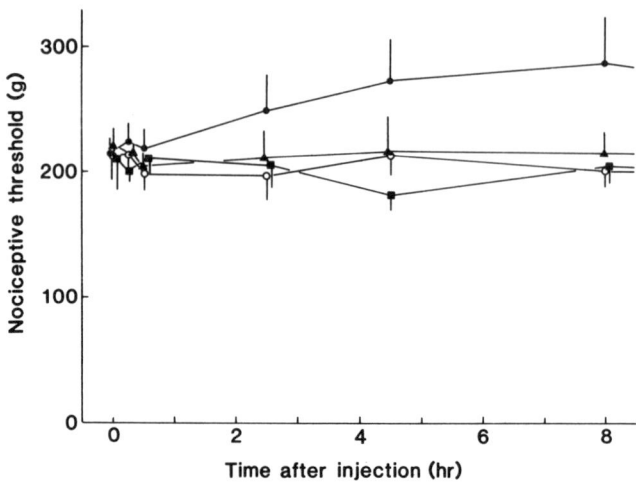

Figure 8. Antinociceptive effect of intrathecal injection of anti-CGRP antiserum in rats. Anti-CGRP antiserum (filled circles), physiological saline (open circles), preimmune serum (filled triangles), or anti-CGRP antiserum absorbed with synthetic CGRP (filled squares) was given in a volume of 10 μl at time 0. The ordinate represents nociceptive threshold of the hind paw for pressure, and values the mean and S.E.M. Four kinds of treatment produced significantly different effects ($F(3, 98) = 7.0434$, $p < .001$, ANOVA). The effects of anti-CGRP antiserum ($n = 4$) were significantly different from those of saline ($p < .001$, $n = 5$), absorbed antiserum ($p < .001$, $n = 5$), and preimmune serum ($p = .010$, $n = 4$) when analyzed by multiple comparisons.

affect the spontaneous release but did markedly potentiate the capsaicin-evoked release of iSP (Figure 9b).

From these findings, it is suggested that endogenous CGRP may act on the capsaicin-sensitive primary afferent terminals to facilitate the activated release of substance P in the spinal dorsal horn; consequently, transmission of noxious pinching-induced nociceptive information, probably mediated by substance P, is enhanced. However, CGRP may not transmit nociceptive information by itself in the spinal dorsal horn.

At the End

As described above, we have revealed individual roles of substance P, somatostatin, and CGRP, which are contained in the small primary afferents separately or together, in nociceptive transmission at the spinal dorsal horn. Further, the author found that the release of substance P

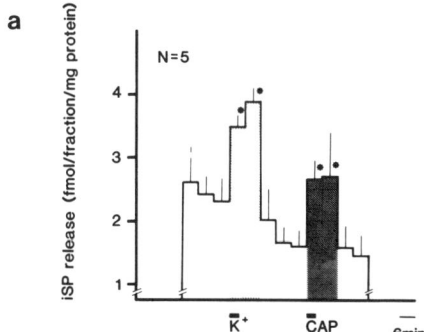

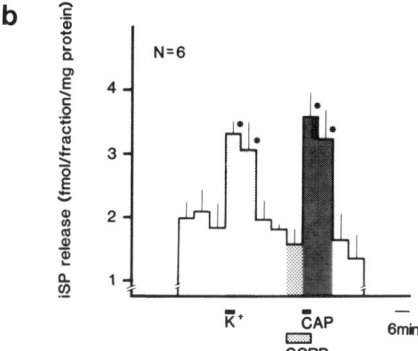

Figure 9a. In vitro release of immunoreactive substance P (iSP) from the spinal dorsal horn of rats by high K^+ (50 mM; K^+) or capsaicin (5×10^{-7}M; CAP). b. the effect of CGRP (1 μM) on the capsaicin-evoked release of iSP. Horizontal black bars indicate the stimulation periods. Horizontal dotted bar shows the superfusion period with CGRP. The hatched columns were regarded as the fractions with iSP released by each stimulation. Vertical bars show S.E.M. The asterisk represents a significant difference ($p < .05$, Student's paired t test) from the fraction immediately before each stimulation.

evoked by noxious pinch of the skin is modulated by the spinal noradrenergic system, while that of somatostatin evoked by noxious heat stimuli by the spinal serotonergic system, although these data are not described in this chapter, owing to limited space. However, none of these three neuropeptides is probably a transmitter in the primary afferents with polymodal nociceptor. Thus, it is of interest to identify it.

ACKNOWLEDGMENTS. The author thanks Professor emeritus H. Takagi, Dr. Y. Kuraishi, Dr. R. Oku, Dr. N. Hirota, Dr. H. Ohno, and Mr. T. Nanayama for their collaboration in this study. Part of this study was supported by Grants-in-Aid for Scientific Research from the Ministry of Education, Science and Culture (Japan), the Ministry of Public Welfare (Japan), and the Naito Foundation Subsidy for Promotion of Specific Research Projects.

References

Amara, S. G., Jonas, V., Rosenfeld, M. G., Ong, E. S., & Evans, R. M. (1982). Alternative RNA processing in calcitonin gene expression generates mRNA encoding different polypeptide products. *Nature (London), 298,* 240–244.
Dodd, J., Jahr, C. E., & Jessel, T. M. (1984). Neurotransmitters and neuronal markers at sensory synapses in the dorsal horn. In L. Kruger & J. C. Liebeskind (Eds.), *Advances in pain research and therapy* (pp. 105–121). New York: Raven Press.
Hökfelt, T., Elde, R., Johansson, O., Luft, R., Nilsson, G., & Arimura, A. (1976). Immunohistochemical evidence for separate populations of somatostatin-containing and substance P-containing primary afferent neurons in the rat. *Neuroscience, 1,* 131–136.
Kuraishi, Y., Hirota, N., Sugimoto, M., Satoh, M., & Takagi, H. (1983). Effects of morphine on noxious stimuli-induced release of substance P from the rabbit dorsal horn in vivo. *Life Sciences, 33*(Suppl. I), 693–696.
Kuraishi, Y., Hirota, N., Sato, Y., Hino, Y., Satoh, M., & Takagi, H. (1985). Evidence that substance P and somatostatin transmit separate information related to pain in the spinal dorsal horn. *Brain Research, 325,* 294–298.
Kuraishi, Y., Nanayama, T., Ohno, H., Minami, M., & Satoh, M. (1988). Antinociception induced in rats by intrathecal administration of antiserum against calcitonin gene-related peptide. *Neuroscience Letters, 92,* 325–329.
Nance, P. W., Sawynok, J., & Nance, D. M. (1987). Modality specific analgesia produced by intrathecal anti-substance P antibody. In J. L. Henry, R. Couture, A. C. Cuello, G. Pelletier, R. Cuirion, & D. Regoli (Eds.), *Substance P and neurokinins* (pp. 282–284). New York: Springer-Verlag.
Ohno, H., Kuraishi, Y., Minami, M., & Satoh, M. (1988). Modality-specific antinociception produced by intrathecal injection of anti-somatostatin antiserum in rats. *Brain Research, 474,* 197–200.
Oku, R., Satoh, M., Fujii, N., Otaka, A., Yajima, H., & Takagi, H. (1987). Calcitonin gene-related peptide promotes mechanical nociception by potentiating release of substance P release from the spinal dorsal horn in rats. *Brain Research, 403,* 350–354.
Satoh, M., Yasui, M., Fujibayashi, K., & Takagi, H. (1983). Bestatin potentiates analgesic effect of intrathecally administered dynorphin in rats. *IRCS Medical Science, 11,* 965–966.
Wiesenfeld-Hallin, Z., Hökfelt, T., Lundberg, J. M., Frossmann, W. G., Reinecke, M., Tschopp, F. A., & Fischer, J. A. (1984). Immunoreactive calcitonin gene-related peptide and substance P coexist in sensory neurons to the spinal cord and interact in spinal behavioral responses of the rat. *Neuroscience Letters, 52,* 199–204.
Willis, W. D. (1985). *The pain system.* Basel: Karger.

CHAPTER 16

Evidence for the Role of the Cerebral Cortex in Acupuncture Analgesia

Lang Yan Xia, J. Peter Rosenfeld, and Kun Hou Huang

Introduction

Current views on acupuncture mechanisms are represented by Pomeranz (1987) in his recently published book and emphasize the role of spinal, brainstem, midbrain, and hypothalamic mechanisms, but no one in the West has emphasized the role of cerebral cortex in acupuncture analgesia (AA).

In this chapter we review two areas. First, we introduce the indirect evidence for the role of cortex in AA that documents the involvement of cortex in painful sensation. Second, direct evidence of cortical involvement in acupuncture analgesia is presented and will include both experimental and clinical studies in animals and humans.

Indirect Evidence

There has long been indirect evidence that cortex may be involved both in painful sensation and in pain-inhibitory mechanisms. There was once a view that cortex is not related to painful sensation since thalamus was felt to be the highest level of the neuraxis related to pain. More

---

Lang Yan Xia • Beijing College of Traditional Chinese Medicine, 100013 Beijing, People's Republic of China.   J. Peter Rosenfeld • Cresap Neuroscience Laboratory, Northwestern University, Evanston, Illinois 60208, USA.   Kun Hou Huang • Chinese Academy of Traditional Chinese Medicine, 100700 Beijing, People's Republic of China.

recently, clinical observation (Huang, Xu, Xia, Meng, Tan, Chen, He, Chen, Liang, & Liu, 1979) showed that there was a difference between the painful sensation on the two sides in patients with unilateral cerebral lesion or with one side of the somatosensory area surgically removed; in this work, stimulation of the middle finger was used to produce pain perception. In an earlier study (Xia, Chen, and Gou, 1978), the injection of morphine (5 mg/kg i.v.) caused a marked decrease in the amplitude of cortical potentials evoked by nociceptive stimulation of dental pulp in awake cats with implanted cerebral evoked potential (CEP) recording electrodes and pulpal stimulation electrodes. However, it produced no definite effect on the CEP of "Hegu" acupoint with subnoxious stimulation by electroacupuncture.

Recently, Dong, Xu, Chen, Xie, Rong, Xu, and Zhang (1984) reported that there are neurons responsive to noxious stimuli in the cerebral cortex. The responses of neurons in the primary somatosensory area (SI) of the cerebral cortex to noxious stimuli were recorded. In all, 570 unit discharges were observed 1 to 2000 μ mm, beneath the cortical surface in 51 cats. The frequency of discharge was increased by noxious stimuli in 66 units and was decreased in 32 units; these cells constitute 17.2% of the total 570 cells. The remaining cells were unaffected by noxious stimulation. Also, the injection of fentanyl reduced the responses to noxious stimuli in the two kinds of neurons.

Gao, Xie, Lu, Liang, and Li (1984) reported the effects of intracortical stimulation of somatic area II on the nociceptive neuronal activities in the mesencephalic reticular formation. Fifty-five rabbits were anesthetized with chloralose and urethane. As soon as the animal recovered consciousness it was immobilized with flaxedil and given artificial respiration. The electrical activities of the nociceptive neurons were recorded with glass microelectrodes with the aid of a stereotaxic apparatus. Eighty-one of the nociceptive units responded to noxious electrical stimulation, which was applied to the peroneal nerve. Among them, 65 units (80%) responded with an increase in discharge frequency to noxious stimuli (pain-excitation neuron, PEN). In contrast, there were 16 units (20%) that responded to noxious stimuli with a decrease in the frequency of the discharge (pain-inhibition neuron, PIN). Similar results were obtained with the stimulation of area SII of the cortex with the same train of pulses. That is, an excitatory effect was observed in PEN and an inhibitory effect was observed in PIN. However, after Dolantin (an opiate) was given intravenously, under the same conditions used above, both the peroneal nerve and area SII were stimulated again, eliciting an inhibitory effect on PEN, and a reduction of inhibition or release from it on PIN.

Most recently, Willis's group (Yezierski, Gerhart, Schrock, & Willis, 1983) extended their earlier (Coulter, Maune & Willis, 1974) study of the effects of cortical stimulation on the responses of spinothalamic neurons. They found that as long as intermediate (200 msec) or long (2 sec) duration cortical conditioning stimulation trains were used, inhibitory effects on responses to noxious stimulation could be demonstrated with stimulation particularly of the primary somatic sensory cortex, as opposed to motor areas. Also, Sessle, Hu, Dubner, and Lucier (1981) and Saade, Tekian, Tamari, Banna, and Jabbur (1981) found that cortical and cerebral peduncular stimulation inhibited orofacial nociceptive responding of neurons, including trigeminal nuclear responses to tooth pulp stimulation. Dubner and Sessle (1971) had earlier shown presynaptic depolarization of trigeminal primary afferents, including A-*delta* fibers, correlated with trigeminal neuronal inhibition produced by cortical stimulation. These are the only studies of direct cortical involvement in descending pain modulation. They clearly support the notion that cortex is involved in analgesia. Less direct support comes from the fact that cortical projections to various brainstem nuclei involved in descending inhibition are well documented, and inhibitory effects on spinothalamic neurons can be obtained by stimulating areas that receive cortical projections (Geisler, Yezierski, Gerhart, & Willis, 1981; Haber, Martin, Chung, & Willis, 1980; Yezierski *et al.*, 1983). Also, work from Rosenfeld's lab has shown that operantly conditioned modifications in the somatosensory cortical evoked response in rats produces orofacial analgesia showing somatotopic specificity and submodality specificity, which is probably mediated by endogenous opiate processes (Dowman & Rosenfeld, 1985; Rosenfeld, Dowman, Heinricher, & Silvia, 1984).

Direct Evidence

Direct support for cortical mediation of Electroacupuncture (EA) analgesia comes from preliminary work by L. Y. Xia, K. H. Huang, and others in the People's Republic of China:

1. Stimulation specific acupoints evoke robust somatosensory cortical evoked potentials (SEPs) at moderate stimulation intensities at which nonacupoints produce no response (Zhang, Cui, and Liu, 1986). The experiments were performed on 20 adult cats anesthetized with a single dose of alpha (a)-chloralose. Concentric acupoint bipolar electrodes were used to stimulate at the acupoint Hegu, the Wangu, and the nonacupoint that was midway between the two acupoints. Side-by-side stimulating electrodes were used to elicit S1 somatosensory evoked potentials, using the computer to average. Twenty cats were observed for

98 trials. Stimulating the Hegu in all of the cats produced the evoked potential from contralateral cortex. The same stimulation on the nonacupoint (1 cm from Hegu) failed to evoke the potential, but during stimulation of the Wangu, the evoked potential appeared again in all of the cats (see Table 1).

The cortex evoked potential of Hegu was a biphasic positive-negative wave, of peak latency 43.32 ± 1.29 msec. The cortex evoked potential of Wangu was also a biphasic positive-negative wave, of peak latency 49.40 ± 1.41 msec, amplitude 44.57 ± 1.89 μv, and duration 44.70 ± 1.48 msec. Analysis of these data showed that the peak latency of Hegu significantly differed ($p < .01$) from the peak latency of Wangu, and the amplitudes were also significantly different ($p < .05$) between the two acupoints, but the duration showed no significant difference (see Table 2).

These results suggest that the cortex evoked potentials of acupoint Hegu were different from those of Wangu and the evoked potential differences were even greater between the acupoints (Hegu, Wangu) and the nonacupoint. Consequently, there is relative cortical connective specificity not only between the acupoint and nonacupoint but also between the two acupoints.

2. Cats were anesthetized with a-chloralose (40 mg/kg). As soon as the animal recovered it was immobilized with flaxedil and given artificial respiration. During supramaximal electrical stimuli delivered to the pulps of the canine teeth, distinct action potentials were recorded from ipsilateral inferior alveolar nerve. Conduction velocity of inferior alveolar nerve recorded in 10 of these 11 cases (91%) was below 15 m/sec, (A-*delta* range). In 2 of these 11 cases (18%) it was below 2 m/sec, the C-fiber velocity also subserving pain. A comparison of the different results of various stimulating intensities showed that some components of cortical potentials evoked by tooth pulp stimulation are related to the activities of small-diameter afferent fibers subserving pain (see Table 3).

Next it was shown that the cortical potentials evoked from painful stimulation of the tooth pulp afferents were markedly inhibited by EA

Table 1. *The Responses of SEPs of Acupoints Hegu, Wangu, and Nonacupoint (in 20 cats, N = 98)*

	Total	Response	Nonresponse	P between acupoint and nonacupoint
Acupoint Hegu	98	98	0	$p < .01$
Nonacupoint	98	0	98	$p < .01$
Acupoint Wangu	98	98	0	

Table 2. Duration, Amplitude, and Latency of SEPs Evoked by Hegu and Wangu (Mean ± SE, N = 98 in 20 cats)

	P-P latency (ms)	Amplitude (v)	Duration (ms)
Acupoint Hegu	43.39 ± 0.74	51.98 ± 2.26	42.73 ± 1.29
Acupoint ± Wangu	49.40 ± 1.41	44.57 ± 1.89	44.70 ± 1.48

stimuli of the Hegu acupoint. When 0.25% atropine was topically applied to the cortical area representative of the Hegu acupoint for 15 minutes, the cortical potentials evoked by Hegu acupoint stimulation were markedly augmented to twice the control group amplitude. On the basis of atropine-induced changes of excitability in this cortical area, the *inhibitory* effect on pulp-evoked cortical potentials due to EA stimulation of the Hegu acupoint was augmented by 13%. In the absence of EA, atropine minimally affects the pulp-evoked responses. Analysis of these data showed that after application of atropine, the potent effect of EA significantly differed ($p < .005$) from the EA effect in the nonatropinized state (see Tables 4–6).

These results strongly suggest that cholinergic mechanisms in cerebral cortex are implicated in EA (Xia et al., 1978).

3. The amplitude of the pain-related C component of the compound action potential in the peroneal nerve is dramatically reduced by EA, and the temporal pattern of attenuation strongly correlates with the time course of attenuation seen in a specific component of the simultaneously recorded cortical evoked response (Huang et al., 1981).

In this work, the evoked potentials of cerebral somatosensory area and the thalamic centromedian nucleus (CM), and the action potentials of peroneal common nerve were recorded simultaneously, while unilateral peroneal common nerve was stimulated by noxious electric stimuli in rabbits. The responses of the three structures before and after EA were observed and compared. The change of the evoked responses was also observed when nucleus CM was damaged by electrolytic lesion. Furthermore, the interaction of the three structures and their roles in acupuncture analgesia were analyzed.

The amplitude of components of cerebral evoked potentials after 70 msec, and N21, P180 components of the evoked potentials of CM were decreased while Sanyinjioao and Yinlinquan were stimulated by EA for 5 minutes (13 rabbits, 22 times). It obtained that the decrease of amplitude was significant ($p < .05$). Twenty minutes after ceasing EA, the

Table 3. Analyses of Components of Action Potential from Inferior Alveolar Nerve in Cats

Cat I.D.	Length of nerves (mm)	Wave 1		Wave 2		Wave 3		Wave 4	
		Latency (ms)	Conductive velocity (m/s)	Latency (ms)	Conductive velocity (m/s)	Latency (ms)	Conductive velocity (m/s)	Latency (ms)	Conductive velocity (m/s)
161	28	—[a]	—	10.0	2.8	15.0	1.8	18.7	1.5
157	24	—	—	2.0	12.0	3.9	6.2	7.3	3.3
155	19	—	—	6.6	2.9	10.0	1.9	13.5	1.4
146	27	—	—	1.8	15.4	—	—	—	—
147	25	—	—	4.3	5.8	7.3	3.5	10.0	2.5
145	26	—	—	1.1	23.7	—	—	—	—
141	22	—	—	3.1	7.1	—	—	—	—
139	27	—	—	2.7	10.0	—	—	—	—
136	21	—	—	1.7	12.6	3.4	6.3	—	—
134	26 (left)	—	—	3.8	6.9	6.4	4.1	—	—
134	26 (right)	—	—	2.5	10.4	6.1	4.3	—	—

[a]Not measured. The conductive velocity of A fiber is below 15 m/s and C fiber is below 2 m/s.

Table 4. *The Change of P-P Amplitude of Hegu SEPs after 0.25% Atropine Topically Applied at Cortical Hegu Area*

Cat I.D.	After atropine %			After atropine average %
	16–23 min	24–30 min	31–37 min	
218	+52	−a	−	+52
221	+460	+440	−	+450
223	+34	−	−	+34
224	+35	+32	−	+34
222	+10	−	+7	+9
225	+70	+70	+25	+55
226	+60	+43	−	+52
227	+117	+146	+142	+135
228	+93	−	−	+93
229	+138	+67	+59	+88
230	+176	+170	+45	+130
Average	+113	+138	+56	+103

^aNot measured.

Table 5. *The Effects of Atropine Topically Applied at Cortical Hegu Area on the EA Analgesia (Compared with the Amplitude of SEPs during EA before Atropine)*

Cat I.D.	After atropine %					After atropine average %
	1–7 min	8–15 min	16–23 min	24–30 min	31–37 min	
218	−20	−16	−a	−	−	−18
221	−19	−30	−	−16	−5	−18
223	−21	−12	−	−43	−	−26
222	−8	−18	−25	−	−25	−20
226	−10	−28	−21	−84	−	−36
228	−18	−7	−22	−	−	−16
229	−2	−2	−32	−15	−13	−13
224	−55	+20	+9	−27	−20	−15
230	+4	−27	+15	−10	−12	−6
225	+24	+31	+9	−22	−	+11
227	−10	+28	+5	+28	+23	+15
Average	−12	−6	−6	−24	−9	−13

^aNot measured.

Table 6. The Effects of Artificial Cerebrospinal Fluid Topically Applied at Cortical Hegu Area on EA Analgesia (Compared with the Amplitude of SEPs during EA before Artificial Cerebrospinal Fluid)

Cat I.D.	After atropine %					After atropine average %
	1–7 min	8–15 min	16–23 min	24–30 min	31–37 min	
232	+7	−4	+4	+4		+2
233	+14	+19	+16	−16		+16
234	+6	+3	−5	+1		+2
238	−10	−19	−10	+51	+42	+10
237	+4		+4	+6	−4	+3
239	−4	0	−8	−22	−6	−8
Average	+3	0	0	+9	+10	+4

amplitude of the P354 component of the CM response was decreased significantly ($p < .02$) (see Tables 7 and 8). The amplitude of the C wave of the action potentials simultaneously recorded from peroneal common nerve was decreased.

The amplitude of the evoked potentials of cortex and residual CM were decreased after partial electrolytic lesion of CM, but the amplitude of the C wave of the action potentials of peroneal common nerve was increased.

The results suggest that the hypothetical higher EA centers may exert, through the descending pathway, a tonic inhibitory control on the transmission of peripheral noxious afferent impulses.

4. The fentanyl- or ketamine-induced depression of somatosensory evoked potentials (SEPs) induced by noxious middle-finger stimulation

Table 7. The Effect of EA Inhibition on Amplitude of SEP ($N = 22$)

Components of SEP (mean ± SE)	EA for 5'	15–20' after ceasing EA
N 72.4 ± 3.3 ms	$p < .05$	$p < .01$
P 160.2 ± 8.8 ms	$.05 < p < .1$	$p = .02$
N 202.8 ± 8.6 ms	$p < .025$	$p < .001$
P 354.7 ± 9.0 ms	$p < .02$	$p < .005$

Table 8. The Effect of EA Inhibition on Amplitude of EP (N = 19)

Components of SEP (mean ± SE)	EA for 5'	15–20' after ceasing EA
N 21.2 ± 3.1 ms	$p < .05$	$p < .01$
P 180.4 ± 10.8 ms	$p < .025$	$p < .02$
N 353.5 ± 22.4 ms	$p < .5$	$p < .02$

correlated with the depression of pain ratings in behavioral data simultaneously collected from human subjects. The effect of EA on SEPs and pain ratings was the same with the fentanyl or ketamine (Xu, Huang, Xia, Meng, Chen, He, Chen, Liu, & Liang, 1979).

This investigation was carried out on human subjects. Painful stimulation of the middle finger was used and the cerebral evoked potentials were recorded at the contralateral scalp. Acupoint loci Neiguan and Jianshi were stimulated by EA. The evoked potentials were transferred to the computer for averaging and plotting. Two studies were done: First, we analyzed the component of the cerebral evoked potential related to pain. The potentials evoked by nonpain and pain stimuli were observed. Observations were also made on general surgery cases using fentanyl and ketamine. Second, we obtained observations of acupuncture effects on the cerebral evoked potentials and pain ratings in healthy adults, and in patients undergoing brain operations.

When we compared the cerebral potentials evoked by nonpain and pain stimulation, we observed that the shape of the potential evoked by nonpain stimulation was simple and the amplitude of the wave was small. However, the shapes of potentials evoked by pain stimulation were complex and the amplitudes were high. In 23 cases of normal adults we observed that the amplitude of Wave P2 (latency is about 200 msec) was significantly different between nonpain and pain stimulation.

In order to exclude the effect of stimulus intensity apart from painful and nonpainful levels of stimulation, the influence of fentanyl (0.1 mg/adult i.v., 16 cases) and ketamine (50 mg/adult i.v., 8 cases) on cerebral potentials evoked by pain stimulation was observed—i.e., before and after intravenous injection. The amplitudes of Wave P2, a positive wave, were decreased after fentanyl, a pain-killer, was injected. Also after administration of ketamine, the same result obtained. This shows that the Wave P2 (latency about 22 msec) was related to pain perception.

The amplitudes of cerebral evoked potentials of healthy adults were decreased during EA, but only the change in amplitude of Wave P2 was significant. The depression of evoked potentials paralleled that of pain ratings. Effects of EA on cerebral evoked potentials were also observed in patients going through brain operation. When the evoked potentials before and after EA from scalp and cerebral cortex were simultaneously recorded, we could see that the shapes of evoked potentials were the same before EA and after EA. We also found the depression by acupuncture on cerebral evoked potential amplitude specifically on P2.

5. Cortical lesions in humans reduce EA effects specific to the lesioned side (Huang et al., 1979).

This study was carried out on eight patients, five with unilateral cerebral lesion, three with one side of the somatosensory area having been surgically removed. One middle finger was stimulated and pain perception was produced. The acupoints used were Neiguan and Jianski. Cortical evoked potentials were recorded bilaterally.

The effect of EA between the intact side and the diseased side showed a significant difference, $p < .05$. The amplitude of cortical evoked potentials decreased 14.5% when the intact side was activated by EA, but when the diseased side was activated, the evoked potential decreased only 4.3%. At the same time, the pain rating was also depressed after activating the intact side. These results suggest that the cerebral cortex participated in EA analgesia.

6. The pure pain-representing components of SEP were inhibited by EA in humans (Huang & Xia, 1985; Xia & Huang, 1980, 1981; Xia, Huang, Zhao, & Rong, 1981; Xia, Huang, Zhao, Xu, Liang, & Rong, 1984a; Xia, Huang, Zhao, Rong, Xu, & Liang, 1984b; Xia, Huang, Rong, Zhao, & Liang, 1984c; Xia, Huang, Zhao, Rong, Xu, & Liang, 1984d).

It is known that certain components of complex cerebral potentials evoked by painful stimulation are highly correlated with pain. The inverse average technique was designed according to the view that the SEPs are complex potentials and the computer averaging technique could be used to reveal the pure pain-related components. We made the model graph of cerebral pain evoked potentials in the human by using the method of group inverse average, and performed appraisal of the recovery of the potentials to guard against possible artifacts of exterior origin during separation of the potentials.

It is also known that some components of the SEP are suppressed by EA. In the past research, only the complex cerebral evoked potentials after and before EA were compared; it was hard to see the complete picture of each component inhibited by EA. So in this work we were able to obtain the visual graph of the waves specifically inhibited by EA in order to analyze the analgesic effects.

The normal volunteers totaled 70, aged 21 to 48. The pain components were separated into 24 cases by using the inverse average technique; the separation of the group inverse average was done in 6 cases, the recovery of the potentials was done by using the group inverse average technique in 6 cases, the effects inhibited by EA were observed in 24 cases, and the visual graph of the potentials inhibited by EA was made in 10 cases.

The right middle finger was stimulated by painful or subpainful stimulation (1 Hz). Average cerebral evoked potentials were recorded from left scalp corresponding to hand area of cerebral cortex. Two acupoints, Neiguan and Tianshi, were stimulated by EA for 5 minutes. The effects of EA (for 5 minutes, and for 10 minutes after ceasing EA) on SEPs were observed.

When the stimulation intensity reached and exceeded pain threshold, the amplitudes of the components (latency about 50–160 msec) of SEP were clearly increased ($p < .05$); the amplitude of the components (latency about 160–300 msec) were also significantly increased ($p < .01$); the inhibitory effect of EA on initial early components was not ($p > .1$). The components of latencies 160 to 300 msec indicated an inhibitory tendency after EA for 5 minutes ($p < .1$). A significant inhibition was indicated on the components of latencies 50 to 160 msec and 160 to 300 msec 10 minutes after ceasing EA ($p < .05$). These main results from the analyses of individual data were reflected in the group (10 cases) visual graph of the potentials inhibited by EA. The wave form of the components inhibited by EA accorded with that of the pure pain components separated on the whole; i.e., there was a dramatic wave from 50 to 300 msec; the latencies of all components also were similar.

The recovery potentials accorded highly with the original potentials. This indicated that the model graph was not caused by nonphysiological interference. It is physiological, real, and reliable. It demonstrated the objective physiological difference of both complex potentials evoked by painful and subpainful stimulation.

The results indicated that there was the inhibitory effect of EA on the components relating to pain of CEP. Acupuncturing Neiguan and Jianshi reduced pain evoked by stimulating the middle finger. The potential graph inhibited by EA was separated by using the method of inverse average and group inverse average. This graph could reflect the complete picture of the inhibitory part of cerebral potentials evoked by painful stimulation after EA.

Several studies have shown that in patients with congenital insensitivity to pain, the amplitudes of P2 are temporarily elevated after naloxone administration; in this condition the subject's pain sensitivities were also temporarily elevated. It was known that P2 is related to pain.

We observed that the main wave of the model graph of cerebral pain evoked potential of humans was placed at the latency of P200; this main wave was also inhibited by acupuncture. It was also known that the acupuncture analgesia can be antagonized by naloxone. The results suggest that endorphine release might be influenced by the cerebral cortex on lower centers; endorphine might be elevated by acupuncture to produce analgesia. This hypothesis implies that superior acupoints have stronger CNS connections to brainstem opiate analgesia centers than do nonacupoints. Direct evidence of these connections has begun to be collected by Li Hongxun (1984) and colleagues at Henan Medical College in the People's Republic of China. They have found that EA at three known acupoints does modify spontaneous neuronal activity of nucleus raphe magnus of the cat.

The datum cited above about acupoints but not nonacupoints evoking cortical potentials is important. Pomeranz's (1987) comprehensive review includes a discussion on the specificity of acupoints. There was no question that acute laboratory pain is differentially affected by acupoints and nonacupoints; however, no clear structural or electrical correlates of the point specificity could be adduced. Citing an extensive Japanese literature (from Takeshige, 1985), Pomeranz (1987) suggests that acupoints and nonacupoints may have *distinct central connections.* This is quite consistent with the SEP specificity seen in cortex.

It is not now known *how* cortex might be involved in acupuncture analgesia, but presumably there would be a descending influence on brainstem structures with known roles in analgesia mechanisms. Xu, Lin, Chen, and Zhang (1984a) reported that the inhibitory effect of EA on the neurons of nucleus parafascicularis (Pf) was abolished by topical administration of GABA on SII, and the inhibitory effect by EA on the nociceptive response of Pf neurons is prolonged after topical administration of glutamate on SII. Also, Lin and Xu (1984) reported that after topical administration of lidocaine on SII, the inhibitory effects of EA on CM neurons was abolished.

All these results consistently support the notion that cortex is importantly involved in the mechanism of acupuncture analgesia.

ACKNOWLEDGMENTS. This work was supported by NIH grant DE07905 and an MoPH grant from the People's Republic of China.

References

Coulter, J. D., Maunz, R. A., & Willis, W. D. (1974). Effects of stimulation of sensorimotor cortex on primate spinothalamic neurons. *Brain Research, 65,* 351–356.
Dong, W. C., Xu, W., Chen, Z. Q., Xie, J. N., Rong, X. D., Xu, W. B., & Zhang, Y. F. (1984).

The influence of acupuncture on response of neurons in the cerebral cortex to noxious stimuli and the effect of naloxone. *Second National Symposium on Acupuncture and Moxibustion and Acupuncture Anesthesia* (Beijing), *357*, 331.

Dowman, R., & Rosenfeld, J. P. (1985). Operant conditioning of somatosensory evoked potential (SEP) in rats. I. Specific changes in SEP amplitude and a naloxone-reversible, somatotopically specific change in facial nociception. *Brain Research, 333*, 201–212.

Dubner, R., & Sessle, B. J. (1971). Presynaptic excitability changes of primary afferent and corticofugal fibers projecting to trigeminal brain stem nuclei. *Experimental Neurology, 30*, 223–238.

Gao, M. L., Xie, H. M., Lu, Y. X., Liang, Y.F., & Li, D. J. (1984). The effect of intracortical stimulation of somatic area II on the nociceptive neuronal activities in the mesencephalon reticular formation and its relation to the acupuncture effect. *Second National Symposium on Acupuncture and Moxibustion and Acupuncture Anesthesia* (Beijing), *356*, 330–331.

Geisler, G. J., Jr., Yezierski, R. P., Gerhart, K.D., & Willis, W. D. (1981). Spinothalamic tract neurons that project to medial and/or lateral thalamic nuclei: Evidence for a physiologically novel population of spinal cord neurons. *Journal of Neurophysiology, 46*, 1285–1308.

Haber, L. H., Martin, R. F., Chung, J. M., & Willis, W. D. (1980). Inhibition and excitation of primate spinothalamic tract neurons by stimulation in region of nucleus reticularis gigantocellularis. *Journal of Neurophysiology, 43*, 1578–1593.

Huang, K. H., & Xia, L. Y. (1985). The advance of painful cerebral evoked potential research in recent years. *Physiological Sciences, 5*(6), 355–357.

Huang, K. H., Xu, W., Xia, L. Y., Meng, Z., Tan, Y., Chen, Y., He, K., Chen, Z., Liang, R., & Liu, J. (1979). The influence of lesion of unilateral cerebral somatosensory area on the cortical evoked potentials and effect of acupuncture in human body. *National symposium of acupuncture and moxibustion and acupunture anaesthesia* (Beijing), *319*, 325–326.

Huang, K. H., Meng, Z. H., Liang, R. Z., Tan, Y. L., Chen, Y., & Xu, W. (1981). The effect of electroacupuncture on evoked potentials of cerebral somatosensory area, nucleus centrum medianum thalami (CM) and nervi peronaeus communis in rabbits. *Acupuncture Research, 6*(2), 107–112.

Lin, Y., & Xu, W. (1984). The function of corticofugal impulses of SII on the inhibitory effect of acupuncture at CM. *Second National Symposium on Acupuncture and Moxibustion and Acupuncture Anesthesia* (Beijing), *354*, 329.

Pomeranz, B. (1987). Scientific basis of acupuncture. In G. Stux & B. Pomeranz (Eds.), *Acupuncture: Textbooks and atlas*. Berlin, Heidelberg: Springer-Verlag, New York.

Rosenfeld, J. P., Dowman, R., Heinricher, M., & Silvia, R. (1984). Operantly controlled somatosensory evoked potentials: Specific effects on pain processes. In B. Rockstroh, T. Elbert, W. Lutzenberger, & N. Birbaumer (Eds.), *Self-regulation of the brain and behavior* (pp. 164–179). Berlin: Springer-Verlag.

Saade, N. E., Tekian, A., Tamari, J. W., Banna, N. R., & Jabbur, S. J. (1981). Stimulation of the cerebral peduncles modulates tooth pulp-evoked firing of trigeminal caudalis neurons. *Experimental Neurology, 4*, 930–934.

Sessle, B. J., Hu, J. W., Dubner, R., & Lucier, G. E. (1981). Functional properties of neurons in cat trigeminal subnucleus caudalis (medullary dirsal horn). II. Modulation of responses to noxious and non-noxious stimuli by periaqueductal gray, nucleus raphe magnus, cerebral cortex, and afferent influences, and effect of naloxone. *Journal of Neurophysiology, 45*, 193–207.

Takeshige, C. (1985). Differentiation between acupuncture and non-acupuncture points by association with an analgesia inhibitory system. *Acupuncture and Electrotherapy Research, 10*, 195–203, 1985.

Xia, L. H., Huang, K. H. (1980). A study of the cerebral average evoked potential as a method of objective pain measurement in human body and its development. *Acupuncture Research, 5*(3), 238–242.

Xia, L. Y., & Huang, K. H. (1984). The somatosensory evoked potential and its use. *Acupuncture Research, 9*(1), 1–5.

Xia, L. Y., Chen, X., & Guo, R. (1978). Beijing Institute of Traditional Chinese Medicine, Institute of Automation, Academia Sinica: Effect of topically changing functional activity of cerebral cortex on acupuncture analgesia in cats. *Acupuncture Anaesthesia, 3*(2), 21–31.

Xia, L. Y. Huang, K. H., Zhao, W., & Rong, X. (1981). Using computer technique to separate the components of pain from cerebral pain evoked complex potential from scalp in humans. *Acupuncture Research, 6*(1), 17–25.

Xia, L. Y., Huang, K. H., Zhao, W., Xu, W., Liang, X., & Rong, X. (1984a). Effects of electro-acupuncture on cerebral pain evoked potential of normal man. *Second National Symposium on Acupuncture and Moxibustion and Acupuncture Anesthesia* (Beijing), 347, 323.

Xia, L. Y., Huang, K. H., Zhao, W., Rong, X., Xu, W., & Liang, X. (1984b). The inhibitory effect of electro-acupuncture on cerebral evoked potential and the model graph of cerebral pain evoked potential of humans. *Second National Symposium on Acupuncture and Moxibustion and Acupuncture Anesthesia* (Beijing), 348, 324–325.

Xia, L. Y., Huang, K. H., Rong, X., Zhao, W., & Liang, X. (1984d). The painful components of cerebral evoked complex potential and model graph of cerebral pain evoked potentials of humans. *Physiological Sciences, 4*(5,6), 89.

Xia, L. Y., Huang, K. H., Zhao, W., Rong, X., Xu, W., & Liang, X. (1984d). The recovery of the potentials separated by group inverse average technique. *Second National Symposium on Acupuncture and Moxibustion and Acupuncture Anesthesia* (Beijing), 349, 325–326.

Xu, W., Huang, K. H., Xia, L. Y., Meng, Z., Chen, Y., He, K., Chen, Z., Liu, J., & Liang, R. (1979). Relationship between cerebral cortex and acupuncture analgesia. *Chinese Journal of Neurology and Psychiatry, 12*(2), 68–72.

Xu, W., Lin, Y., Chen., Z. Q., & Zhang, Y. F. (1984a). The influence of changing the functional state of SII by GABA on the acupuncture effect of Pf neurons. *Second National Symposium on Acupuncture and Moxibustion and Acupuncture Anesthesia* (Beijing), 352, 327–328.

Xu, W., Lin, Y., Chen, Z. Q., Zhang, Y. F. (1984b). The influence of changing the functional state of SII by glutamate on the acupuncture effect of Pf neurons. *Second National Symposium on Acupuncture and Moxibustion and Acupuncture Anesthesia* (Beijing), 353, 328–329.

Yezierski, R. P., Gerhart, K. D., Schrock, B. J., & Willis, W. D. (1983). A further examination of effects of cortical stimulation on primate spinothalamic tract cells. *Journal of Neurophysiology, 49,* 424–441.

Zhang, J., Cui, R., & Liu, G. (1986). The relative specificity of the cortex evoked response elicited by stimulation of acupoints and non-acupoints on forelimb in cats. *Acupuncture Research, 11*(2), 146–150.

Index

A-beta fiber, nociception and, 228
  transcutaneous electrical stimulation effects, 233–234
Acetylcholine, seizure effects, 134
Acupuncture, cerebral cortex involvement, 12–13, 206, 267–280
  cholinergic mechanisms, 271
  direct evidence, 269–278
  gamma-aminobutyric acid and, 278
  glutamate and, 278
  indirect evidence, 267–269
  pain-excitation neurons, 268
  pain-inhibition neurons, 268
  somatosensory cortical evoked potentials, 269–275, 276, 278
  thalamic centromedian nucleus evoked potentials, 271, 274, 278
A-delta fiber, nociception and, 224, 227, 228
Adenosine, seizure inhibitory effects, 134
Adenosine monophosphate, cyclic(cAMP), long-term potentiation and, 101
Adrenergic receptor, opioid analgesia and, 213–214, 215–216
α_2-Adrenergic receptor agonist, 211
β-Adrenergic response, in Raynaud's disease, 60
Adrenocortical steroid, 163
Adrenocorticotrophic hormone(ACTH)
  activation, 192
  dexamethasone-mediated inhibition, 203
  emotion-related secretion, 191
  precursor, 209

Afferent nervous system
  epicritic, 224
  protopathic, 224
Affine-mapping, 112
Alanine, seizures and, 134
  gamma-aminobutyric acid receptor modulators and, 137, 138, 141
γ-Aminobutyric acid. See Gamma-aminobutyric acid
Analgesia. See also Pain control
  acupuncture-related, 12–13, 206, 267–280
    cholinergic mechanisms, 271
    direct evidence, 269–278
    gamma-aminobutyric acid and, 278
    glutamate and, 278
    indirect evidence, 267–269
    pain-excitation neurons, 268
    pain-inhibition neurons, 268
    somatosensory cortical evoked potentials, 269–275, 276, 278
    thalamic centromedian nucleus evoked potentials, 271, 274, 278
  α_2-adrenergic agonist-related, 211
  clonidine-related, 211
  glutamate-related, 213
  opioid-related, 205, 207–221
    action mechanisms, 209
    action sites, 210–212
    norepinephrine-mediated, 211
    receptors and, 208, 209–210, 211
    serotonin-mediated, 211
    stimulation-produced, 209, 212–214, 230–232

281

Analgesia (cont.)
    transcutaneous electrical stimulation-related, 233–234
Angina pectoris, surgical placebo therapy, 183–184
Antiarrhythmic drugs, long-term potentiation and, 101
Anticonvulsants, slow cortical potentials and, 88–89
Antigen, hypothalamic neuron response, 163
Antilymphocyte serum immunoconditioning stimuli, 165, 197, 198, 203
    with lithium chloride, 200–201
    with saccharin, 199–200
Anxiety
    of heart disease patients, 36
    progressive relaxation therapy, 127–128, 131
Aspartic acid, seizures and, 134
    gamma-aminobutyric acid receptor modulators and, 138, 140
Autoimmune disease, conditioned immunosuppression, 165–178
    adaptive response, 167–169
    central nervous system involvement, 177, 178
    homeostasis, 168–169, 177–178
    learning ability deficits and, 166–167, 173, 176
Autonomic nervous system, cognitive function and, 122, 123
Avoidance response. See also Taste aversion, conditioned
    in immune complex disease, 164

Bacille Calmette-Guerin, as immunoconditioning stimuli, 197, 198
Baclofen, seizure effects, 134, 135–136, 137–139, 140, 141
Baroreceptor, in blood pressure reduction, 19
Behavioral intervention
    disease mechanisms and, 183–195
        guided imagery, 186–190
        miraculous healing, 186
        physiological processes, 190–192
        placebo response, 183–184, 185, 186
    for pain control, 234

Beta-antagonist, event-related slow potentials and, 101
Beta-blocker
    hyperventilation effects, 33
    respiratory sinus arrhythmia effects, 24–27
Biofeedback. See Feedback
Blood flow
    coronary, hyperventilation effects, 34
    in Raynaud's disease, 43
Blood pressure
    autonomic blockade effects, 96
    baroreceptors and, 19
    in Raynaud's disease, 43, 45
    diastolic, 50, 51
    systolic, 44, 50, 51
    sex factors, 44
Blood viscosity, in Raynaud's phenomenon, 42–43
Blood volume, in Raynaud's phenomenon, 44
Brain. See also specific areas of brain
    cardiovascular system regulation by, 16, 95–99
    opioid receptor content, 208
    opioid sensitivity, 210
    stimulation-produced analgesia, 213
Brainstem, descending pain control system, 214

Calcitonin gene-related peptide, dorsal horn content, 256
    in nociception, 262–265
Calcium, opioid interaction, 209
Cancer
    emotional factors, 184–185
    imagery therapy, 186–190
        adverse effects, 188–190
    placebo therapy, 183
    stress and, 164
β-Carboline, seizure excitatory effects, 134
Carbon dioxide
    end-tidal, 66
    hyperventilation and, 32–33, 35, 37
Cardiac output
    hyperventilation effects, 34
    in Raynaud's disease, 44, 45, 52, 53, 54, 59–60
    sex factors, 44

Cardiovascular disease. *See also* specific
  types of cardiovascular disease
    event-related potentials and, 101
Cardiovascular system
  cerebral mediation, 16, 95–99
  hyperventilation effects, 4, 32–37
    anxiety disorders and, 36
    beta-blocker effects, 33
    carbon dioxide levels, 32–33, 35, 37
    cardiac output, 34
    coronary blood flow, 34
    in coronary disease, 34, 35–37
    ECG, 34, 35–36
    respiratory rate, 34
    tidal volume, 34
  respiratory mediation, 3–4, 17–39
    biobehavioral framework, 17–21
    hyperventilation, 4, 32–37
    nonadaptive responses, 4, 21–32
    processes affecting, 19
    respiratory sinus arrhthymia, 4, 21–32
Catecholamines, immune system effects, 163
Central nervous system
  immune system relationship, 163, 190–192
  conditioned immunosuppression, 177, 178
  opioid effects, 209
Cerebral cortex
  acupuncture analgesia involvement, 12–13, 206, 267–280
    cholinergic mechanisms, 271
    direct evidence, 269–278
    gamma-aminobutyric acid and, 278
    glutamate and, 278
    indirect evidence, 267–269
    pain-excitation neurons, 268
    pain-inhibition neurons, 268
    somatosensory cortical evoked potentials, 269–275, 276, 278
    thalamic centromedian nucleus evoked potentials, 271, 274, 278
    seizure-related amino acid content, 136–137, 138, 139–141
C fiber, in nociception, 224, 227, 228, 229
  transcutaneous electrical stimulation effects, 233–234

Chaos theory. *See* Olfactory bulb, as neocortical model
Cholinergic mechanisms, of acupuncture analgesia, 271
Clonidine, 211
Cognitive function, relaxation-related control, 121–132
  autonomic nervous system, 122, 123
  brain function, 122, 123
  emotional control, 128–129
  eye response, 122–123
  imagery, 123, 124, 128
  neuromuscular circuits/model, 6–7, 122–125, 126
  reflexes, 129
Cognitive therapy, for pain control, 234
Cold response, in Raynaud's disease, 42, 43
Complement C3a, 191
Conditioning. *See also* Immunosuppression, conditioned
  for seizure control, 66
Coronary artery occlusion, autonomic blockade and, 96–97
Coronary disease, hyperventilation and, 34, 35–37
Corticosterone, 192
Cortisol, 191
Cyclophosphamide, as immunoconditioning stimuli, 8, 197, 198, 202–203
  in autoimmune disease, 166–178
  taste aversion learning, 170–173
  voluntary consumption, 173–175
Cysteic acid, seizure excitatory effects, 134
Cysteine sulphuric acid, seizure excitatory effects, 134

Depolarization, nociception and, 226–227
Depression, progressive relaxation therapy, 126–127
Descartes, Rene, 185
Descending pain control system, 230–232
  dorsolateral funiculus and, 230, 231
  hypothalamic, 214, 215–216
  opioid analgesia and, 207–221
  organization, 215–217
  stimulation-produced analgesia and, 212–214

Desensitization, systemic, 127
  for seizure control, 66
Dexamethasone, conditioned immunosuppression effects, 202–203
Diazepam, seizure effects, 135–136, 137, 138, 140–141
Disease. *See also* specific diseases
  behavioral interventions, 183–195
    guided imagery, 186–190
    miraculous healing, 186
    physiological processes, 190–192
    placebo response, 183–184, 185, 186
  emotional factors, 184–185, 191
Dopamine, seizure effects, 134
Dorsal horn
  in nociception
    clonidine effects, 211
    gate control theory, 225, 226, 228–230, 231, 232, 233–234
    morphine effects, 211
    neuropeptides and, 255–266
    stimulation-produced analgesia, 212
    transcutaneous electrical stimulation, 233–234
  structure, 228, 229
Dorsolateral funiculus, descending pain control system and, 230, 231
Dreams, 121, 122
Dynorphin
  dorsal horn content, 230
  precursor, 209

Edinburgh Masker, 152
Electrocardiogram(ECG), hyperventilation effects, 34, 35–36
Electroencephalogram(EEG)
  of chaotic processes, 103
  gamma-aminobutyric acid receptor modulator effects, 137–139, 141
  instrumental modification, 67–68
Emotion, disease and, 184–185, 191
β-Endorphin
  activation, 192
  dexamethasone-mediated inhibition, 203
  precursor, 209
Enkephalin
  dorsal horn content, 230, 231, 232
  spinal cord neuron content, 214
Epilepsy. *See also* Seizure control

Epilepsy (*cont.*)
  anticonvulsant-refractory, 65
  prevalence, 65
Ethmozine, 101
Excitatory amino acids, in epileptic seizures, 7, 134, 136
  gamma-aminobutyric acid receptor modulator effects, 137–138, 139–142
Extinction, for seizure control, 66
Eye response, cognitive function and, 122–123

Feedback
  in slow cortical potential self-regulation, 68–91
    age factors, 89
    EEG synchronization, 81, 84, 85, 87
    seizure frequency effects, 79–82, 83–84, 85, 87, 88
  in speech production
    delayed auditory, 119–120, 148, 149, 150, 152, 153
    sensory, 150–151
Fibrillation, ventricular, autonomic blockade, 97
Fifth cranial nerve, orofacial pain involvement, 239, 240
  subnucleus caudalis, 239, 240–243, 247–249
  subnucleus interpolaris, 239, 240, 249
  subnucleus oralis, 239, 240, 241, 242, 243, 244–248, 249
Finger pulse amplitude, in Raynaud's disease, 52, 55, 59
Frontal lobe
  as antiarrhythmia drug action site, 101
  autonomic activity regulation by, 95–97
  event-related slow potentials
    blockade, 101
    in cardiovascular disease, 16, 101–102
    electrochemical events, 97, 98
  learning-dependent noradrenergic mechanisms, 96, 97
Frontocortical-brainstem pathway, 96, 101

Galen, Claudius, 184–185
Gamma-aminobutyric acid (GABA)
  acupuncture analgesia and, 278

Gamma-aminobutyric acid (*cont.*)
  receptor modulators
    EEG response, 137–139, 141
    seizure effects, 133–144
Gamma-aminobutyric acid, γ-vinyl, seizure control effects, 135–136, 137, 138, 140
Gastrointestinal tract, opioid effects, 208
Gate control theory, of pain control, 10–11, 223–237
  clinical implications, 232–235
  depolarization, 226–227
  descending pain control system and, 230–232
  dorsal horn and, 225, 226, 228–230, 231, 232, 233–234
  hyperpolarization, 226–227
  T-cells and, 225–226, 232
Geometric affine-mapping, 112
Glutamate, analgesic effects, 213
  in acupuncture analgesia, 278
Glutamic acid, seizures and, 134
  gamma-aminobutric acid receptor modulators and, 136, 138, 140
Glutamine, gamma-aminobutyric acid receptor modulators and, 137, 138
Glycine, seizure inhibitory effects, 134
Graft-versus-host response, 165
Growth hormone, 191, 192
Guilt, imagery-related, 188–189, 190

Hallucinations, 121–122
Healing, miraculous, 186, 186
Heart rate
  in Raynaud's disease, 52–53, 54, 59
  in respiratory sinus arrhythmia, 28–29
Heart size, sex factors, 44
Herpes virus, 192
Hippocrates, 185
Histamine, conditioned release, 165
Homeostasis, in autoimmune disease immunosuppression, 168–169, 177–178
Homocysteic acid, seizure excitatory effects, 134
Hormones. *See also* specific hormones
  stress-related production, 190
Hyperactivity, 192
Hyperpolarization, nociception and, 226–

Hyperpolarization (*cont.*)
  227
  primary, 227–228
Hypersensitivity, delayed-response, 165
Hyperventilation
  cardiovascular function effects, 15, 32–37
  anxiety disorders and, 36
  beta-blocker effects, 33
  carbon dioxide levels, 32–33, 35, 37
  cardiac output, 34
  coronary blood flow, 34
  in coronary disease, 34, 35–37
  ECG, 34, 35–36
  respiratory rate, 34
  tidal volume, 34
  definition, 32
Hypnosis, for pain control, 234
Hypotaurine, seizure inhibitory effects, 134
Hypothalamus
  descending pain control system, 214, 215–216
  immunologic reactivity and, 163
  stimulation-produced analgesia, 213

Imagery
  as cognitive process component, 123, 124, 128
  guided
    adverse effects, 188–190
    as cancer therapy, 186–190
Immune complex disease, avoidance response in, 164
Immune system, central nervous system relationship, 163, 190–192
Immunity
  cell-mediated, conditioned changes, 165
  conditioned, 161–162. *See also* Immunostimulation; Immunosuppression
  stress effects, 164
Immunostimulation, taste aversion conditioning, 197, 201–202
Immunosuppression, conditioned
  in autoimmune disease, 163–178
  adaptive response, 167–169
  central nervous system involvement, 177, 178
  homeostasis, 168–169, 177–178

Immunosuppression, conditioned (*cont.*)
  in autoimmune disease (*cont.*)
    learning ability deficits and, 166–167, 173, 176
    conditioned stimuli, 165, 166–169, 198, 199–202
    unconditioned stimuli
      antilymphocyte serum, 165, 197, 198, 199–201, 203
      Bacille Calmette-Guerin, 197, 198
      cyclophosphamide, 8, 166–178, 197, 198
      levamisole, 197, 198, 201–202
      lithium chloride, 167, 169–170, 173, 198, 200–201
Injury, nociception during, 223
Inosine, seizure inhibitory effects, 134
Interbeat interval, in Raynaud's disease, 56–59
Interferon, 191
Interleukin 1, 191, 192

Jenner, Edward, 185

Krebiozen, 183

Larynx, in stuttering, 146–147, 150
Leucine-enkephalin
  precursor, 209
  seizure excitatory effects, 134
Levamisole, as immunoconditioning stimuli, 197, 198
  with saccharin, 201–202
Lithium chloride, as immunoconditioning stimuli, 198
  with antilymphocyte serum, 200–201
  in autoimmune disease, 167, 169–170, 173
Locus coeruleus
  descending pain control system, 214, 215
  stimulation-produced analgesia, 213
Lourdes, 186, 186
Luteinizing hormone, 192
Luteinizing hormone-releasing hormone, 192
Lymphoid tissue, sympathetic nervous innervation, 163
Lymphokines, 191, 192

Mammary artery, internal ligation, 183–184
Medulla
  caudal, stimulation-produced analgesia, 213
  rostral ventral
    descending pain control system, 214, 215, 230
    opioid sensitivity, 210, 211
Melanocyte-stimulating hormone, 209
Metastases, immune function and, 164
Methionine-enkephalin
  precursor, 209
  seizure excitatory effects, 134
Methysergide, morphine analgesia effects, 210
Midbrain
  descending pain control system, 214
  stimulation-produced analgesia, 213
Mind, concept of, 121–122
  Descartes', 185
Miracles, 186, 186
Monoamines, seizure effects, 134
Morphine
  action mechanisms, 207, 210–212
  nucleus raphe magnus administration, 213
  serotonin interaction, 210
Muscarinic agonists, long-term potentiation and, 101
Muscimol, seizure control effects, 135–136, 137, 138
Musculature, cognitive process involvement, 119, 124–125
  during stress, 128, 129
Myocardial performance, in Raynaud's disease, 43–61
  blood pressure, 44, 45, 50, 51
  cardiac output, 44, 45, 52, 53, 54, 59–60
  contractility, 15
  digital blood flow, 44
  impedance cardiographic data, 48, 49
  sex factors, 44–45
  stress response, 46

Naloxone, 211, 212
Natural killer cell, conditioned changes, 165
Neocortex, biological model, 95–117
  behavioral paradigm, 104–105

Neocortex, biological model (*cont.*)
  chaotic attractor, 102–104, 106–113
  dimensional analysis, 103–104
  event-related slow potentials, 101–102, 105, 113
  field potential dimension analysis, 97, 99, 102–113
  long-term potentiation, 101
  parallel processing, 112–113
  surface potentials, 99, 100, 102, 105–113
Neuralgia
  postherpetic, 234–235
  trigeminal, 241
Neuromusculature model, of self-regulation, 119, 124–125, 128, 129
Neuropeptides
  nociceptive transmission and, 12
  seizures and, 134
  spinal, 206
Neurotransmitters. *See also* specific neurotransmitters
  seizure involvement, 133–144
Newcastle disease virus, 192
Nociception
  dorsal horn involvement, 255–266
  during injury, 223
  spinothalamic tract neurons and, 228–229
  suppression, 223. *See also* Pain control
  wide-dynamic range neurons and, 228–229
Noradrenaline, seizure effects, 134
Norepinephrine
  as analgesia depressant, 230
  event-related slow potentials and, 97, 98
  locus coeruleus production, 214
  as opioid analgesia mediator, 211
  spinal, 216
Nucleus cuneiformis, stimulation-produced analgesia, 213
Nucleus paragigantocellularis, opioid sensitivity, 210
Nucleus raphe magnus
  descending pain control system, 215, 216–217, 230, 231
  opioid sensitivity, 210
  stimulation-produced analgesia, 212–213

Nucleus reticularis
  paragigantocellularis, descending pain control system, 230, 231

Olfactory bulb, as neocortical model, 16, 97–113
  behavioral paradigm, 104–105
  chaotic attractor, 102–104, 106–113
  dimensional analysis, 103–104
  event-related slow potentials, 101–102, 105, 113
  field potential dimension analysis, 97, 99, 102–113
  long-term potentiation, 101
  parallel processing, 112–113
  surface potentials, 99, 100, 102, 105–113
Opioids, 207–221
  action mechanisms, 209
  action sites, 210–212
  endogenous, 207, 209–210
    distribution, 230
  receptors
    classification, 208
    opioid selectivity, 10, 209–210
Orofacial pain, trigeminal nuclear complex involvement, 239–254
  fifth cranial nerve, 239, 240
  subnucleus caudalis, 239, 240–243, 247–249
  subnucleus interpolaris, 239, 240, 249
  subnucleus oralis, 239, 240, 241, 242, 243, 244–248, 249
  main sensory trigeminal nucleus, 239, 240, 241, 242, 243, 244–248, 249
  submodality segregation model, 241, 243, 252
Oxygen consumption, sex factors, 44

Pain, definition, 255
Pain control, 10–13
  descending systems
    dorsolateral funiculus and, 230, 231
    hypothalamic, 214, 215–216
    opioid analgesia and, 207–221
    organization, 215–217
    stimulation-produced analgesia and, 212–214
  gate control theory, 10–11, 223–237
    clinical implications, 232–235

Pain control (cont.)
  gate control theory (cont.)
    depolarization, 226–227
    descending pain control system and, 230–232
    dorsal horn and, 225, 226, 228–230, 231, 232, 233–234
    hyperpolarization, 226–227
    T-cells and, 225–226, 232
Parabrachial area, stimulation-produced analgesia, 213
Parasympathetic nervous system, respiratory sinus arrhythmia involvement, 21–22, 23, 24, 25, 27, 29–32
Periaqueductal gray matter
  descending pain control system, 214, 215
  opioid sensitivity, 210–211
  stimulation-produced analgesia, 212–214, 230, 231
Phencyclidine, 208
Phobia, progressive relaxation therapy, 127
ω-Phosphono-α-aminocarboxylic acid, seizure effects, 135–137, 139–140
Pituitary-adrenal axis, in brain-immune system relationship, 190, 191
Placebo therapy, 8–9
  adverse effects, 184
  for cancer, 183
  emotional basis, 186
  for pain control, 234
  for psychiatric disorders, 184
  surgical, 183–184
Plaque-forming cell, suppression, 165
Pons, descending pain control system, 214
Potassium
  event-related slow potential effects, 97, 98
  opioid interaction, 209
Potentiation, long-term, 101
Potentials
  event-related, 16, 97, 98, 101–102
  slow cortical
    contingent negative variation, 68, 69
    as cortical excitability indicators, 68–70
    EEG synchronization, 81, 84, 85, 87
    in epileptic patients, 73–91
    paroxysmal depolarization shifts, 70
    reinforcement, 71

Potentials (cont.)
  slow cortical (cont.)
    seizure frequency effects, 79–82, 83–84, 85, 87, 88
    self-regulation, 70–91
    somatosensory cortical evoked, 269–275, 276
    thalamic centromedian nucleus evoked, 271, 274, 278
Precision Fluency Shaping Program, 151–152
Problem-solving, 121
Prodynorphin, 209, 210
Proenkephalin, 209, 210
Progabide, seizure effects, 135–136, 138, 140
Prolactin, 192
Proopiomelanocortin, 209
Propranolol, frontal lobe action site, 100, 101
Prostaglandins, seizure inhibitory effects, 134
Psychiatric disorders
  immune system relationship, 192
  placebo therapy, 184
Psychoneuroimmunology, 8, 161–162
Pulse transit time, in Raynaud's disease, 52, 55, 56

Raynaud's disease, 41
  beta-adrenergic blockade, 45
  cold response, 42, 43
  digital blood flow, 43
  pathophysiological theories, 42–43
  stress-related myocardial performance, 43–61
    beta-adrenergic response, 60
    blood pressure, 43, 44, 45, 50, 51
    cardiac output, 44, 45, 52, 53, 54, 59–60
    contractility, 15
    digital blood flow, 44
    finger pulse amplitude, 52, 55, 59
    heart rate, 52–53, 54, 59
    impedance cardiographic data, 48, 49
    interbeat interval, 56–59
    left ventricular ejection time, 52, 53, 54–55
    preeinjection period, 52, 53–54, 55–59, 60

Raynaud's disease (cont.)
stress-related myocardial performance (cont.)
pulse transit time, 52, 55, 56
sex factors, 44–45
stress response, 43, 46
stroke volume, 52–53, 54
Raynaud's phenomenon
definition, 41
myocardial contractility, 4–5
primary. See Raynaud's disease
secondary, 41, 42, 43
Reflexes, in progressive relaxation, 129
Relaxation, progressive
as anxiety therapy, 127–128, 131
as cancer therapy, 186, 187
cognitive function control by, 121–132
autonomic nervous system, 122, 123
brain function, 122, 123
emotional control, 128–129
eye response, 122–123
imagery, 123, 124, 128
neuromuscular circuits, 122, 123, 124, 126
reflexes, 129
for seizure control, 66
Respiratory depression, opioid-related, 208, 211
Respiratory rate
hyperventilation effects, 34
in respiratory sinus arrhythmia, 23–24, 27–28, 29
Respiratory sinus arrhythmia, 4, 21–32
definition, 21
respiratory mediation, 15, 21–32
beta-blocker effects, 24–27
heart rate, 28–29
parasympathetic control, 21–22, 23, 24, 25, 27, 29–32
respiratory rate, 23–24, 27–28, 29
during task performance, 28–32
tidal volume, 23–24, 27
vagal tone, 21–22, 23, 24–25, 27–32

Saccharin, as conditioned taste stimulus
with antilymphocyte serum, 199–200
in autoimmune disease, 165, 166–169
with cyclophosphamide, 198, 202
with levamisole, 201–202

Scleroderma, Raynaud's phenomenon-related, 41
Seizure control
behavioral, 65–91
biofeedback of end-tidal CO_2, 66
classical conditioning, 66
desensitization, 66
EEG instrumental modification, 67–68
extinction, 66
relaxation therapy, 66
self-control, 66
neurotransmitter-related, 119, 133–144
aspartic acid, 134, 138, 140
gamma-aminobutyric acid, 133–144
slow cortical self-regulation, 5, 73–91
age factors, 89
anticonvulsant effects, 88–89
EEG synchronization, 81, 84, 85, 87
seizure frequency effects, 79–82, 83–84, 85, 87, 88
single case reports, 82–88
Serotonin
analgesic role, 230
descending pain control system and, 213–214, 215–216
morphine interaction, 210
as opioid analgesia mediator, 211
seizure inhibitory effects, 134
spinal, 216
Sex factors, in Raynaud's disease, 44–45
Sheep red blood cells, as immunoconditioning stimuli, 197, 198
Slow cortical potentials, 5, 68–91
contingent negative variation, 68, 69
as cortical excitability indicators, 68–70
event-related
blockade, 101
in cardiovascular disease, 16, 101–102
definition, 97
electrochemical events, 97, 98
paroxysmal depolarization shifts, 70
self-regulation, 70–91
age factors, 89
EEG synchronization, 81, 84, 85, 87
in epileptic patients, 73–91
reinforcement, 71
seizure frequency effects, 79–82, 83–84, 85, 87, 88
Smallpox, vaccination, 185

Somatostatin
  dorsal horn content, 206, 255–256
  in nociception, 259–262
  seizure excitatory effects, 134
Speech production model, 150–151
Spinal cord. *See also* Dorsal horn
  α_2-adrenergic receptors, 211
  enkephalin-containing neurons, 214
  opioid receptors, 208, 211
Spinothalamic tract, neurons, 228–229
ST-91, 211
Stimuli
  conditioned, in immunosuppression, 165, 166–169, 198, 199–202
  hallucinations and, 121–122
  perceptual processes and, 122
  unconditioned, in immunosuppression
    antilymphocyte serum, 165, 197, 198, 199–201, 203
    Bacille Calmette-Guerin, 197, 198
    cyclophosphamide, 8, 166–178, 197, 198
    levamisole, 197, 198, 201–202
    lithium chloride, 167, 169–170, 173, 198, 200–201
Stress
  cancer and, 164
  immune system effects, 164, 191
  muscle response, 128, 129
  Raynaud's disease and, 43
    beta-adrenergic response, 60
    blood pressure, 43, 44, 45, 50, 51
    cardiac output, 52, 53, 54, 59–60
    cardiovascular measures of, 43–61
    finger pulse amplitude, 52, 55, 59
    heart rate, 52–53, 54, 59
    interbeat interval, 56–59
    left ventricular ejection time, 52, 53, 54–55
    preejection period, 52, 53–54
    pulse transit time, 52, 55, 56
    stroke volume, 52–53, 54
Stroke volume, in Raynaud's disease, 52–53, 54
Stuttering
  definition, 146
  fluency enhancement, 7, 119–120, 148–159
    conditions related to, 148–150

Stuttering (*cont.*)
  fluency enhancement (*cont.*)
    delayed auditory feedback, 148, 149, 150, 152, 153
    metronome system, 149, 152
    Precision Fluency Shaping Program, 151–152
    voice feedback system, 153–157
    white noise masking, 148, 149, 152, 153
  measurement, 146–148
Substance P
  dorsal horn content, 206, 255, 256
  in nociception, 259–265
  inhibition, 231
Substantia caudalis, orofacial pain involvement, 239, 240–243, 247–249
Substantia gelatinosa, in pain suppression, 224, 228, 231, 232
Substantia interpolaris, orofacial pain involvement, 239, 240, 249
Substantia oralis, orofacial pain involvement, 239, 240, 241, 242, 243, 244–248, 249
Sympathetic nervous system
  lymphoid tissue innervation, 163
  in Raynaud's phenomenon, 42, 43–44
Systemic lupus erythematosus, conditioned immunosuppression, 165–178
  adaptive response, 167–169
  central nervous system involvement, 177, 178
  homeostasis, 168–169, 177–178
  learning abililty deficits and, 166–167, 173, 176
  taste aversion, 166–178

Taste aversion, conditioned, 8–10, 197–203
  in autoimmune disease, 165–178
    adaptive response, 167–169
    central nervous system involvement, 177, 178
    homeostasis, 168–169, 177–178
    learning ability deficits and, 166–167, 173, 176
    conditioned stimuli, 165, 166–169, 198, 199–202

Taste aversion, conditioned (*cont.*)
  unconditioned stimuli
    antilymphocyte serum, 165, 197, 198, 199–201, 203
    Bacille Calmette-Guerin, 197, 198
    cyclophosphamide, 8, 166–178, 197, 198
    levamisole, 197, 198, 201–202
    lithium chloride, 167, 169–170, 173, 198, 200–201
Taurine, seizures and, 134
  gamma-aminobutyric acid receptor modulators and, 138
T-cell, in nociception, 225–226, 232
Terbutaline, 45
Thalamus, inferior peduncle, 96
Thought, rational, 121
Thymosin alpha 1, 187–188
Thymosin peptides, 191–192
Thyrotropine-releasing hormone, 134
Tic douloureux, 241
Tidal volume
  hyperventilation effects, 34
  in respiratory sinus arrhythmia, 23–24, 27

Transcutaneous electrical stimulation(TENS), 233–234
Trigeminal nuclear complex, orofacial pain involvement, 11–12, 206, 239–254
  fifth cranial nerve, 239, 240
  subnucleus caudalis, 239, 240–243, 247–249
  subnucleus interpolaris, 239, 240, 249
  subnucleus oralis, 239, 240, 241, 242, 243, 244–248, 249
  main sensory trigeminal nucleus, 239, 240, 241, 242, 243, 244–248, 249
  submodality segregation model, 241, 243, 252

Vascular abnormalities, in Raynaud's phenomenon, 42
Vasoconstriction, in Raynaud's disease, 46
Ventricular ejection time, in Raynaud's disease, 52, 53, 54–55
Voice feedback system, for fluency enhancement, 153–157

White noise masking, 148, 149, 152, 153